Detection and Measurement of Visual Impairment in Pre-Verbal Children

Documenta Ophthalmologica
Proceedings Series volume 45

Detection and Measurement of Visual Impairment in Pre-Verbal Children

Proceedings of a workshop held at the Institute of Ophthalmology, London on April 1–3, 1985, sponsored by the Commission of the European Communities as advised by the Committee on Medical Research

Edited by Barrie Jay

1986 **MARTINUS NIJHOFF/DR W. JUNK PUBLISHERS**
a member of the KLUWER ACADEMIC PUBLISHERS GROUP
DORDRECHT / BOSTON / LANCASTER

IV

Distributors

for the United States and Canada: Kluwer Academic Publishers, 190 Old Derby Street, Hingham, MA 02043, USA
for the UK and Ireland: Kluwer Academic Publishers, MTP Press Limited, Falcon House, Queen Square, Lancaster LA1 1RN, UK
for all other countries: Kluwer Academic Publishers Group, Distribution Center, P.O. Box 322, 3300 AH Dordrecht, The Netherlands

Library of Congress Cataloging in Publication Data

```
Detection and measurement of visual impairment in
  pre-verbal children

    (Documenta ophthalmologica  proceedings series ;
45) (EUR ; 10217 EN)
    1. Vision disorders in children--Diagnosis--
Congresses.  2. Vision--Testing--Congresses.
3. Infants--Medical examinations--Congresses.
I. Jay, Barrie.  II. Commission of the European
Communities.  III. Series: Documenta ophthalmologica.
Proceedings series ; v. 45.  IV. Series: EUR ;
10217 EN.
RE48.2.C5D47  1986     618.92'0977     85-31938
```

ISBN-13:978-94-010-8393-5   e-ISBN-13:978-94-009-4263-9
DOI: 10.1007/978-94-009-4263-9

EUR 10217 EN

Book information

Publication arranged by: Commission of the European Communities, Directorate-General Information Market and Innovation, Luxembourg

Copyright/legal notice

INTRODUCTION

Over the past few years there have been considerable advances in our understanding of the normal development of vision and in our ability to detect and measure visual impairment in early childhood. It was appropriate, therefore, that a workshop, sponsored by the European Communities, should be held on the 'Detection and Measurement of Visual Impairment in Pre-verbal Children.'

This workshop, which was held at the Institute of Ophthalmology, London, between 1 and 3 April 1985, brought together visual physiologists and ophthalmologists who exchanged and discussed ideas of mutual interest. After an introductory session when the normal development of vision and the causes of visual impairment were reviewed, there were sessions devoted to the theoretical aspects of electrophysiological and psychophysical tests, the measurement of visual acuity in pre-verbal children, the measurement of other visual functions, and visual screening of pre-verbal children.

This volume contains the papers presented at the workshop, and transcripts of the various discussions that took place. It was a measure of the success of the workshop that participants from several different disciplines were able to have fruitful discussions and to suggest areas of common interest where collaborative ventures could usefully be pursued. It is hoped that this venture will be followed by others where a multi-disciplinary approach will improve both our knowledge of visual handicap in childhood and our management of this important group of sensorily impaired children.

Barrie Jay

CONTENTS

VIII

X

LIST OF PARTICIPANTS

APKARIAN, Dr Patricia A, Netherlands Ophthalmic Research Institute,
P.O. Box 12141, 1100 AC Amsterdam, The Netherlands

ARDEN, Professor Geoffrey B, Institute of Ophthalmology, Judd Street,
London WC1H 9QS, England

ATKINSON, Dr Janette, Department of Experimental Psychology, Downing
Street, Cambridge CB2 3EB, England

BAGLEY, Miss Pauline, Royal Berkshire Hospital, London Road, Reading,
Berkshire RG1 5AN, England

BOERGEN, Professor Klaus-Peter, Augenklinik der Universitat Munchen,
Mathildenstrasse 8, 8000 Munchen 2, West Germany

BRADDICK, Dr Oliver J, Department of Experimental Psychology, Downing
Street, Cambridge CB2 3EB, England

CAMPOS, Professor Dr Emilio C, Clinica Oculistica d'ell'Universita,
Via Del Pozzo 71, 41100 Modena, Italy

CHARLIER, Dr Jacques, Centre de Technologie biomedicale INSERM,
13-17 Rue Camille Guerin, 59800 Lille, France

DUBOWITZ, Dr Lilly MS, Department of Paediatrics, Royal Postgraduate Medical
School, Hammersmith Hospital, Ducane Road, London W12 0HS, England

EMILIANI, Dr Pier Luigi, IROE, CNR, Via Panciatichi 64, 50127 Firenze,
Italy

FELLS, Mr Peter, Moorfields Eye Hospital, City Road, London EC1V 2PD,
England

FIELDER, Mr Alistair R, Department of Ophthalmology, Clinical Sciences
Building, Leicester Royal Infirmary, Leicester LE2 7LX, England

FIORENTINI, Professor Adriana, Istituto di Neurofisiologia del CNR,
Via San Zeno 51, 56100 Pisa, Italy

HAASE, Professor Dr Wolfgang, Universitats-Augenklinik, Martinistrasse 52,
2000 Hamburg 20, West Germany

HACHE, Professor Jean-Claude, 221 Boulevard de la Liberte, 59000 Lille,
France

HARCOURT, Mr Brian, Leeds General Infirmary, Great George Street,
Leeds LS1 3EX, England

HOF-VAN DUIN, Dr Jackie van, Department of Physiology, Erasmus University,
PO Box 1738, 3000 DR Rotterdam, The Netherlands

HYVARINEN, Dr Lea, Harmaaparrankuja 3, SF-02200 Espoo, Finland

JAY, Professor Barrie, Institute of Ophthalmology, 17-25 Cayton Street, London EC1V 9AT, England

KOMMERELL, Professor Guntram, Universitats-Augenklinik, Killianstrasse 5, 7800 Freiburg, West Germany

LAEY, Professor Jean-Jacques De, Akademisch Ziekenhuis, De Pintelaan 135, 9000 Gent, Belgium

LEE, Mr John, Moorfields Eye Hospital, City Road, London EC1V 2PD, England

LENNERSTRAND, Dr Gunnar, Karolinska Sjukhaset, Box 605 00, 140 01 Stockholm, Sweden

LITH, Professor Dr Fried van, Oogziekenhuis, Schiedamse Vest 180, 3000 LM Rotterdam, The Netherlands

LOEWER-SIEGER, Dr D Hetti, Netherlands Ophthalmic Research Institute, P.O. Box 12141, 1100 AC Amsterdam, The Netherlands

LOULY, Miss M, Service d'Ophtalmologie, Hopital Regional, Place de Verdun, 59037 Lille, France

MAFFEI, Professor Lamberto, Istituto di Neurofisiologia del CNR, Via San Zeno 51, 56100 Pisa, Italy

MEHDORN, Dr Ekkehard, Augenklinik der Universitat, Ratzeburger Allee 160, D 2400 Lubeck, West Germany

MINOGUE, Mr Conor, Bio-medical Research Ltd, Shannon Industrial Estate, Shannon Airport, Co Clare, Ireland

MOHN, Dr Gesine, Department of Physiology, Erasmus University, PO Box 1738, 3000 DR Rotterdam, The Netherlands

MOLONEY, Dr Jane, Research Foundation, Royal Victoria Eye and Ear Hospital, Adelaide Road, Dublin 2, Ireland

MUSHIN, Dr Joan, 935 Finchley Road, London NW11 5PE, England

NOEL, Dr P, Departement de Neurologie Pediatrique, Hopital Universitaire St Pierre, 322 rue Haute, 1000 Bruxelles, Belgium

NORREN, Dr D van, Institute for Perception TNO, Kampweg 5, P.O. Box 23, 3769 ZG Soesterberg, The Netherlands

PORCIATTI, Dr Vittorio, Divisione Oculistica, Spedali Riuniti USL N. 13, Viale Alfieri 36, 57100 Livorno, Italy

PSILAS, Professor Konstantinos G, Department of Ophthalmology, University of Ioannina, Ioannina, Greece

SARGENTINI, Dr A, Laboratorio di Ingegneria Biomedica, Istituto Superiore Sanita, Via Regina Elena 299, 00161 Rome, Italy

SCHULZ, Dr Elizabeth, Universitats-Krankenhaus, Eppendorf-Augenklinik, Martinistr 52, 2000 Hamburg 20, West Germany

SIRETEANU, Dr Ruxandra, Max-Planck-Institut fur Hirnforschung, Deutschordenstr 46, Postfach 710409, 6000 Frankfurt a. M. 71, West Germany

SKUPINSKI, Dr W, CEC P 6 XII, Recherche Medicale, 200 Rue de la Loi, 1049 Bruxelles, Belgium

SPEKREIJSE, Professor Henk, Netherlands Ophthalmic Research Institute, P.O. Box 12141, 1100 AC Amsterdam, The Netherlands

TAYLOR, Mr David, Hospital for Sick Children, Great Ormond Street, London WC1, England

TSIKOULAS, Dr I, 1st Paediatric Clinic, Aghia Sophia Hospital, Thessaloniki, Greece

VERRIEST, Dr Guy, Oogheelkunde, Akademisch Ziekenhuis, De Pintelaan 135, B-9000 Gent, Belgium

VITAL-DURAND, Dr Francois, INSERM Unite 94, 16 avenue du Doyen Lepine, 69500 Bron, France

WARBURG, Dr Mette, Eye Clinic for the Mentally Retarded, 40 Sognevej, 2820 Gentofte, Denmark

ORGANIZATION, DEVELOPMENT AND EARLY MANIPULATIONS OF PRIMATE'S VISUAL PATHWAYS

Francois VITAL-DURAND

Laboratoire de Neuropsychologie Expérimentale
INSERM U 94, 16 avenue du doyen Lépine
69500 BRON- France

INTRODUCTION

Monkeys and humans are primate of extremely close proximity as far as visual system organization and functions are concerned. What is known about gross and detailed anatomy in these two groups suggests that they have reached an evolutionary level which allow them to live in a similar large and unspecific niche. Monkeys and men seem to be fairly well adapted to a variety of living conditions and this assertion is comforted by comparison of their sensory capacities. It is well known that resolution power, contrast sensitivity, color discrimination, spatial and temporal modulation sensitivities can attain similar values provided patience is afforded when dealing with animals (De Valois, Morgan, Polson, Mead and Hull, 1974 ; De Valois, Morgan and Snodderly, 1974). The same holds for the fine control of eye position whose role in tracking and capture of the visual object should not be overlooked. This does not intend to imply that perceptual and cognitive capacities are equivalent as well. But as far as sensory and oculo-motor equipement is under scrutiny, the monkey visual system can be taken as a good model of that of the human.

Starting from the output cells of the retina, we will describe the three physiological channels processing visual messages to different sets of targets organized in a network subserving specialized analysis of every component of the message. It is well accepted that the visual cortex, also called area 17, striate cortex or V1, constitutes the hub of the machinery responsible for the detailed analysis of the visual scene. But it should be clear that it can only be considered as a privileged site in a network of structures performing this task with the help of the dozen or so visual areas and several subcortical structures. It is also self evident that perception of an object includes its location in the visual field, based upon a system of spatial references contributing to the sense of position in which the whole body is included. There would be no need to detect a snake if you had no control of its location relative to your limbs. Several subcortical structures seem to be happy candidates to perform such a role. Firstly, because their ancestry suggest that they serve the more basic function of localization rather than the more complex function of identification. Secondly, less neuronal circuitry is required and there is not much need for an extensive cortical template to achieve these tasks that we often consider as unconscious, automatic or reflexive. These considerations mean that the visual system, as a constituent of a behavioural set supporting the harmony between the individual and its external world, has no intrinsic limits. For practical purposes only, these limits are commonly drawn at the stage of cellular processing at which the visual message becomes mixed with a fair amount of other sensory modalities.

As it can be described in the adult, the visual system is the final form of the compromise between genetic forces scaffolding the networks of structures programmed to take advantage of sensory interactions with the outside world and the actual history of the individual who has accumulated visual experiences sharpening the functional capacities of the neuronal circuits. Emphasis on the crucial role of early visual stimulation is especially important as the two eyes would be competing to death, actually to functional elimination at the level of the striate cortex , if no proper collaborative relationship is established. The therapist will be the mediator whose role is to prevent or limit the damages brought about by interocular imbalance which might eventually express a deleterious effect in terms of acuity loss or misalignment.

THE THREE RETINAL OUTPUTS

Three main categories of retinal ganglion cells are morphologically distinguished. Their physiological identification is due to Enroth Cugell and Robson (1966) who described opposite responses in two categories of cells, linear versus non-linear, that they called X and Y. A third category was discovered later which could not fit with either of these two types and was celled W (Stone and Hoffmann 1972). An excellent up-to-date account of this topic is to be found in Stone (1983). In the monkey, Perry and Cowey (1984) and Perry, Oehler and Cowey (1984) have given an extensive anatomical description.

P gamma or C cells, which correspond to physiological W type, are characterized by a small cellular body and a few long dendrites sparsely ramified. Their axones reach the Superior Colliculus (SC) and eventually send a collateral branch to the Lateral Geniculate Body (LGN). Physiologically, their slow conduction velocity and sluggish responses hamper definition of the functional role of this heterogenous group which constitutes about 10% of the ganglion-cell population.
P alpha or A cells have the biggest cellular bodies surrounded by regularly radiating branching dendritic arborizations. They project mainly to the magnocellular layers of the LGN and form about 10% of the total population. Some project to the SC. P alpha cells correspond to the physiological Y type, whoses main features are achromatic broad band responses, with short latency and non linearity of the receptive field components. Very sensitive to low contrast, but not to high spatial frequency gratings (i.e. they have low acuity), they have been attributed a role in coding the movement or detection of visual objects on the ground that their responses are fast and brisk.
P beta or B cells have a rather small cellular body giving rise to one, occasionally two or three, stout primary dendrites which then branch to form a dense bushy dendritic tree. These cells form the great majority of ganglion cells (80%). They correspond to the X type which project mainly to LGN parvocellular layers, where cells are color opponent, have medium latencies and sum linearly the responses from the constituent sub-regions of the receptive field. Their high resolution power indicates that they could subserve fine discrimination tasks.

For all three ganglion-cells categories, the size of the dendritic field increases with excentricity and the cell density decreases. These physiological groups of cells do not lose their specificities when they reach their first target. Indeed the LGN is sharply divided between parvocellular layers, whose axones arborize in sublayers IVa and IVc beta of the visual cortex, and magnocellular layers whose axones arborize inbetween in layer IVc alpha, hence maintaining the specificity of its input streams.

THE CENTRAL NETWORK

In addition to defining a large number ot retinotopically and
functionnally distinct subcortical relays, each receiving its own set of
retinal afferents, recent research has shown that there are a number of
parallel independent pathways from the retina to the mammalian cortex
apart from the retino-hypothalamic pathway that we shall ignore here.
Three main pathways dispatch different qualities of message to the
Accessory Optic Tract, the Pretectum and Superior Colliculus and the
Lateral Geniculate Body.

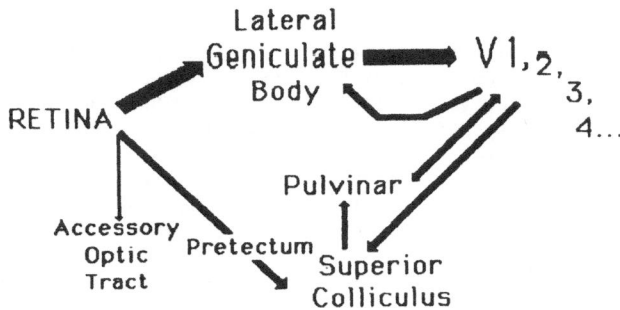

Fig 1 Visual pathways in primates.

This template is intended to draw attention to the different routes
leaving the retina, their relative numerical importance and their
distribution on interconnected structures. The visual part of the
Pulvinar includes the lateral and inferior nuclei. Vl, 2, 3, 4 are the
occcipital visual areas. They are heavily interconnected.

Despite its name, the **Accessory Optic Tract** is a primary visual
system arising from retinal ganglion cells. Its first relay is made of
three nuclei located in the mesencephalon, close to Substantia nigra and
Pretectum. It contributes fundamentally to the stabilization of the
retinal image, a prerequisite to the normal functions of the other
visual systems. A comprehensive review of its anatomy and physiological
properties is to be found in Simpson (1984).

The **Pretectum** is the next larger target of retinal ganglion cell
axons. Their terminals arborize in five different nuclei located in the
rostral part of the brainstem. What is known of the physiological
properties of the neurones recorded there indicates that they deal with
eye movements, particularly when vestibulo-ocular or optokinetic
reflexes are involved (see Precht 1982 for review).

The **Superior Colliculus** (SC) receives about 10 per cent of
ganglion- cells axons, largely of the W type. They are precisely
distributed to convey retinotopic representation of the entire visual
field. But it should be noted here that a very dense projection to the
upper layers of the SC also arises from the depth of the primary visual

cortex (area 17). This double input system means that the very function of the SC cannot be restricted to a simple task of detection or localization exemplified by the generation or modulation of eye movements (review by Wurtz and Albano 1980). In any case the SC gives rise to a substantial retinotopic projection to the inferior and lateral nuclei of the Pulvinar, and it could be so considered as no more than a relay structure in the subcortical visual network. The other significant output of the SC is to the Tectospinal Tract which plays a role in adjusting body position to the external world as perceived through proprioceptive, vestibular and auditory channels.

Although they do not receive direct input from the retina the **lateral and inferior Pulvinar** deserve special mention as a major relay nucleus of the visual system. The main afferent pathways originate in the visual cortices and Superior Colliculus. Three retinotopic representations of the visual field have so far been demonstrated in two parts of this nucleus, and from there projections reach several non-visual cortical areas in addition to an ascending projection upon the visual cortices. It is not yet clear what functional role could be assigned to this structure but its connections, dimensions and organization deserve consideration as a major visual element.

Finally, the retino-geniculo-striate pathway is the largest of all. 90% of its fibers terminate in two sets of geniculate layers, parvocellular or magnocellular. The **Lateral Geniculate Body** or Nucleus is made of six layers, most commonly numbered from one to six starting from the hilus. Half of these layers receive their input from each eye , layers 1, 4 and six from the contralateral eye, layers 2, 3 and 5 from the ipsilateral one. The two ventral layers are magnocellular and the four dorsal layers derive from a doubling of two ancestral parvocellular layers. This point is worth noticing because the physiological properties of these two groups of layers are different.

The ventral layers contain relay cells of the Y pathway among a dominant population of X type cells. This point is a bit controversial as it relies on a single, however very discriminative criterion for assigning the X or Y character to a cell : the linear summation of the responses from the subfields constituent of the receptive field. If response latencies are used as the discriminative criterion, then the magnocellular layers only contain Y cells, as it is clear that they diplay shorter latency responses. In any case, color sensitivity is a property of the parvocellular layers where the cells also tend to have better resolution for smaller stimuli. On the other hand contrast sensitivity and movement sensitivity are greater in the ventral laminae.

From there most geniculate neurones send their axons to arborize within layer IV of the striate area where they terminate in distinct sublayers according to their parvo or magnocellular origin. Furthermore, terminals from each eye are laid in an organized pattern of stripes in which terminals from the right and left eye alternate. This design has been called **ocular dominance columns** or slabs by D H Hubel and T N Wiesel who discovered them (Fig 2). In addition to a fair sharing of the cortical mantle by the two eyes, each retinal point is represented in this cortex to form a complete retinotopic map of the visual field, most of the space of the cortex being devoted to central vision. The magnification factor defines the extent of cortical surface devoted to each unit of visual space. It is very high for central vision, low for peripheral vision.

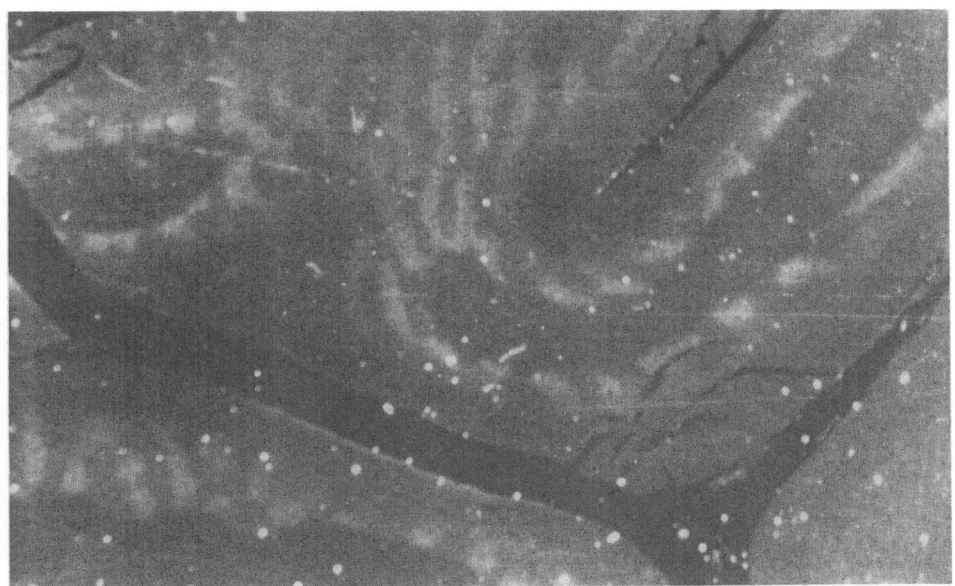

Fig 2 Ocular dominance columns in a gibbon.

Tritiated amino-acids were injected in the vitreous of the right
eye two weeks before sacrifice of the animal. The white grains are
situated were terminals from this eye reach layer IV of the visual
cortex. In this normal animal, spacing between columns equals the width
of the column. In visually deprived animals, the relative size of the
columns and their intervals indicates the loss of cortical territory.

Area V1 should not be considered as an end-point of the major
visual pathway. On the contrary, a number of intracortical pathways
interconnect V1 with at least some of the dozen or so other visual
areas (Van Essen 1979, Van Essen and Maunsell 1983) and subcortical
projections feed their messages to structures like the Superior
Colliculus or the Pulvinar. Furthermore, the striate cortex send down
to the Lateral Geniculate Body a huge feed-back loop as is the rule
between the cortex and thalamic structures.

Three considerations can be proposed at this point. One points out
the fact there is no clear anatomical evidence to divide the network of
visual structures into subsystems independently devoted to the
processing of parameters of the visual message, although on the input
side the X, Y and W channels are truly independent and specific. It
had been proposed that a subcortical system could be concerned with
target localization and body orientation, a role easily granted to
the tectal network (Superior Colliculus and Pretectum) and a cortical
machinery whose evolutionnary development gives upper mammals the
privilege of fine form recognition (Ingle 1982).
However heuristic this view has been, supported by studies in
animals specialized for very specific categories of tasks, it appears
that when several mammalian species are compared, cortical development
results in a new balance of functions among cortical and subcortical
structures. It appears particularly odd to grant a crucial role to the

retino-tectal pathway if one remembers that the largest input to the Superior Colliculus is not retinal but has its origin in the striate cortex. Taking the monkey as an example, Superior Colliculus lesions lead to discrete alteration of spatial behaviour, nothing comparable to the dramatic deficit observed after a similar lesion in mammals deprived of extensive cortical visual areas (Collin and Cowey 1980). As a consequence, the hypothesis of a double visual system appears now obsolete at least as far as higher mammals and primates are considered.

Another comment deals with the hierarchical hypothesis proposed by Hubel and Wiesel (1962) to explain the processing of visual information along the geniculo-striate pathway. In this hypothesis the input cells of the striate area present Simple receptive fields, resulting from convergent excitatory inputs from a set of similar geniculate cells whose circular receptive fields are distributed in overlapping fashion over a straight line. Response of this receptive field is the simple addition of the elements of response generated by each constitutent zone. The next set of cells was called Complex because their properties cannot be derived in a single logical step from those of the lateral geniculate cells. It was proposed that they would be the product of the next stage of processing, adding together several Simple-cell receptive fields. The reponse is no more the simple addition of responses from each component. According to this hypothesis, the message is progressively elaborated in a sequential way. New research has brought several drawbacks to this appealing proposition. One is that it would require a direct and unique projection from the Lateral Geniculate Body to the Simple cells and from them to the Complex cells. It is now clear that this is not the case and that some Complex cells definitely receive a direct geniculate input (Bullier and Henry 1980). It is also demonstrated that a projection from the LGN directly reaches V2, shunting V1.

Also, from the X, Y and W ganglionic cells of the retina emerge at least three categories of fibers making their route toward different targets in the Tectum or toward specific layers of the Lateral Geniculate Body. The best known of these sytems, X and Y, carry messages coded according to very different principles, and arguments accumulate to attribute specific properties to each of these streams of information.

DEVELOPMENT

The primate visual system is fairly immature at birth. Newborn babies, both human and monkey have grating resolution acuities of only 1-2 c/deg (cycle per degree of visual angle), about 25-50 times less than grating acuity in adults (Teller, Morse, Borton and Regal 1974; Teller, Regal, Videen and Pulos1978) and it could be asked if maturation obeys a gradient from the ocular globe to the striate area and beyond. At birth, ocular media are clear enough so that the macular region is discernable, but clearing of optical media and packing of photoreceptors is still in progress. It seems that at this stage the limiting factor of visual acuity does not sit in the eye (Boothe 1982). Nothing is known of the physiology of retinal ganglion cells near birth but in the Lateral Geniculate Body neurones respond to visual stimuli and can be classified as linear (X) or non-linear (Y) (Blakemore and Vital-Durand in prep.). In many aspects maturation of their receptive fields correlates well with behavioural data on visual acuity.

Over the first year or more of life there is a remarkable change in the spatial properties of LGN cells. Improvement of spatial resolution of LGN cells matches, in general form, the gradual

improvement in behavioural acuity tested by the preferential looking
technique (Teller et al 1978), (Fig 3). It is conceivable that the
preferential looking technique tends to under-estimate the ultimate
behavioural capacity, especially in very young animals, in which the
number of trials is obviously limited. It could also be postulated that
the response is limited by slower development of striate cortical
neurones. However, in a study of striate cortical neurones from the
same animals we found that at every stage the best of them can resolve
just about as well as the best cell in the LGN (Blakemore and
Vital-Durand 1982).

Many other parameters of striate neurone reponses are also very
immature at birth. Some mature within a few weeks after birth, others
need a year or more to reach adult level.
When they are recorded on the day of birth, no more than about
forty per cent of the cells in area V1 display orientation selectivity
for an elongated stimulus. About ten per cent present a bias in their
response in favor of one orientation but are not completely
unresponsive to the orthogonal orientation. The rest of the cells are
either undiscriminative for orientation or visually unresponsive. It is
very striking that within two weeks after birth, orientation
selectivity among cortical neurones reaches adult characteristics, the
bulk showing tuning curves very specific for a limited range of
stimulus orientations.

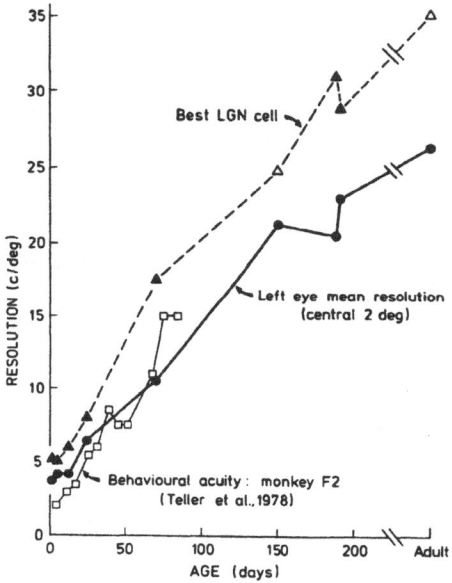

Fig 3 Development of spatial resolution.

The time course of the improvement of neuronal acuity. Each filled
circle is the mean resolution for all cells recorded in the LGN laminae
connected to the left (normal) eye from a series of monkeys whose other
eye was deprived. Only cells whose receptive fields lay in the central
2 deg of the visual field were considered. For comparison the unfilled
squares show behavioural determinations of visual acuity as a function
of age for an individual monkey tested by the preferential looking
technique (Teller et al 1978).

Most striate area neurones can be activated through stimulation of either eye, and hence are called binocular. Detailed analysis of the strength of the response to stimulation of either eye shows a complete range of ocular dominance as some are activated more readily trough one eye than the other. At birth, just less than half of the responsive neurones have already developed enough synaptic contacts to be binocularly driven so that the other half of the cells remain monocular. Again this proportion changes very quickly in normal conditions, and by the end of a fortnight nearly all the cells, except those in layer IV, have become binocular.

The same timescale does not hold for other cortical cell properties investigated. Grating resolution only begins to improve significantly from its neonatal values after two or more weeks and is not yet fully mature at the end of the first year (Fig 3). This delayed increase in spatial resolution takes place in a comparable length of time in humans. Indeed this function, the most commonly evaluated because of testing handiness, is known to achieve adult level around the fourth year. In infant monkeys, it has been argued that poor acuity in young infants cannot be attributed primarily to either poor optical quality or receptor sampling frequency (Boothe 1982). Unit recording in the LGN representation of the central visual field suggests that normal development of acuity depends on the maturation of neural elements that lie in the retina, LGN and possibly visual cortex. Similarity between behavioural performances obtained with the preferential looking technique in monkeys and electrophysiological data favors the proposition that neural maturation is the limiting factor of visual acuity in monkey and human infants (Blakemore and Vital-Durand in prep).

Given these basic data two questions are addressed to implement our knowledge of the processes involved. The first one deals with the role of time and existence of a critical or sensitive period, the other one with localization in the brain of the sites concerned with specific deficits consecutive to early manipulations of individuals' visual experience. Visual deprivation studies bring some answers to these questions. As excellent reviews of this vast body of litterature are available (Hubel, Wiesel and LeVay 1977; Blakemore 1978; Mitchell and Timney 1984; Boothe, Dobson and Teller 1985), a few examples from monkey experiments will be described to illustrate crucial features.

VISUAL DEPRIVATION

Since the original paradigm of early monocular deprivation was introduced by Wiesel and Hubel (1963) the period during which cortical neurones are sensitive to deprivation is known to span the first few months of life. Monocular lid suture affects cellular growth in the corresponding layers of the LGN, but receptive field properties (Hubel, Wiesel and LeVay 1977) and spatial resolution of these same cells is not affected (Blakemore and Vital-Durand 1981). In the visual cortex, lid suture dramatically impairs binocularity , ocular dominance and spatial resolution. Indeed, the affected cells lose their excitatory input from the deprived eye and can only be activated through the experienced one. This condition can be reversed up to a certain age by the procedure of reverse suturing, reopening the initially deprived eye and suturing the other (Blakemore and Van Sluyters 1974). The latest age at wich this procedure is followed by a recovery of excitability through stimulatioin of the initially deprived eye is the end of the critical or **sensitive period for ocular dominance**. In the monkey it occurs around the 9th week of age although

some effect on cells outside layer IV is still observed at a later age
(Blakemore , Garey and Vital-Durand 1981).

These data and others illustrate the concept of binocular
competition, a phenomenon known to play a role in human amblyopic or
strabismic patients. The fact is that anatomical study of the relative
width of ocular dominance slabs as evidenced by autoradiographic
transport of tritiated aminoacids show a fairly good correlation
between deprivation amblyopia measured behaviourally (Harwerth, Smith,
Boltz, Crawford and von Noorden 1983) or electrophysiologically and
attrition of columns normally dominated by the altered eye (
Blakemore, Vital-Durand and Garey 1981 ; Swindale, Vital-Durand and
Blakemore 1981). The dramatic effect of these manipulations is to be
sought at the cortical level, as it appears that smaller cell size
observed in the layers of the LGN connected to the deprived eye
(Vital-Durand and Garey1978) does not impede signal transmission, but
could altogether be a consequence of the alteration of the
cortico-geniculate feed-back loop.

Reverse suture experiments demonstrate that the simple reopening
of a deprived eye is not followed by any anatomical, physiological or
behavioural recovery as long as the experienced eye is not deprived in
turn (Blakemore et al 1981).

The nature of the deleterious effect of visual deprivation on
message transmission in cortical layer IV is still unclear. Anatomical
studies fail to show obvious synaptic distributon changes which could
explain why few striate cortex cells respond to visual stimulation of
the deprived eye, even in layer IV. Terminals from this eye are not
evidenced by autoradiographic techniques, but a few days of reverse
suturing are enough to restore excitability in these handicaped cells.
In cats, it has been shown that some very powerful treatments like
pharmacological manipulation, enucleation of the non-deprived eye or
electrical stimulation can instantly rehabilitate the excitability of
the deprived cortical cells (see review in Sherman and Spear 1982). The
most reasonable explanation is that axone terminals from the deprived
eye are still at least partially there but lack adequate metabolic
activity or the precise pattern of spatial distribution or temporal
firing requisite to trigger generation of action potentials in the
postsynaptic cell. Their functional properties are altered although
their fine anatomical features appear normal. The term "synaptic
efficiency" has been forged to describe this condition.

CONCLUSION

These facts have been put together to substantiate some basic
principle of organization of the visual system that we could summarize
as follows.

Vision is one among many processes by which the organism senses
its position in the outside world. Audition, vestibular sense,
proprioception and muscular sense combine with vision to supply the
necessary spatial informations to stabilize the relative position of
the body in space. Each captor and its processing features can only be
considered as one element of a structure. Any local deficit would
affect the global behaviour of the individual.

The same principle holds at the next smaller stage of analysis.
The visual system is the sum of partial functions which, for clarity,
could be called resolution capacity, contrast sensitivity, movement
detection and analysis, color discrimination, depth sensitivity and
stereopsis, form discrimination. Anatomical considerations support this

10

view exemplified by the existence of several parallel channels coding and carrying varieties of messages to different parts of the central network. On the basis of current physiological knowledge, it would be premature to assign precise function to each of them.

This description of the normal adult system is the end-product of complex developmental interactive processes during which genetic programing and epigenetic factors have sculptured the capacities of the adult individual. These developmental processes are by nature irreversible and discontinuous, some stages being particularly critical because of their increased sensitivity to external influence.

The sensitive period for ocular dominance is only one demonstrative example of crucial interference between a developmental process and visual experience. There are probably many other sensitive periods pertaining to other visual, visuo-motor or perceptual functions, but not much is known of their possible interdependence.

Finally, we have already alluded to the basic role of eye movements in the management of visual information by the individual; much more needs to be done to understand how their development fits in the maturation of the whole process of vision.

Aknowledgements. This work was supported by INSERM. D J Perkel revised the english text.

REFERENCES

Blakemore C. Maturation and modification in the developing visual system. In: Held R, Leibowitz HW, Teuber HL., eds. Handbook of sensory physiology vol. VIII, Perception. Berlin: Springer, 1978:377-436.

Blakemore C, Van Sluyters RC. Reversal of the physiological effects of monocular deprivation in kitten : further evidence for a sensitive period. J. Physiol 1974;237:195-216.

Blakemore C, Vital-Durand F. Postnatal development of the monkey's visual system. In: Ciba Foundation Symposium n°86. The fetus and independent life, 1981: 152-171.

Blakemore C, Vital-Durand F. Development of contrast sensitivity by neurons in monkey striate cortex. J Physiol (London) 1982;334:18-19P.

Blakemore C, Vital-Durand F, Garey LJ. Recovery from monocular deprivation in the monkey. I. Reversal of physiological effects in the visual cortex. Proc Roy Soc Lond B 1981;213:399-423.

Boothe RG. Optical and neural factors limiting acuity development : evidence obtained from a monkey model. Current Eye Res 1982;2:211-215.

Boothe RG, Dobson V, Teller DY. Postnatal development of vision in human and nonhuman primates. Ann Rev neurosci 1985;8:495-545.

Bullier J, Henry GH. Ordinal position and afferent input of neurons in monkey striate cortex. J Comp Neurol 1980;193:913-935.

Collin NG, Cowey A. The effect of ablation of frontal eye-field and superior colliculi on visual stability and movement discrimination in rhesus monkey. Exp Brain Res 1980;40:251-260.

De Valois RL, Morgan HC, Polson MC, Mead WR, Hull EM. Psychophysical studies of monkey vision. I. Macaque luminosity and color vision tests. Vision Res 1974;14:53-67.

De Valois RL, Morgan H, Snodderly DM. Psychophysical studies of monkey vision. III. Spatial luminance contrast sensitivity tests of macaque and human observers. Vision Res 1974;14:75-81.

Enroth-Cugell C, Robson JG. The contrast sensitivity of retinal ganglion cells of the cat. J Physiol 1966;187:517-552.

Harwerth RS, Smith III EL, Boltz RL, Crawford MLJ, Von Noorden GK. Behavioral studies on the effect of abnormal early visual experience in monkeys : spatial modulation sensitivity. Vision Res 1983;23:1501-1510.

Hubel DH. Exploration of the primary visual cortex, 1955-1978. Nature 1982;299:515-524.

Hubel DH, Wiesel TN. Receptive fields, binocular interaction and functional architecture in the cat's visual cortex. J Physiol

1962;160:106-154.

Hubel DH, Wiesel TN. Functional architecture of macaque monkey visual cortex. Proc R Soc London B 1977;198:1-59.

Hubel DH, Wiesel TN, Le Vay S. Plasticity of ocular dominance columns in monkey striate cortex. Phil Trans R Soc Lond B 1977;278:377-409.

Ingle DJ. Organization of visuomotor behaviors in vertebrates. In: Ingle DJ, Goodale MA, Mansfield RJW, eds. Analysis of visual behavior. Cambridge, Mass. : MIT Press, 1982: 67-109.

Mitchell DE, Timney B. Postnatal development of function in the mammalian visual system. In: Handbook of Physiology, The Nervous System III. Bethesda, Md : American Physiological Society, 1985:507-555.

Perry VH, Cowey A. Retinal ganglion cells that project to the superior colliculus and pretectum in the macaque monkey. Neuroscience 1984;1125-1137.

Perry VH, Oehler R, Cowey A. Retinal ganglion cells that project to the dorsal lateral geniculate nucleus in the macaque monkey. Neuroscience 1984;12:1101-1123.

Precht W. Anatomical and functional organization of optokinetic pathways. In: Lennerstrand G, Zee DS, Keller EL, eds. Functional basis of ocular mobility disorders. Oxford : Pergamon Press, 1982:291-302.

Shermann SM, Spear PD. Organization of visual pathways in normal and visually deprived cats. Physiol Rev 1982;62:738-855.

Simpson JI. The accessory optic system. Ann Rev Neurosci 1984;7:13-41.

Stone J. Parallel processing in the visual system. New York : Plenum Press, 1983:(XVI) + 438 p (index).

Stone J, Hoffmann KP. Very slow conducting ganglion cells in the cat's retina : a major new functional type ? Brain Res 1972;43:610-616.

Swindale NV, Vital-Durand F, Blakemore C. Recovery from monocular deprivation in the monkey : III. Reversal of anatomical effects in the visual cortex. Proc Roy Soc Lond B 1981;213:435-450.

Teller DY, Morse R, Borton R, Regal D. Visual acuity for vertical and diagonal gratings in human infants. Vision Res 1974;14:1433-1439.

Teller DY, Regal DM, Videen TO, Pulos E. Development of visual acuity in infant monkeys (Macaca nemestrina) during the early postnatal weeks. Vision Res 1978;18:561-566.

Van Essen DC. Visual areas of the mammalian cerebral cortex. Am Rev Neurosci 1979;2:227-263.

Van Essen DC, Maunsell HR. Hierarchical organization and functional streams in the visual cortex. Trends Neurosci 1983;6:370-375.

Vital-Durand F, Garey LJ, Blakemore C. Monocular and binocular deprivation in the monkey : morphological effects and reversibility. Brain Res 1978;158:45-64.

Wiesel TN. Postnatal development of the visual cortex and the influence of environment. Nature 1982;299:583-591.

Wiesel TN, Hubel DH. Effects of visual deprivation on morphology and physiology of cells in the cat's lateral geniculate body. J Neurophysiol 1963;26:978-993.

Wurtz RH, Albano JE. Visual motor function of the primate superior colliculus. Ann Rev Neuroscience 1980;3:189-226.

OCULAR GROWTH AND THE NORMAL DEVELOPMENT OF VISION
CLINICAL ASPECTS

Alistair R. Fielder

Leicester University Medical School, Leicester.

INTRODUCTION

Since the late 1950's when Fantz showed that infants preferred to look at a patterned rather than a non-patterned stimulus there has been a tremendous growth in interest in the vision of the pre-verbal child. Psychologists, neurophysiologists, physicists and paediatricians have all contributed to our present level of understanding of infant vision. New techniques, such as preferential looking (PL) and the visually evoked potential (VEP) have been developed enabling the detailed study of visual function. Until very recently the ophthalmologist, has kept relatively remote from these developments and even today, in Britain, these new methods have yet to make a significant impact on clinical practice.

There are a variety of reasons for this. First, simple observations on visual alertness, fixation and reaching are often thought to suffice and the finding of an ocular anomaly such as optic nerve hypoplasia, atrophy or absent pupillary reflex is confirmation enough of a visual problem. Quantitation has not been required by parent or colleague; but this situation is now changing. Second, the ophthalmologist, having at his disposal retinoscopy, biomicroscopy and ophthalmoscopy can examine the eye in great detail and by undertaking surgical or orthoptic correction, if feasible, may feel that all that can be done for vision has been done and a prolonged laboratory test, which will not influence management is clinically irrelevant. Third, the expense incurred and technical expertise required for some investigations prohibits their general use. Fourth, clinical workload does not permit devoting 20 to 30 minutes per child for acuity testing, particularly if the result will not influence management.

Inevitably articles reflect the interest and discipline(s) of the workers involved and sometimes details not directly within their sphere of expertise are poorly presented or inappropriately emphasised. An obvious example would be to consider VEP acuity in infancy without considering foveal development. To an extent this is inevitable: no single person can be aware of all recent developments, but it does indicate the need for a multidisciplinary approach.

In this article I will review certain aspects of ocular
growth of which an understanding is a mandatory
pre-requisite to the study of visual development. I will
then briefly consider the refractive status of the infant,
the visual evoked potential and preferential looking
techniques and delayed visual maturation. References will
be selective rather than comprehensive.

OCULAR GROWTH

With the current level of interest in the vision of
full-term and preterm infants it is pertinent to briefly
consider certain developmental aspects of the eye and
visual pathways. After birth the eyeball increases in
weight by a factor of 3 to reach its adult size whereas
the corresponding change in bodyweight is 20. The power
of the eye decreases from its neonatal 85 D to 58 D in the
adult. Not all ocular tissues grow equally, the major
increase affecting the posterior segment. During
pregnancy there is a linear increase in the sagittal
length of the globe to reach 16.0 to 17.7mm at 40 weeks of
gestation (Luyckz 1966; Harayama et al 1981), this being
proportional to birth weight (Blomdahl 1979). Most of the
subsequent increase takes place in the first three years,
following this there is only a small increase to reach the
adult length of 24 mm by the mid-teens (Weale 1982).

The cornea is relatively fully developed at term (Sorsby
and Sheridan 1960), only small changes in corneal diameter
occur after birth (Weale 1982) and these in the first year
of life. In contrast, corneal radius of curvature
increases rapidly after birth (Scammon and Armstrong
1925). Mandell (1967) has suggested that alterations in
corneal contour permit maximum visual acuity during each
phase of ocular growth.

The anterior chamber of the eye increases in depth
steadily up to the mid-teens (Weale 1982). Lens thickness
reaches a maximum of 4 mm by the age of one year, whereas
its diameter increases throughout life (Weale 1982). This
structure, relatively spherical at birth does not assume
its lenticular shape until accommodation is active (Fisher
1969).

Foveal development is incomplete at term. Early work
suggested that it was complete by 4-6 weeks post-natally
(Mann 1964), but a recent detailed study by Hendrickson
and Yuodelis (1984) has shown that this is not so,
maturity not being reached until between 15 and 45 months
of age. The internal foveal depression is developed by 15
months, but the external fovea is not seen until 45
months, by which time the transient layer of Chievitz, a
marker of immaturity, has almost disappeared. Movement
takes place in two directions: central migration of
photoreceptors, particularly cones (completed by 45

months) and the peripheral movement of bipolar, horizontal, ganglion and some Muller cells (completed between 15 and 45 months). Outer segment development occurs almost entirely after birth.

Myelination is first observed in the optic nerve between 6 and 8 months of foetal life (Bembridge 1956; Magoon and Robb 1981) and proceeds centrifugally from the optic tract. Contrary to previous reports Magoon and Robb (1981) noted myelin in only some optic nerve fibres near the globe but by 7 months of post natal life virtually all fibres are myelinated. Myelin around each individual nerve increases rapidly up to the age of two years and thereafter only in small amounts. These authors could not confirm an earlier observation (Bembridge 1956) that foveal fibres become myelinated first.

Garey and de Courten (1983) have recently reviewed the structural development of the lateral geniculate nucleus and visual cortex. Both undergo a rapid increase in volume, between birth and 6 months of age, due to dendrite and spine formation, accompanied by an increase in complexity of the cerebral convolutions. Thereafter volume stabilises but synapses are eliminated massively.

What effect does birth with its attendent changes in internal and external environment have on ocular development? Weale (1982) has recently reviewed a number of factors influencing ocular growth such as genetic factors, sex and diet. Does exposure to light limit ocular growth? This is not entirely academic, as ocular development in the baby born prematurely is inevitably, at the time of birth, at a much earlier stage than if gestation had proceeded for 40 weeks. It is still not known whether ocular development is adversely affected by premature exteriorisation although these persons are liable to develop myopia later in childhood (Fledelius 1976) possibly due to the arrest of corneal curvature development resulting in a relative keratoconus (Weale 1982). That this could be the result of a thermal deficit during a period of rapid ocular growth consequent on premature birth has recently been speculated (Fielder et al submitted). A different mechanism from that causing the myopia of retrolental fibroplasia. Compare this to axial myopia associated with ipsilateral ptosis in the human (Hoyt et al 1981) and the monkey (Wiesel and Raviola 1977), which may result from an increase in local temperature, observed in lid closure (Fielder et al 1981), leading to enhanced growth of the eyeball.

That exposure to light may hasten myelination (Langworthy 1933) has not been confirmed by Magoon and Robb (1981) in the human, or in the cat (Moore et al 1976), neither does increased visual experience appear to advantage the premature baby compared to its full-term counterpart (van Hof-van Duin et al 1983).

REFRACTION

As already noted, the power of the eye lessens in early
life, due to alterations in: corneal curvature, eyeball
axial length, anterior chamber depth and the lens. What
literature is available on refraction in infancy is
difficult to analyse as there is often failure to
distinguish ethnic origin, degree of prematurity or to
exclude ocular pathology.

It is generally accepted that the full-term infant is
hypermetropic, of the order of one to two dioptres (Banks
1980a; Fulton et al 1980), being at its maximum at two to
four months of age (Yamamoto et al 1979) and changing only
a small amount later in the first year (Banks 1980a).
Following this there is a gradual reduction in the degree
of hypermetropia during childhood (Banks 1980a), although
two studies failed to observe a significant decrease
between six months (Shapiro et al 1980) or one year
(Ingram and Barr 1979) and three and a half years.

The incidence of astigmatism in early infancy measured
using cycloplegic refraction, is at least twice that seen
in the adult (Fulton et al 1980). Three studies, using
cycloplegia, have reported incidences (note minimum amount
of astigmatism recorded varies between studies) of between
13.2 % and 50 % (Santonastaso 1930; Ingram 1979 and Fulton
et al 1980), while without cycloplegia this incidence is
almost 60% (Mohindra et al 1978) or 63% (Howland et al
1978). There is a trend for the amount of cylindrical
ametropia to decrease in early childhood (Fulton et al
1980; Ingram and Barr 1979).

Premature infants are often myopic in the neonatal period
(Graham and Gray 1963; Dobson et al 1981 and Scharf et al
1978), its severity related inversely to gestational age.
By six months of age there is a change of refraction
towards emmetropia (Scharf et al 1978) and in one study
(Shapiro et al 1980) at this age there was no difference
between premature and full-term infants.

Infants begin to accommodate at two to three months of age
(Banks 1980b). As the eye grows depth of focus decreases
and the accuracy of accommodation increases (Green et al
1980). Consequently, in the small eye with a relatively
low visual acuity but large depth of focus, i.e. the eye
liable to contain a refractive error, the perceptual
consequences of these errors should be small (Green et al
1980), as has been shown in infants with large astigmatic
errors (Gwiazda et al 1978).

Thus infants, especially if prematurely born, often
exhibit refractive errors particularly astigmatic. There
is a tendency for this ametropia to decrease with age.
This process, emmetropisation, (Banks 1980a; Koole and van
der Heijde 1983) is poorly understood, depends upon the
delicately balanced pattern of different rates of growth

of the various ocular tissues but is also probably
influenced by visual experience (Rabin et al 1981; Wallman
et al 1981). Could this process be interfered with and
explain why children with neurodevelopmental problems
(Gardiner 1963) and certain ocular problems such as
congenital achromatopsia have a high incidence of
hypermetropia?

VISUAL EVOKED POTENTIAL

Surely one of the most exciting developments in paediatric
ophthalmology in recent years has been the introduction of
the visual evoked potential. VEP methodology is
progressing rapidly, increasing the already huge gulf
between research worker and clinician: the latter often
using this test so crudely that little reliance can be
placed on the result. Thus the precise role of the VEP in
routine clinical paediatric ophthalmological practice has
yet to be defined.

Early VEP studies employed a flash stimulus. Lacking an
edge it is not suitable for acuity measurement and also
being prone to both intra- and inter-individual variation
(Fielder et al 1983) has become largely superseded by the
VEP to a patterned stimulus. But the flash VEP is simple
to perform, robust, and in infancy does exhibit certain
reliable features: the simple neonatal shape becomes more
complex between 42 and 84 days of life, and both N1 and P2
latency decrease with increasing age in a highly
statistically significant manner. Amplitude measurements
are not reliably related to age (Fielder et al 1983). A
recent study (de Vries-Khoe and Spekreijse 1982) has
stated that the decrease in VEP latency can be entirely
attributed to the increase in EEG frequency in the first
year of life and state of alertness, but not to visual
pathway maturation, observations not in agreement with
Ellingson (1970). As P2 latency decreases more rapidly
than would be expected from the change in background EEG
frequency (Hagne 1972), de Vries-Khoe and Spekreijse
(1982) suggest that this corresponds to the completion of
optic nerve myelination at this age, although as we have
already seen full myelination of the optic nerves is not
achieved until two years of age (Magoon and Robb 1981).
Provided only modest requirements are made concerning
latency and morphology the flash VEP together with a
non-corneal ERG is useful clinically: in distinguishing
retinal and more central visual pathway pathology, as a
base-line reading in the blind infant who may improve and
as a base-line for the infant who may later regress
neurologically.

Processing of different stimulus types is probably
subserved by separate neural substrates and although the
VEP to a flash stimulus does have some clinical value it
cannot be used to estimate acuity. For this a patterned
stimulus is required. Both Marg and colleagues (1976) and

Sokol (1978) using different stimuli reported that EP acuity reached adult levels by six months, whereas PL acuity at this age is approximately 6/45 (Fulton et al 1981; Dobson 1983). In a recent study (Sokol et al 1984) in which VEP's and FPL were compared in the same children, the former was consistently higher than the latter except for three patients with nystagmus. This discrepancy often being considerable. Results from separate laboratories utilising different stimulus parameters cannot be equated, but it is relevant to note that foveal development takes much longer than previously thought (Hendrickson and Yuodelis 1984), corresponding closer to PL than EP techniques. The one exception to this is the EP study of de Vries-Khoe and Spekreijse (1982), the results of which correlate with both anatomical and behavioural data.

PREFERENTIAL LOOKING

Over the past decade or so PL procedures have been used extensively in the study of visual development (reviews Teller 1983; Dobson 1983). During development PL acuity is consistently lower than VEP acuity not reaching 6/6 until about three years of age (Fulton et al 1981). The possible anatomical reasons for this have already been discussed, although Held and associates (1979) claimed that PL acuity is underestimated because gratings near threshold are not preferentially fixated. Unfortunately, althugh th apparatus is relatively simple and cheap, the procedure is both tedious and time-consuming to perform and has not been widely incorporated into routine paediatric ophthalmic practice despite having been demonstrated to be of value (Jacobson et al 1982; Dobson 1983). Procedural modifications have been introduced: forced choice and diagnostic stripe procedure (Dobson et al 1978; and Teller 1979), and operant FPL (Mayer and Dobson, 1980). Recently a rapid test procedure has been described using a portable apparatus in which gratings are presented on cards rather than on televisions (McDonald et al in press). This test can usually be completed in two or three minutes. Contact can be maintained with the infant through the aperture in the screen between stimulus presentations and fixation checked by a small sideways movement of the hand-held card containing the grating (personal observations).

Recognition and PL grating acuities may differ significantly in certain conditions (Mayer et al 1984). This disparity in which PL is better than recognition acuity, may be large and is found in children with dense amblyopia and macular anomalies. In those non-amblyopic patients with cataracts, optic nerve anomalies, generalized retinal degenerations etc. both tests correlate well. Thus in albinism (i.e. foveal hypoplasia), PL grating acuities are significantly better than in generalized retinal degenerations (Mayer et al in press). This phenomenon has not been fully explained as yet, but Weale noted in 1982 "few contemporary grating measurements are confined to the foveal region". Other

factors to be considered include stimulus complexity and
the crowding phenomenon. Clearly it is mandatory that the
clinician is aware that the PL acuity in amblyopia may be
greater than that obtained by traditional means.

Both EP's and PL have advantages and disadvantages. The
VEP has the advantage of being a relatively fast procedure
to perform and does not rely on a sensory response,
furthermore it provides valuable information on visual
pathway function, apart from acuity, which cannot
otherwise be obtained. But it is not cheap and requires a
level of technical expertise not currently generally
available; nor, taking populations as a whole, is likely
to be in the forseeable future. The attachment of
electrodes is unacceptable to some children and
occasionally also to a parent. The VEP is often
unsatisfactory in the presence of nystagmus. PL has the
advantage of being cheap, simple and now rapid to perform.
It is unsuitable in certain oculomotor disturbances, such
as congenital ocular motor apraxia and often fails between
the ages of 12 to 24 months.

There are unexplained discrepancies between EP, PL and
recognition acuities, of which the clinician should be
aware. In some studies EP acuity is reported to reach 6/6
long before the fovea is fully developed. PL and
recognition acuities are discrepant in certain conditions,
notably amblyopia. All tests of acuity may fail in the
hyperactive or retarded. No test is infallible in the
clinically important period between 18 months and two and
a half years.

DELAYED VISUAL MATURATION

That the sight of a child blind in infancy may
subsequently improve has been known to clinicians for many
years, although only relatively recently has it received
attention in the literature (Illingworth 1961; Mellor and
Fielder 1980; Hoyt et al 1983 and Cole et al 1984).
Uemera and colleagues (1981) were the first to state, a
point previously only alluded to, that delayed visual
maturation (DVM) is not a homogenous condition and these
authors subdivided DVM into three categories: 1, DVM as an
isolated anomaly, 2, DVM in association with mental
retardation, and 3, ocular abnormalities accompanied by
DVM.

A recent study of 53 cases (Fielder et al in press)
further subdivided group 1 into A those without and B
those infants with problems in the neonatal period. Group
2 infants presented with severe developmental problems and
poor vision. The distinctive feature of group 3 was a
visual defect greatly out of proportion to the ocular
condition. All infants in this ocular/nystagmus group had
nystagmus, either of the congenital or albino types and in

one case there was also an early cataract. Nystagmus was
never seen in group 1 and only in one infant in group 2.
With the exception of infants in group 3 and the presence
of a convergent squint in seven, no ocular abnormality was
detected other than could be attributed to reduced vision.

Electroretinography was performed in 33 and was normal in
all. Of the 41 on whom flash VEP's were obtained only
nine were unequivocably normal. VEP abnormalities
included: a flat response which later improved, delay of
P2, or amplitude reduction. The temporal relationship
between the presence of VEP abnormalities and visual
status is not clearly established, but preliminary studies
do not show them to be precisely related.

Two interesting features of DVM, have received no
attention so far. First, time of recovery. For group 1A
this occurred at a median age of 14 weeks (range 9-19),
and although the median age of improvement was also 14
weeks for group 1B the range was greater (range 11-40),
presumably reflecting the coexisting systemic problems.
In group 1 visual improvement in preterm babies
corresponded closer to corrected rather than chronological
ages. For group 2, mentally retarded infants, the median
age of recovery was 60 weeks (range 26- 100) and for group
3 the corresponding figures were 20 (range 16-36).
Second, speed of recovery. For all of group 1 this was
rapid usually within 14 days, but always within a month.
Improvement was always slow for group 2, often taking
months to decide whether any visual change had taken
place. The pattern of improvement for group 3 was
variable. Thus time and speed of improvement are
dramatically different between isolated DVM and that
associated with severe developmental delay.

Once improvement has occurred in isolated DVM, visual
development appears to be on course, e.g. no response to
PL acuity of 3 cycles/degree within one month. To date,
with a maximum follow-up of eight years, no child of any
group has suffered either a visual relapse or a permanent
bilateral visual defect.

It is now apparent why isolated DVM is not well known to
the non-clinical visual scientist; most are likely to have
improved by the time detailed investigation is
contemplated (delay in referral). It could be sensibly
argued that further study is unnecessary. Clinically this
may be so, but scientifically surely DVM must contain many
secrets of visual development? Its pathogenesis is
unknown (Mellor and Fielder 1980; editorial Lancet 1984):
as the ERG is normal a retinal origin is unlikely. A
delay in myelination cannot be excluded but in isolated
DVM neither the time or rapid speed of improvement
correlate well with previous studies of normal
myelogenesis. Furthermore pupillary responses are
unaffected. The analogy between DELAYED visual
maturation with NORMAL myelination may not necessarily be

appropriate. Another possibility is a disturbance of posterior visual pathway development during the period of rapid dendrite and spine formation (Garey and de Courten 1983) in either or both the lateral geniculate nucleus and visual cortex. This theory is currently the most attractive: visual improvement, in isolated DVM, occuring in the latter part of this period of rapid dendrite growth. It is relevant to note that 26 of 53 had problems in the perinatal period, and of these 11 sustained permanent neurological sequelae of varying severity, possibly indicating an insult to the central nervous system in this crucial period. Only two infants (of the remaining 27) not suffering perinatal difficulties had neurodevelopmental problems and one of these had tuberous sclerosis.

Although the indications so far are that most infants with isolated DVM have, superficially, no further visual problems, the possibility of learning or perceptual difficulties persisting into later childhood has not been explored. The study of infants with DVM must surely provide further insight into the understanding of visual development.

REFERENCES

Banks MS. Infant refraction and accommodation. Int Ophthalmol Clin 1980a;20:205-232.

Banks MS. The development of visual accommodation during early infancy. Child Dev 1980b; 51:646-666.

Bembridge BA. The problem of myelination in the central nervous system with special reference to the optic nerve. Trans Ophthalmol Soc UK 1956;76;311-321.

Blomdahl S. Ultrasonic measurements of the eye in the newborn infant. Acta Ophthalmol 1979;57:1048-1056.

Cole GF, Hungerford J, Jones RB. Delayed visual maturation. Arch Dis Child 1984;59:107-110.

Dobson V. Clinical applications of preferential looking measures of visual acuity. Behav Brain Res 1983;10:25-38.

Dobson V, Teller DY, Lee CP, Wade B. A behavioural method for efficient screening of visual acuity in young infants. Invest Ophthalmol Visual Sci 1978;17:1142-1150.

Dobson V, Fulton AB, Manning K, Salem D, Petersen RA. Cycloplegic refractions of premature infants. Am J Ophthalmol 1981;91:490-495.

Editorial. Delayed visual maturation. Lancet 1984;1:1158-1159.

Ellingson RJ. Variability of visual evoked responses in the human newborn. Elecroencephalogr Clin Neurophysiol 1970;29:10-19.

Fielder AR, Winder AF, Cooke DE, Bowcock SA. Arcus senilis and corneal temperature in man. Proc Eur Congr Ophthalmol ed PD Trevor-Roper Royal Soc Med 1981; 1015-1020.

Fielder AR, Harper MW, Higgins JE, Clarke CM, Corrigan D. The reliability of the VEP in infancy. Ophthal Paed Genet 1983;3:73-82.

Fielder AR, Levene MI, Russell-Eggitt IM, Weale RA. Temperature-a factor in ocular development? submitted.

Fielder AR, Russell-Eggitt IM, Dodd KL, Mellor DH. Delayed visual maturation. Trans Ophthalmol Soc UK in press.

Fisher RF. The significance of the shape of the lens and capsular energy changes in accommodation. J Physiol 1969; 201: 21-47.

Fledelius H. Prematurity and the eye. Acta Ophthalmol 1981;Suppl 128:1-239.

Fulton AB, Dobson V, Salem D, Mar C, Petersen RA, Hansen RM. Cycloplegic refractions in infants and young children. Am J Ophthalmol 1980;90:239-247.

Fulton AB, Hansen RM, Manning KA. Measuring visual acuity in infants. Surv Ophthalmol 1981;25:325-332.

Gardiner PA. Refractive errors and cerebral palsy. In: VH Smith, ed. Visual disorders and cerebral palsy. Little Club Clinics in Developmental Medicine No 9. Wm Heinemann Medical Books Ltd London, 1963:44-47.

Garey LJ, de Courten C. Structural development of the lateral geniculate nucleus and visual cortex in monkey and man. Behav Brain Res 1983;10:3-14.

Graham MV, Gray OP. Refraction of premature babies' eyes. Brit Med J 1963;1:1452-1454.

Green DG, Powers MK, Banks MS. Depth of focus, eye size and visual acuity. Vision Res 1980;20:827-835.

Gwiazda J, Brill S, Mohindra I, Held R. Infant visual acuity and its meridional variation. Vision Res 1978;18:1557-1564.

Hagne I. Development of the EEG in normal infants during the first year of life. Acta Paediatr Scand Suppl 1972;232:1-53.

Harayama K, Amemiya T. Nishimura H. Development of the eyeball during fetal life. J Pediatr Ophthalmol Strabismus 1981;18:37-40.

Held R, Gwiazda J, Brill S, Mohindra I, Wolfe J. Infant

visual acuity is underestimated because near threshold gratings are not preferentially fixated. Vision Res 1979;19:1377-1379.

Hendrickson AE, Yuodelis C. The morphological development of the human fovea. Ophthalmology 1984;91:603-612.

Howland HC, Atkinson J, Braddick O, French J. Infant astigmatism measured by photorefraction. Science 1978;202:331-333.

Hoyt CS, Stone RS, Fromer C. Monocular axial myopia associated with neonatal eyelid closure in human infants. Am J Ophthalmol 1981;91:197-200.

Hoyt CS, Jastrzebski G, Marg E. Delayed visual maturation in infancy. Brit J Ophthalmol 1983;67:127-130.

Illingworth RS. Delayed visual maturation. Arch Dis Child 1961;36:407-409.

Ingram RM. Refraction of 1-year-old children after atropine cycloplegia. Brit J Ophthalmol 1979;63:343-347.

Ingram RM, Barr A. Changes in refraction between the ages of 1 and 31/2 years. Brit J Ophthalmol 1979;63:339-342.

Jacobson SG, Mohindra I, Held R. Visual acuity of infants with ocular disases. Am J Ophthalmol 1982;93:198-209.

Koole FD, van der Heijde GL. Alteration in axial length in unilateral posttraumatic pseudophakia. Ophthal Paed Genet 1983;3:187-190.

Langworthy OR. Development of behaviour patterns and myelination of the nervous system in the human fetus and infant. Contr. Embryol 1933;139:1-57.

Luyckx J. Mesure des composantes optiques de l'oeil du nouveau-ne par echographie ultrasonique. Arch Opht (Paris) 1966;26:159-170.

Magoon EH, Robb RM. Development of myelin in human optic nerve and tract. Arch Ophthalmol 1981;99:655-659.

Mandell RB. Corneal contour of the human infant. Arch Ophthalmol 1967;77:345-348.

Mann I. The Development of the Human Eye. 3rd ed. London: Brit Med Assoc. 1964.

Marg E, Freeman DN, Peltzman P, Goldstein PJ. Visual acuity development in human infants: evoked potential measurements. Invest Ophthalmol 1976;15:150-153.

Mayer DL, Dobson V. Assessment of vision in young children: a new operant approach yields estimates of acuity. Invest Ophthalmol Vis Sci 1980;19:566-570.

Mayer DL, Fulton AB, Rodier D. Grating and recognition acuities of pediatric patients. Ophthalmology 1984;91:947-953.

Mayer DL, Fulton AB, Hansen RM. Visual acuity of infants and children with retinal degenerations. Ophthal Paed Genet in press.

McDonald MA, Dobson V, Sebris SL, Baitch L, Varner D, Teller DY. The acuity card procedure: a rapid test of infant acuity. Invest Ophthalmol Vis Sci in press.

Mellor DH, Fielder AR. Dissociated visual development: electrodiagnostic studies in infants who are "slow to see". Develop Med Child Neurol 1980;22:327-335.

Mohindra I, Held R, Gwiazda J, Brill S. Astigmatism in infants Science 1978;202:329-331.

Moore CL, Kalil R, Whitman R. Development of myelination in optic tract of the cat. J Comp Neurol 1976;165:125-136.

Rabin J, Van Sluyters RC, Malach R. Emmetropization: a vision-dependent phenomenon. Invest Ophthalmol Vis Sci 1981;20:561-564.

Santonastaso A. La rifrazione oculare nei primi anni di vitra. Ann Ottal Clin Ocul 1930;58:852-885

Scammon RE, Armstrong EL. On the growth of the human eyeball and optic nerve. J Comp Neurol 1925;38:165-219.

Scharf J, Zonis S, Zeltzer M. Refraction in premature babies: a prospective study. J. Pediatr Ophthalmol Strabismus 1978;15:48-50.

Shapiro A, Yanko L, Nawratzki I, Merin S. Refractive power of premature children at infancy and early childhood. Am J Ophthalmol 1980;90:234-238.

Sokol S. Measurement of infant visual acuity from pattern reversal evoked potentials. Vision Res 1978;18:33-39.

Sokol S, Hansen VC, Moskowitz A, Greenfield P, Towle VL. Evoked potential and preferential looking estimates of visual acuity in pediatric patients. Ophthalmology 1983;90:552-562.

Sorsby A, Sheridan M. The eye at birth: measurement of the principle diameters in forty-eight cadavers. J Anat 1960; 94:192-195.

Teller DY. The forced-choice preferential looking procedure: a psychophysical technique for use with human infants. Infant Behav Dev 1979; 2:135-153.

Teller DY.   Measurement of visual acuity in human and
monkey infants: the interface between laboratory and
clinic.   Behav Brain Res 1983;10:15-24.

Uemera Y, Oguchi Y, Katsumi O.   Visual developmental
delay. Ophthal Paed Genet 1981;1:49-58.

Van Hof-Van Duin J, Mohn G, Fetter WPF, Mettau JW, Baerts
W. Preferential looking acuity in preterm infants.   Behav
Brain Res 1983;10:47-50.

de Vries-Khoe LH, Spekreijse H.   Maturation of luminance
and'pattern EP's in man.   Docum Ophthal Proc Series Vol
31, ed G. Niemeyer and Ch Huber. 1982:461-475.

Wallman J, Adams JI, Trachtman JN.   The eyes of young
chickens grow toward emmetropia.   Invest Ophthalmol Vis
Sci 1981; 20:557-561.

Weale RA. In A Biography of the Eye: Development, Growth,
Age. London: HK Lewis and Co Ltd. 1982.

Wiesel TN, Raviola E. Myopia and eye enlargement after
neonatal lid fusion in monkeys.   Nature 1977;266: 66-68.

Yamamoto M, Tatsugami H, Bun J.   A follow-up study of
refractive errors in premature infants.   Jpn J. Ophthalmol
1979;23:435-443.

GENETIC CAUSES OF VISUAL IMPAIRMENT IN CHILDHOOD

Mette Warburg

Gentofte Hospital, Eye Clinic for the Multiply
Handicapped, 40, Sognevej, DK-2820 Gentofte

INTRODUCTION

In this review I shall discuss the progress in understanding of
the genetic causes of visual impairment, beginning with the
studies in the 1960's on the prevalence and morphological
classification of the genetic disorders; I shall proceed to
discuss the studies on genetic heterogeneity which were the
main issues in the 1970's and shall eventually mention studies
on mapping the human genome with an emphasis on information
about ophthalmic disorders.

PREVALENCE OF VISUAL IMPAIRMENT

In the 1950's and 60's almost all educationally normal
children with visual impairment were notified and educated at
Blind schools and schools for the partially sighted. It was
therefore possible to study the national prevalence of such
impairments. Prevalence figures from England and Wales,
British Columbia and the small European countries were rather
similar (Fraser & Friedman 1967, Robinson et al 1968, Schappert-
-Kimmijser et al 1979) presenting a prevalence of 20 per 100.000
of severe visual impairment, and the prevalence of moderate
visual impairment was assumed to be slightly larger (Jay 1979).

In the 1970's the scientific interest in mental retardation increased, and it was found that retarded children had a prevalence
of severe visual impairment 200 times as great as that observed
in the educationally normal children (Warburg 1983). The total
prevalence of severe visual impairment in childhood was estimated to be 40 per 100.000, the sum prevalence of moderate and
severe visual impairment thus being of the order of 80 per
100.000.

The four most common causes of visual impairment in childhood
are congenital or juvenile cataracts, retinal disorders, optic
atrophy and congenital malformations, including aniridia, each
comprising 15 - 20 per cent of all (Fraser & Friedman 1967, Jan
et al 1977). Genetic causes comprised 40 percent of all cases,
but it was suggested (Jay 1979) that further knowledge would
increase this fraction.

MORPHOLOGICAL CLASSIFICATION

In the early years ophthalmo-genetics was dominated by the important works of Sorsby (1951, 1970), Waardenburg (1932, 1961, 1963), Francois, and Franceschetti (1958, 1963). These early studies were almost exclusively based upon data from pedigree studies, and the disorders were classified by very accurate morphological descriptions of findings in the slitlamp, the ophthalmoscope and the light microscope. It was surmised that lesions which looked similar had similar aetiology, and it was rare for ophthalmologists to classify disorders according to findings in other tissues than the eye, optic atrophy being an obvious exception.

Prevention

Since most visually impaired children were living in Blind schools, few ophthalmologists were knowledgeable about the causes of blindness. Genetic counselling was rarely given, partly because the children met the experts when their siblings had already been born, and partly because it was considered harmful to counsel the young persons themselves in case they had autosomal dominant or X-linked disorders, because counselling is only possible if the counsellee receives full information about the prognosis even if he has a progressive disorder.

GENETIC HETEROGENEITY

Pedigree studies

Genetic heterogeneity has been the main issue of the 1970's. It was observed that clinically similar (ie phenotypically similar) disorders were often genetically distinct. In other words, the eye would react with only limited morphological changes to numbers of genetic and environmental influences. Initially genetic heterogeneity was documented when the same phenotype had dissimilar inheritance or when there was only normal offspring of a couple who both have a recessive phenotypically similar trait. Examples are plenty, and I need only mention the cases of autosomal dominant, recessive and X-linked retinitis pigmentosa or cataract, and the pedigree, originally described by Trevor-Roper (1952 and 1963) in which two albino parents had four normally pigmented children.

Syndromes

It was also observed that a number of rare genetic disorders of the eye were part of generalised syndromes, and that although the patients suffered from the classical causes of blindness, the generalised signs indicated new heterogeneities. Examples of systemic genetic syndromes with visual impairment are the cryptophthalmos syndrome where renal aplasia is the leading sign, the Marfan syndrome, and the holoprosencephaly syndromes wherein the cerebral anomalies are associated with cyclopia, microphthalmos or hypotelorism.

Cytogenetics

Human cytogenetics is a discipline now 30 years old (Thio &
Levan 1956). The first chromosome preparations gave information
about the trisomies, most of which are of ophthalmological as
well as of systemic interest. With the banding techniques
(Casperson 1970) it became possible to identify all chromosomes
and for some chromosomes to demonstrate whether a given case
of trisomy was due to errors in the meiosis of the father or
the mother. It is also possible to identify small translocations
and duplications and to see which band is missing in small
deletions.

High resolution techniques have recently demonstrated that some
cases of aniridia are associated with deletions on the short
arm of chromosome 11 (11p13) (Francke et al 1979). These patients
also have Wilm's tumor or gonadoblastoma (Andersen et al 1978)
and varying degrees of mental retardation depending upon the
length of the deletion.

Deletions on the long arm of chromosome 13 (13q14) have been observed in some patients with retinoblastoma, and this finding
has given rise to the assignment of the locus of retinoblastoma
to a recessive gene at 13q14 (surveyed by Murphree & Benedict
1984). In the genetic type of retinoblastoma the patients have
a germinal mutation of one allele at 13q14, and a "second hit"
(Knudson 1971) transforms the other allele either by mutation or
chromosomal rearrangement.

Various deletions and unbalanced translocations are associated with
colobomata and microphthalmos (Warburg 1982) and this is further
evidence of the abundancy of genetic heterogeneity.

Heterogeneity at the gene level

Molecular genetics has shown that at the gene level heterogeneity is the rule rather than the exception. Enzymatic aber-
rations have been discovered in a great number of recessive disorders and many dominant traits are due to abnormal structural
proteins. Decreased enzymatic activity can be measured in
amniotic cells and chorionic villus biopsies, and couples who
would previously have had only statistical counselling can now
be told antenatally if their child is affected or not. Prenatal
diagnosis and counselling requires that the aberration is identified,
and that the laboratory is informed about the arrival of the
specimens. There are more than 200 genetic disorders wherein the
metabolic defect has been identified (McKusick 1982). Routine
assays are run only in few laboratories and no single laboratory
can cover all the assays. It is therefore necessary to know
where to send the samples. A survey of such laboratories within
the EEC is badly needed.

In 1902 Garrod described the first known inborn error of metabolism, alcaptonuria (ochronosis), which presents in the eye as a
discoloration of the sclera, but since then it is astonishing
how few of these disorders have been identified in ophthalmology.

Notable examples are albinism, galactosaemia, homocystinuria and
ornithinuria, but the majority of enzymatic disorders with ocular
signs are assessed in paediatric departments, such as cases of
mucopolysaccharidoses, mucolipidoses, gangliosidoses and neuro-
lipidoses.

Anomalies of structural proteins are being studied intensively
these days. The structure of the haemoglobin molecule has been
known for many years, and several haemoglobinopathies have
been found to be due to substitutions of single aminoacids in
the haemoglobin molecule. Insulin and neuropeptides are in
focus now, and from an ophthalmological point of view it is
interesting that studies of collagen are in the vanguard of
research. The collagen in some cases of glaucoma contains abnormal
aminoacids (Tengroth & Ammitzbøll 1984), and studies of the
Ehlers-Danlos and the osteogenesis imperfecta syndromes (reviewed
by Prockop & Kirivikko 1984, Prockop 1984), have shown anomalies
of the structure of procollagen and collagen. I believe that
such studies will strongly influence our understanding of dominant
malformations of the anterior part of the eye because the sclera,
cornea and iris are derived from collagen secreted by differentiat-
ing neural crest cells (surveyed by Bahn et al 1984).

Malformations of the sclera, cornea, iris and zonules of the
lens are poorly understood in biochemical terms and it is quite
possible that analyses of procollagen and collagen produced
during the genetically determined migration and differentiation
of neural crest cells will improve our understanding.

MAPPING THE HUMAN GENOME

Assignment of some genetic disorders to genes on the X-chromosome
has been performed by pedigree analyses in a number of cases.
Genes on the autosomes have been localised ia by cell hybrid-
ization, mostly man-rodent hybrid cells. The hybrids preferentially lose human chromosomes in a random manner, and if
the character, often an enzyme, is expressed, it can be
assigned to a specific chromosome by studying a panel of different
man-rodent hybrids.

Enzymatic activity or immunological markers may be lost,or
present reduced activity in patients with chromosomal deletions,
and it was possible in this way to localise the genes for the HLA
types to chromosome 6.

When a polymorphic marker, such as blood groups, complement, HLA
types or enzymes has been located, it is possible to analyse
whether a dominant trait is closely linked to the marker. Linkage
analyses require more than one generation and more than one
affected person, and large families are much more informative than
numbers of small ones, because it is important to exclude heterogeneity.

Linkage analyses with polymorphic markers have been used for the
mapping of some ocular disorders. Autosomal dominant anterior
segment dysgenesis was linked to the MNS system on chromosome 4.
In the same way linkage was found between dominant posterior
polar cataract and haptoglobin on chromosome 16;

aniridia was linked to acid phosphatase-1 on chromosome 2 (surveyed by Hittner & Farrell 1982), thus showing yet an example of heterogeneity, since aniridia and Wilm's tumor are located on chromosome 11. In a large family with Kjer's autosomal dominant optic atrophy, Kivlin et al (1983) found evidence for close linkage to the Kidd blood group locus on chromosome 2. The dominant nuclear pulverulent cataract (the Coppock cataract) has been assigned to chromosome 1, linked to the Duffy blood group locus, but in another family with congenital pulverulent dominant cataracts such linkage was not apparent (Stabile et al 1983). There has been much controversy about linkage relations of dominant retinitis pigmentosa. Loose linkage was originally found with the Rhesus blood group locus on chromosome 1, but extended studies failed to verify the results (Field et al 1982).

DNA TECHNOLOGY

Restriction   fragment length   polymorphisms

Human DNA can be broken down into millions of fragments by restriction endonucleases which cut at specific base sequences. Each restriction fragment length can be purified (cloned) in bacterial vectors, and will hybridize exclusively to homologous DNA regions in the human genome when used as a probe. Thus, radioactive labelled probes can be used for the visualization of homologous regions in the genome. A great number of restriction fragment length polymorphisms (RFLPs) have been detected throughout the genome by this method, and they can be applied in linkage analyses as can other polymorphic markers such as blood groups.

Once it has been shown that a probe is closely linked to a certain dominant or X-linked gene locus, family studies may reveal whether a specific DNA fragment segregate with the trait in that particular family. For those disorders which have been mapped to a particular chromosome or even part of a chromosome, as in X-linked diseases, RFLP analyses can be used to assess whether a member of a family carries the mutant gene or the normal one without knowledge of the basic molecular defects. In informative families RFLP analyses may thus reveal not only who will become affected but also indicate heterozygous carriers of the (X-linked) disorder.

One of the most fascinating examples of the use of RFLPs is Huntington's disease. This is a disorder that presents with progressive choreatic movements and dementia in all gene carriers. The age of manifestation varies from the first to the 6th decade of life, and the issue today is whether individuals at risk for this dominant disease should be offered a prospective diagnostic analysis of their RFLP-pattern, an opportunity existing at present (reviewed by Conneally 1984).

In some families this may tell the individual whether he or she will suffer from the disease, and evidently each son or daughter of a patient with Huntington's disease speculates about the risk of having affected children and about what may happen to themselves.

In ophthalmology identical problems are awaiting once linkage relations of autosomal dominant retinitis pigmentosa have been resolved.

RFLPs have been applied to localize the loci on the X-chromosome for ocular albinism, retinoschisis, choroideraemia, X-linked retinitis pigmentosa (Friedrich et al 1985), Norrie's disease and many non-ocular disorders (Wieacker et al 1984). The problem with X-linked disorders is that daughters of carriers have a 50 per cent risk of being carriers, but fortunately carriers of ocular albinism, choroideraemia and X-linked retinitis pigmentosa can be assessed clinically. This, however, is not the case for carriers of Norrie's disease who show no clinical signs. It is now possible in informative families of Norrie's disease for daughters of carriers to be assessed as either carriers of the mutant gene or of the wild type allele (Gal et al 1985). Since RFLPs can also be shown in amniotic fibroblasts and chorionic villi cells, prenatal diagnosis is a possibility. The precision of the prenatal diagnosis depends upon the frequency of recombination between the mutant gene locus and the probe.

DNA banks

The application of RFLPs for the assessment of gene carriers in dominant and X-linked disorders requires information about the polymorphisms in affected and healthy relatives. It is therefore important for young individuals to have access to information about the DNA-restriction fragment lengths of their parents and grandparents when they consider having a family. This has given rise to DNA banks wherein individuals from families with dominant disorders have donated DNA extracts or in rare cases deep-frozen fibroblast cultures for future use strictly within the family (Conneally 1984).

DNA technology

Linkage relations with RFLPs are used in families where it is easy to delineate gene carriers from other relatives. In recessive disorders other probes have been more useful. If the deficient enzyme or another polypeptide has been identified, its messenger RNA (mRNA) can be purified and used for the synthesis of complementary DNA (cDNA), that is a DNA which contains the nucleotides from which the mRNA is transcribed. The cDNA can then be used as a probe which will hybridize with both the mutant and the normal alleles of individuals in the family. Individuals with recessive disorders carry two copies of the mutant allele while the heterozygotes carry one mutant and one normal allele, and for some defects this can be demonstrated electrophoretically. Application of cDNA in prenatal determination of affected foetuses has been used in families with phenylketonuria (surveyed by Güttler 1984).

In ophthalmology there is so far no similar information, but when the inborn errors of metabolism for retinal degenerations have been resolved, it will be possible to synthesize cDNA probes from their respective mRNAs.

TREATMENT OF GENETIC EYE DISORDERS

Surgical treatment of genetic disorders has improved markedly
over the last ten years. Congenital cataracts are removed early,
and congenital glaucoma which was previously associated with
severely impaired vision can now be surgically treated with
good result.

Photocoagulation and vitreous microsurgery has greatly improved the prognosis for patients with vitreous vascular prolifera-
tion due to the genetic haemoglobinopathies. Retinoblastoma is
cured in 80 - 90 per cent of cases by high-voltage irradiation
and cytostatica. The prognosis for the late appearing second
primary tumours in these patients, however, is unknown.

Dietary treatment for genetic disorders has been introduced
for patients with glactosaemia, Refsums's disease, gyrate atrophy,
and in other non-ocular genetic disorders, notably phenylketonuria.

Some enzymatic disorders can be treated with drugs that either
enhance the activity of the deficient enzyme or promote alternative pathways. This is observed i.a. in patients with homocystinuria, but due to heterogeneity at the molecular level
(Skovby et al 1982), some patients fail to react.

In Wilson's disease the high copper level can be reduced by
treatment with penicillamide or trientine hydrocholoride (Walshe
1982), but treatment of the fundamental errors in genetic disorders
is only beginning to appear for the majority of genetic traits.

DNA technology is expected to provide some of the drugs needed.
Insulin, human growth hormone and some of the blood clotting
factors can be synthesized by reverse DNA technology, but the
initial step in such projects, of course, is identification of
the metabolic error. It is this information that makes it possible to purify mRNA and synthesize cDNA. The cDNA must then be
inserted into an organism together with a promotor gene to induce
the genetic transcription. Finally the problem is to administer
the synthetic protein in such way that it reaches the tissue
for which it is needed.

Ophthalmo-genetics is entering this field. It has for a long
time been possible to assess inborn errors of metabolism from
conjunctival fibroblast cultures. Corneal and retinal pigment-
epithelial cells are also cultured in several laboratories and
it will presumably not be very long until the molecular genetics
of some causes of congenital malformations of the cornea and
anterior chamber and of retinal degenerations are identified at
the gene level.

CONCLUSION

There are approximately 3500 inherited diseases described in the
last edition of McKusick's catalog, and many will be described
in the years to come. Assessment of genetic disorders requires

multidiscplinary work comprising many clinical specialities,
cytogenetics, electron- and light microscopy of specimens,
determination of rare enzymatic deficiencies, analysis of the
molecular structure of polypeptides and DNA technology. This
need has given rise to the appearance of a number of genetic
units, mainly associated with pediatric departments and in-
stitutes for human genetics.

In ophthalmology genetic units are rare and genetics are part
of the syllabus in only few ophthalmic training centres. Therefore pediatric geneticists are often unaware of the assistance
they might have from expert ophthalmological examination of their
patients, and newly described genetic disorders are often discussed without emphasis on ocular features, even when such have
been described. Ocular pathology is rarely mentioned in the
abstracts of genetic papers, and therefore do not appear in
literature retrieval systems. It is therefore difficult for the
ophthalmogeneticist to keep abreast of clinical development.

There is a need for a genetic catalogue, revised with regard
to the ophthalmological signs of monogenic disorders. Such could
be produced under the aegis of the EEC.

Acknowledgement

I am grateful for the comments of Dr. N. Tommerup and Dr.
G. Hertz. I thank Mrs. D. Aagaard and Mrs. L. Rappeport for
typing the manuscript.

REFERENCES

Andersen SR, Geertinger P, Larsen H-W, Mikkelsen M, Parving A, Vestermark S, Warburg M. Aniridia, cataract and gonadoblastoma in a mentally retarded girl with deletion of chromosome 11: a clinico-pathological case report. Ophthalmologica 1978;176: 171-177.

Bhattacharya SS, Wright AF, Clayton JF et al. Close genetic linkage between X-linked retinitis pigmentosa and a restriction fragment length polymorphism identified by recombinant DNA probe L1. 28. Nature 1984;109:251-255.

Bahn CF, Falls HF, Varley GA, Meyer RF, Edelhauser HF, Bourne WM. Classification of corneal endothelial disorders based on neural crest origin. Ophthalmol. 1984;91:558-563.

Caspersson T, Zech L, Johansson C, Modest EJ. Identification of human chromosome set by aid of DNA-binding fluorescent agents. Exper Cell Res 1970;62:490-492.

Conneally PM. Huntington disease. Genetics and epidemiology. Am J Hum Genet 1984;36:506-526

Conneally PM. 1984. Personal Communication.

Field LL, Heckenlively JR, Sparkes RS, Garcia CA, Farson C, Zedalis D, Sparkes MC, Crist M, Tideman S, Spence MA. Linkage analysis of five pedigrees affected with typical autosomal dominant retinitis pigmentosa. J Med Genet 1982;19:266-270.

Franceschetti A, Francois J, Babel J. Les Hérédo-dégenérescences chorio-rétiniennes. Masson et Cie. Paris 1963.

Francois J. L'Hérédité en ophthalmologie. Masson et Cie. Paris 1958.

Francke U, Holmes LB, Atkins L, Riccardi VM. Aniridia-Wilm's tumor association: Evidence for specific deletion of 11p13. Cytogent Cell Genet 1979;24:185-192.

Fraser F, Friedmann AI. The Causes of Blindness in Childhood. The Johns Hopkins Hospital Press. Baltimore 1967.

Friedrich U, Warburg M, Wieacker P, Wienker TF, Gal A, Ropers H-H. X-linked retinitis pigmentosa: Linkage with the centromere and a cloned DNA sequence from the proximal short arm of the X-chromosome. Hum Genet 1985 In press

Gal A et al. Norrie's disease: Close linkage with genetic markers from the proximal short arm of the X-chromosome. Clin Genet. In press.

Garrod AE. The incidence of alkaptonuria: A study in chemical individuality. Lancet 1902;ii:1616-1620.

Güttler F. Phenylketonuria: 50 years since Følling's discovery and still expanding our clinical and biochemical knowledge. Acta Paediatr Scand 1984;73:705-716.

Hittner HM, Ferrell RE. Autosomal dominant ophthalmologic disorders and linkage. J Ped Ophthalmol Strab 1982;19:40-46.

Jay B. Genetic causes of visual handicap: Prevalence and prevention. In: Smith V and Keen J. Eds. Visual Handicap in Children. Clinics in Developmental Medicine No. 73. Spastics International Med Publ with W. Heinemann Medical Books. London, Philadelphia 1979:94-101.

Kivlin JD, Lovrien EW, Bishop DT, Maumenee IH. Linkage analysis in dominant optic atrophy. Am J Hum Genet. 1983;35:1190-1195.

Knudson AG jr. Mutation and cancer: Statistical study of retinoblastoma. Proc Nat Acad Sci 1971;68:820-823.

McKusick VA. Mendelian inheritance in man. Catalogs of autosomal dominant, autosomal recessive and X-linked phenotypes. The Johns Hopkins University Press, Baltimore, London. 6th ed. 1983.

Murphree L, Benedict WF. Retinoblastoma: Clues to human onco-genesis. Science 1984;223:1028-1033.

Prockop DJ. Osteogenesis imperfecta:Phenotypic heterogeneity, protein suicide, short and long collagen. Am J Hum Genet 1984;36:499-505.

Prockop RE, Kirivikko KI. Heritable diseases of collagen. New Engl J Med 1984;311:376-

Robinson GC. Epidemiological studies of congenital and acquired blindness in blind children born in British Colombia 1944-1973. Proc. first National Multidisciplinary Conf. Blind Children Vancouver, Brit. Columbia. 1974:1-21.

Schappert-Kimmijser J. Causes of severe visual impairment in children and their prevention. (J.Schappert-Kimmijser, ed.). Documenta Ophthalmologica 1975;39:224-228.

Skovby F, Kraus J, Redlich C, Rosenberg LE. Immunochemical studies on cultured fibroblasts from patients with homocystinuria due to cystathionine beta-synthase deficiency. Am J Hum Genet 1982;34:73-83.

Stabile M, Amoriello A, Capobianco S, Cavaliere ML, Conte N, De Rosa C, Ruoppo S, Sorrentino V, Ventruto V. Study of a form of pulvurulent cataract in a large kindred. J Med Genet 1983;20:419-421.

Sorsby A. Ophthalmic genetics. 2nd ed. London. Butterworths 1970. First ed. 1951.

Tjio JH, Levan A. The chromosome number of man. Hereditas 1956;42:1-6.

Tengroth B, Ammitzbøll. Changes in the content and composition of collagen in the glaucomatous eye - basis for a new hypothesis for the genesis of chronic open angle glaucoma. Acta Ophthalmol (Kbh) 1984;62:999-1008.

Trevor-Roper PD. Marriage of two complete albinos with normally pigmented offspring. Br J Ophthalmol 1952;36:107-110 and Proc Roy Soc Med 1963;56:21-24.

Walshe JM. Treatment of Wilson's disease with trientine (triethylene tetramide) dihydrochloride. Lancet 1982;i:643

Warburg M. Congenital blindness. In Emery AE, Rimoin DL. Principles and Practice of Medical Genetics, vol 2. Churchill Livingstone, London, Edinburgh, Melbourne, New York 1983:471-481.

Warburg M. Diagnostic precision in microphthalmos and coloboma of heterogeneous origin. Birth Def OAS 1982;18/6:31-50.

Waardenburg PJ. Das menschliche Auge und seine Erbanlagen. M. Nijhoff Haag 1932.

Waardenburg PJ, Franceschetti A, Klein D. Genetics and Ophthalmology. R. Van Gorcum Netherlands, Blackwell Oxford, CC Thomas 1961 and 1963.

Wieacker P, Davies KE, Cooke HJ, Pearson PL, Williamson R, Bhattacharya S, Zimmer J, Ropers H-H (1984). Toward a complete linkage map of the human X-chromosome: regional assignment of 16 cloned single-copy DNA sequences employing a panel of somatic cell hybrids. Am J Hum Genet 36:265-276.

NON-GENETIC CAUSES OF VISUAL IMPAIRMENT IN EARLY CHILDHOOD.

J.J. De Laey and F. Meire

Department of Ophthalmology,University of Ghent,
Belgium

INTRODUCTION

It is by no means easy to analyse the relative importance
of the different causes of visual handicap in children.
Indeed we may be faced with a number of problems.

1. The retrospective diagnosis of prenatal
   disease may sometimes be extremely difficult
   expecially when the child is first seen at
   the age of 1 or 2 years.
2. Extensive and sometimes repeated familial
   examinations may be needed to exclude a
   possible genetic cause. The penetrance of the
   gene may be variable and the clinician must be
   aware of the different modes of presentation
   of a given disease.
3. Some acquired diseases are phenocopies of known
   hereditary diseases.
4. The prevalence of non-genetic versus genetic
   diseases may markedly vary in different periods and different parts of the world.
5. They may also be differences when comparing
   mentally normal with mentally handicapped
   children.

Most important of course in analysing the data is the care with
which the clinician has made the diagnosis. Improved diagnostic
techniques and increased clinical knowledge will lead to more
precise data. This is well illustrated by the following statistics by Cozijnsen & Delleman (1981) who reviewed the causes
of visual handicap in a Dutch center for visually and mentally
handicapped children. (Table I). This table also underlines
the fact that genetic causes of blindness in childhood are by
far more frequent than non-genetic causes.

Causes of the visual handicap

	1969 (n = 211) %	1979 (n = 261) %
non-genetic	10,0	24,1
genetic	46,4	72,4
unknown	34,6	3,5

Table I (from Cozijnsen & Delleman,1981)

MATERIAL & METHODS

In order to assess the prevalence of non-genetic blindness
in childhood in a Belgian population, the files of 242 children
followed in 1984 in a school for children with visual and
hearing impairment (Spermalie, Brugge), were reviewed.
The children were considered as mentally normal if they had an
IQ of at least 90. Grossly retarded children were not seen in
Spermalie and are thus not included in this study.

A genetic cause was accepted in the presence of a positive
family history or if the child presented a known genetic syndrome, such as Crouzon's disease. The cause was considered as
unknown if no positive family history was obtained and if no
direct cause could be determined for the visual handicap. In
this group however a number of cases are possibly of genetic
origin.

RESULTS

The results are summarized in table II, III and IV

N = 242 (september 1984)		
Non-genetic	77	(32 %)
Genetic	132	(54,5%)
Unknown	33	(13,5%)
Total	242	(100 %)

Table II. Causes of visual impairment in Spermalie, Brugge

	IQ ⩾90	IQ < 90
1. Prenatal		
Rubella	2	4
Toxoplasmosis	9	4
Toxic	2	-
Others	-	1
	13	9

Total 22

	IQ $\geq$ 90	IQ $<$ 90
2. Perinatal		
RLF	4	16
Cataract	3	2
Optic atrophy	3	7
Others	-	1
	10	26
		Total 36
3. Postnatal		
Infection	2	2
Trauma	1	6
Tumours	3	2
Others	3	-
	9	10
		Total 19

Table III.Non-genetic causes of visual impairment
in Spermalie Brugge

	IQ $\geq$ 90	IQ $<$ 90
Non-genetic causes	32	45
Genetic causes	93	39
Unknown	27	6

Table IV.Causes of visual impairment in relationship with
mental handicap

DISCUSSION

The different causes will be discussed in function of the period when the child has become primarily affected.

I. Prenatal causes.

1. Infections

Prenatal infections especially during the first 8 weeks
of pregnancy may provoke extensive ocular damage in the child
if the infecting agent is capable of traversing the placental
barrier. The best known agents causing prenatal ocular disease
are toxoplasmosis, rubella, cytomegalovirus and syphillis.
Except for the last, the disease only mildly affects the
mother and may even go by unnoticed. All of them have however potentially disastrous effect on the foetus.

1.a.Rubella.

Ocular manifestations of rubella embryopathy was
first recognizedby Gregg in 1941. The virus is not only teratogenic but may also cause active inflammation. The presence
of the virus in the lens of infected infants has been
demonstrated up to the age of 21 months and this may explain
the greater incidence of complications during cataract surgery
in these children (Scheie & Scheffer,1968). The virus could
occasionally be isolated from the urine of infants up to 10
weeks of age (Blattner,1974). During the worldwide rubella
epidemic of 1964-1965 an estimated 20.000 to 30.000 infants
were born with the congenital rubella syndrome (Blattner,1974).

The essential characteristics of congenital rubella
syndrome are congenital heart defects, deafness and ocular
malformations. They may be associated with mental retardation,
microcephaly, hydrocephaly, encephalitis, growth retardation,
skeletal malformations, anemia, Thrombocytopenic purpura,
hepatosplenomegaly. Abnormal behaviour patterns, suggestive
for autism i.e. mannerism or ritualistic patterns, associated
with sensory loss are not unfrequently found in congenital
rubella children (Desmonsd et al.,1970).

The ocular manifestations have been well described
(Wolff,1973). Various parts of the eye may be affected.
Iridocyclitis is an almost constant feature, cataract, which
is usually bilateral, but not always complete is found in 80 %
of the cases. Microphthalmia is seen in 60 %. Glaucoma may
occur in 20 % and be secondary to the chronic iridocyclitis or
may be of the congenital type. Retinopathy with atypical
course pigmentation, normal retinal vessels and normal optic
disc is seen in 50 % of the cases. If the retinopathy is un-
associated with other eye involvement the vision may be
normal. The ERG is either normal or only mildly affected.
However, macular choroidal neovascularisation may result in
loss of central vision in late childhood (Deutman & Grizzard,
1978).

1.b.Congenital toxoplasmosis.

Toxoplasmosis is a widespread disease and positive
intradermo-toxoplasmin reactions are found between 10 to 48 %
in Europe and in the USA (Huismans,1979). The prevalence of
toxoplasma infection in women of childbearing age in the Paris
area is even as high as 82 % (Desmont & Couvreur,1974). In a
study of 183 pregnant women who were infected during pregnancy
they found 7 cases of abortion (4 %), 55 cases of definite
toxoplasmosis (30 %) and 11 cases of possible toxoplasmosis
(6 %).

Congenital toxoplasmosis is characterized by the
classical triad of internal hydrocephaly, intracerebral calcifications and macular chorioretinits. There may be evidence of
infection in almost all tissues including the liver, lymphnodes,
lungs, heart and skeletal muscles (Martyn,1983). The ocular
and cerebral manifestations may not always be found at birth,
but appear in some cases after several months (Desmont &
Couvreur,1974).

The visual problems of children affected with congenital toxoplasmosis may be the result of the fundus involvement but
may also be primarily due to the encephalomyelitis.

1.c.Congenital syphilis.

Congenital syphilis has been considered for many
years as the major cause of pseudo-retinitis pigmentosa.
However none of the 10 cases of congenital syphilis seen by
Fontaine (1969) presented ocular involvement. Perivascular
infiltration by T.pallidum in cornea, uvea, retina or optic
nerve are consequences of congential syphilis (Martyn,1983).
The classical ocular finding of congenital syphilis which
occurs in 10 to 15 % of the cases is interstitial keratitis.
It is probably immunologically mediated. Interstitial
keratitis appears between the age of 2 and 20 and is associated
with mild anterior uveitis, and marked photophobia. The
condition is characterized by extensive vascular infiltration
of the cornea and corneal haze. It heals spontaneously
leaving irregular infiltrates in the corneal stroma and
ghost vessels. The vision is variably affected depending on
the extent of the nebulae and on the astigmatism. Interstitial
keratitis is associated with other stigmata of congenital
syphilis, such as nerve deafness, depressed nasal bridge
(saddle nose) and deformities of the permanent teeth. The
typical Hutchinson triad consists of nerve deafness, interstitial keratitis and teeth deformity.

1.d.Congenital cytomegalovirus desease.

Cytomegalovirus infections are usually asymptomatic
in healthy adults. The infection may be potentially dangerous
in congenital infections and in immunodepressed patients. CMV
is the most common congenital virus infection. 0,5 to 1 % of
all infants secrete the virus (Blattner,1974). According to
this author every year a minimum of 5.000 infants are born with
some degree of brain damage related to CMV infection in the USA
and 200 to 600 in England and Wales. Congenital CMV infection
may be associated with sensorineural hearing loss anterior uveitis, chorioretinits, optic neuritis and optic atrophy.
Optic nerve hypoplasia and partial colobomata of the optic nerve
have been attributed to congenital CMV infection by Hittner et
al. (1976). Other findings include purpura, respiratory illness, jaundice and hepatosplenomegaly.

1.e.Herpes simplex virus.

Herpes simplex virus infection is sometimes acquired
in utero (Hutchinson et al.,1975), although most cases of neonatal herpetic keratitis were infected from the genital tract
of the mother. It is thus by no way surprising that 80 % of
neonatal herpetic infections are related to type 2 genital herpes (Nohmias et al.,1970). Intra-uterine infection may possibly
provoke microcephaly, periventricular calcifications, micro-
ophthalmia, chorioretinits and cataract.

1.f.Varicella-zoster virus.

Congenital anomalies may exceptionally result from
varicella-zoster infection during the early months of
pregnancy.

The eye is the most commonly affected organ. In a tabulation
of defects in 11 cases from the literature Williamson
(cited by Blattner,1974) found ocular defects in 9 cases
(cataract, microphthalmos, Horner syndrome, anisocoria, optic
atrophy, nystagmus and chorioretinits). Brain damage was found
in 9 cases and hypoplasia of limbs and trunk 5 cases.

2. Toxic causes

2.a. Radiation.
The teratogenic effect of radiation has been demonstrated with dosis far higher than that encountered during diagnostic applications of ionizing radiation (Sternberg,1973).
In children irradiated in utero in Hiroshima with doses between
50 and 100 rads there was a significant degree of microcephaly and mental retardation. This was sometimes associated
with retinal dystrophy. Microphthalmos and coloboma may be
observed with X-ray radiation of the mouse.

2.b. Drugs.
A number of drugs are actually known to be teratogenic
with ocular involvement.
1. Thalidomide (Lenz & Knapp,1962) provokes major malformations of the extremities (phocomelia), malformations of the
gastro-intestinal tract (duodenal stenosis, duodenal atresia),
cardiac anomalies but also anophthalmia and microphthalmos.

2. Coumadin (Warfarin) is known to have caused microphthalmos, optic atrophy and cataracts (Altman,1983).

3. Tetracycline may provoke yellow discoloration of the
cornea and lens in the foetus (Krejci and Brettschneider,1983).

4. Psychofarmaca form a progressively increasing cause of
teratogenic malformations. In our series we observed one
case of high myopia and one of congenital nystagmus in children
of mothers who used psychofarmaca during the pregnancy. The
mother of the child with congenital nystagmus was also
etheromaniac.

5. LSD. Multiple ocular anomalies associated with maternal
LSD ingestion were described by Apple & Bennett (1974) and by
Chan et al. (1978). They include microphthalmos, intraocular
cartilage, cataract, persistent hyperplastic primary vitreous
and retinal dysplasia. LSD may also be the cause of optic nerve
hypoplasia (Margalith et al,1984).

6. Fetal alcohol syndrome. Children of chronic alcoholic
women frequently present growth deficiency, developmental delay,
craniofacial anomalies and limb defects. The frequency is
estimated up to 43 % (Jones & Smith,1975). Ocular manifestations include telecanthus, hypertelorism, epicanthus, moderate
ptosis, hypoplasia of the optic nerve, optic atrophy and
cataract (Stromland,1981).

3.Non-infectious maternal disease

3.a.Maternal diabetes
Neonatal hypoglycemia related or not to maternal diabetes may be associated with optic nerve hypoplasia in childhood (Margalith al.,1984;Skarf & Hoyt,1984). This was also
the case in one child in our series.

3.b.Hypovitaminosis.
Hale (1933) reported that pregnant sows fed on a diet
deficient in vit A produced pigs without eyeballs. If the mother
presents a deficient vit A status, the child may develop
xerophthalmia in utero (Sommer,1982).

II.Perinatal causes

1. Difficulties at birth.

The term perinatal damage syndrome was used by Fraser &
Friedman (1967) to describe the various problems related to
difficulties experienced around the term of birth. They may
be related to a disturbed pregnancy, (maternal toxicosis,
dysmaturity) or to difficulties at birth (traumatic delivery,
asphyxia, hypocalcemia, hypoglycemia, hypothermy).
The visual problems are not unfrequently associated with mental retardation,hearing loss or motoric problems.

1.a.Tears in the corneal endothelium and Descemet's membrane may result from a complicated forceps delivery. This
is associated with corneal oedema, periorbital oedema and
ecchymosis. Improved prenatal care and elective Cesarean
section has now made this complication rare.

2.b.Cataract.
Perinatal cataract may be observed in neonatal hypoglycemia (Merin & Crawford,1971;Bleeker-Wagemakers,1981)
especially in dysmature children. Bleeker-Wagemakers in her
series found 29 neonatal cataracts 17 children were dysmature
and hypoglycemia was demonstrated in 3 cases. Anoxia in the
perinatal period is a possible cause of cataract (Brown,1963).

3.c.Optic atrophy.
Optic atrophy is often associated with traumatic delivery but may also result from meningitis or bloodgroup in-
compatibility (Bleeker-Wagemakers,1981).

1.d.Cerebral involvement.
This is mainly related to prolonged delivery, asphyxia
or cerebral haemorrhage.

2. Perinatal infections.

2.a.Herpes virus infection.
As already mentionned most cases of HSV infections in
the neonatal period are type 2 and the children are most
probably infected from the genital tract of the mother.

2.b.Ophthalmia neonaturum.

Ophthalmia neonaturum has become relatively rare in
Europe and in the USA. The incidence rates for gonococcal
ophthalmia is there about 0,5 per 12.000 live births whereas the incidence of chlamydial ophthalmia neonaturum varies
between 5 to 60 per 1.000 live births. In developing countries
ophthalmia neonaturum is much more common. In Nairobi 8 %
are due to C.trachomatis and 47 % are related to N.gonorrhoeae
(Fransen & Piot,1985).

2.c.Meningitis or encephalitis during the neonatal period
may result in optic atrophy or cerebral blindness. A potential porte d'entrée is the infected navel.
(Bleeker-Wagemakers,1981)

2.d.Candida infections.

It is by no means surprising that candida endophthalmitis, which in the adult is found in compromised patients,
has also been diagnosed in premature infants (Baley et al.,
1981).

2.e.β-streptococcal disease.

β-streptococcal disease may be acquired by passage
through the birth canal. The vagina in as many as 25 % of
all pregnant women is colonized by β-streptococci. This
may result in septicemia, respiratory distress, encephalitis.
Cases of neonatal endophthalmitis in β-streptococcal disease
have been reported (Berger,1981).

3.Retinopathy of prematurity

Retinopathy of prematurity, which was first described
by Terry in 1942 is still one of the major causes of perinatal
visual loss and this despite a better oxygen monitoring in
premature children. This is related to the fact that more
infants with very low birth weight are saved. Retinopathy of
prematurity is often associated with mental retardation and
this is again illustrated in our series.

III.Postnatal causes.

1.Trauma

Ocular trauma may have different origins. It may be
related to accidents at home, on the playground, at school and
especially on the road. Eye injuries may result from chemical
burns, penetrating injuries, ocular contusion... In mental
defective children they may be the result of selfinflicted
injuries and in this population even foveal burns due to sun-
gazing may be observed. The most dramatic cases are due to
physical child abuse. There is an apparent increased incidence
of reports on battered children in the literature, although
the problem is certainly not new. (Harley & Spaeth,1982).
The most common ocular symptoms in battered children are retinal
and subhyaloid haemorrhages, orbital haemorrhages and lid
ecchymosis.

Other signs are subconjunctival haemorrhage; hyphaema, cataract, lensluxation, anisocoria, retinal detachment, optic atrophy.

2.Infectious diseases.

Various causes of ocular infection found in adults may also be diagnosed in early childhood. The anterior segment (especially conjunctivits and keratitis) are affected, although involvement of the posterior segment is also possible. Most cases of bilateral visual loss related to infection result from bacterial or viral encephalitis.

In developing countries trachoma and onchocerciasis are still two of the main blinding diseases even in childhood. Measles which in Europe only exceptionally produced ocular complications is cited as the major cause of childhood blindness for many parts of Africa (Quéré,1964). This is probably related to malnutrition and vit A deficiency (Sommer,1982).

3.Tumours

In our series tumours are the second most important cause of blindness postnatal origin. In 2 patients (one with menigioma and one with astrocytoma) the disease was misdiagnosed as congenital optic atrophy. Unexplained optic atrophy in children must always raise the suspicion of an intracranial tumour and especially of craniopharyngioma. X-rays of the skull will in such cases possibly show the characteristic calcifications.

4.Ocular inflammation

4.a.Vernal conjunctivits is a major cause of ocular handicap in central Africa. The condition is there called tropical endemic limboconjunctivitis (Diallo,1976). 40 % of the patients of the eye department in Dakar under the age of 20 are affected. In itself the disease is relatively benign, however it may be complicated by corneal infections resulting in permanent visual loss.

4.b.Uveal inflammation such as posterior cyclitis, sarcoid, Behcet's disease and Vogt-Koyanagi-Harada's disease are exceptionnal in young children.

5.Nutritional blindness

Xerophthalmia and nutritional blindness still form a major problem in developing countries. More than half a million children are affected each year (Sommer,1982). Night blindness is an early sign; twice as many children examined by Sommer had a history of hemeralopia as had conjunctival xerosis. In extreme situation vit A deficiency may lead to corneal ulceration and corneal necrosis. The condition becomes diastrous in case of surinfection.

6.Toxic causes

Optic atrophy or optic neuritis in childhood may be caused by antituberculosis treatment (streptomycin, isoniacid, ethambutol) but also by sulphonamides and chloramphenicol especially when it has been used during a long period of time in children with fibrocystic disease (Harcourt,1979). Optic atrophy which is partially reversible has been described in children treated with Vincristine for intracranial tumours. These children also received con- comitant radiotherapy, so that possibly the blood-brain barrier was affected. This may have increased the susceptibility of the optic nerve to vincristine (Shurin et al.,1982).

CONCLUSION

Much more frequently than genetic causes of childhood blindness, the non-genetic causes are associated with mental deficiency. A number of the non-genetic causes of visual im- pairment are preventable. This accounts as well for the pre-, peri- or postnatal causes. Prophyllactic measures are thus needed.

Prenatal causes :

- systematic vaccination programmes against rubella
- monitoring of drugs taken by pregnant women
- prevention of drug and alcohol abuse during pregnancy

Perinatal causes :

- prevention of birth trauma
- improved neonatal care
- improved monitoring of premature babies

Postnatal causes :

- improved nutrition and hygiene in third world countries
- prevention of trauma's;especially road- accidents
- early detection of battered children
- early detection of cerebral tumours

ACKNOWLEDGEMENT

L.Standaert MD was of great help in the review of the files at Spermalie Institute in Brugge.

REFERENCES

Altman B. Drugs in pediatric ophthalmology. In: Harley R.D. Pediatric ophthalmology. Second Edition. Philadelphia W.B.Saunders & C°, 1983;82-107.

Apple D.J.,Bennett T.T. Multiple systemic and ocular malformations associated with maternal LSD usage. Arch. Ophthalmol.
1974;92:301-303.

Beley J.E.,Annable W.L.,Kliegman R.M. Candida endophthalmitis
in the premature infant. J.Pediatr. 1981;98:458-461.

Berger B.B. Endophthalmitis complicating neonatal group b
streptococcal septicemia. Am.J.Ophthalmol. 1981;92:681-684.

Blattner R.J. The role of viruses in congenital defects. Am.J.
Dis. Child. 1974;128:781-786.

Bleeker-Wagemakers E.M. On the causes of blindness in the
mentally retarded. With special reference to the genetic
aspect. Bartimeus Foundation Series,the Netherlands. 1981.

Brown C.A. Post-natal cataracts in premature infants. Trans.
Ophthalmol.Soc.U.K. 1963;83:493-504.

Chan C.C.,Fishman M.,Egbert P.R. Multiple ocular anomalies
associated with maternal LSD ingestion. Arch.Ophthalmol.
1978;96:282-284.

Cozynsen M.,Delleman J.W. Causes of the visual handicap in
Bartimeus-Zeist. In: de JongC.V.A. ed. Ophthalmological dis-
order resulting from perinatal damage. Bartimeus Foundation
Series,the Netherlands. 1981;22-30

Desmond M.M., Wilson G.S., Verniaud W.M. et al. The early
growth and development of infants with congenital rubella.
Adv.Teratol. 1970;4:39-63.

Desmonts G.,Couvreur J. Congenital toxoplasmosis. a prospective study of 378 pregnancies. N.Engl.J.Med. 1974;290:1110-
1116.

Deutman A.F., Grizzard W.S. Rubella retinopathy and sub-
retinal neovascularization. Am.J.Ophthalmol. 1978;85:82-87.

Diallo J.S. Tropical endemic limboconjunctivitis. Revue Int.
Trachome 1976;53:67-80.

Fontaine M. Les cécités de l'enfance. Paris,Masson et C°,1969.

Fransen L.,Piot P. Ophthalmia neonaturum. In press.

Fraser G.R.,Friedman A.I. The causes of blindness in childhood. Baltimore: The Johns Hopkins Press. 1967.

Gregg M.M. Congenital cataract following German measles in the
mother. Trans.Ophthalmol.Soc.Aust. 1941;3:35-46.

Hale F. Pigs born without eye balls. J.Hered. 1933;24:105-106.

Harcourt B. Optic atrophy in childhood. In:Smith V.,Keen J.
eds. Visual prognosis in children. Clinics in Developmental
Medicine 1974;73:22-28.

Harley R.D., Spaeth G.L. Ocular manifestations of child
abuse. In:François J.,Maione M. Paediatric ophthalmology.
Chichester: John Wiley & Sons. 1982;141-145.

Hittner H.M.,Desmond M.M.,Montgomery J.R. Optic nerve manifestations of human congenital cytomegalovirus infection. Am.J.
Ophthalmol. 1976;81:661-665.

Huismans H; Tierische Parasiten des menschlichen Auges.
Bücherei des Augenatzen 1979;80:22-35.

Hutchinson D.S.,Smith R.E.,Haughton I.B. Congenital herpetic
keratitis. Arch.Ophthalmol. 1975;93:70-73.

Jones K.L., Smith D.W. The fetal alcohol syndrome.
Teratology 1975;12,1-10.

Krejci L.,Brettschneider I. Congenital cataract due to tetracycline. Animal experiments and clinical observations. Ophthal-
mol.Paed. Genet. 1983;3:59-60.

Lenz W.,Knapp K. Foetal malformations due to thalidomide. Ger.
Med. Mthly. 1962;7:253-258.

Loewer-Sieger D.H. Retrolental fibroplasia. In: de Jong C.V.A.
ed. Ophthalmological disorder resulting from perinatal damage.
Bartimeus Foundation Series,the Netherlands. 1981;

Margalith D.,Jan J.E.,Mc Cormick A.Q., Tze W.J., Lapointe J.
Clinical spectrum of congenital optic nerve hypoplasia: review of 51 patients. Dev.Med.Child.Neurol. 1984;26:311-322.

Martyn L.J. Pediatric neuro-ophthalmology. In: Harley R.D.
Pediatric ophthalmology. Second edition. Philadelphia
W.B. Saunders 1983;767892.

Merin S.,Crawford J.S. Hypoglycaemia and infantile cataract.
Arch. Ophthalmol. 1971;86:459-501.

Nahmias A.J.,Alford C.A., Koronar S.B. Infections of the newborn with herpes virus hominis. Adv.Pediat. 1970;17:185-226.

Quéré M.A. Les complications oculaires de la rougeole cause
majeure de cécité chez l'enfant en pays tropical. Ophthalmologica 1964;148:107-120.

Scheie H.G.,Scheffer D.B. Congenital cataracts. In: Symposium
on surgical and medical management of congenital anomalies of
the eye. Trans.New Orleans Acad.Ophthalmol. St Louis: C.V.Mosby
1968;322-341.

Shurin S.B.,Rekate H.L.,Annable W. Optic atrophy induced by Vincristine. Pediatrics 1982;70:288-291.

Skarf B.,Hoyt C.S. Optic nerve hypoplasia in children. Association with anomalies of the endocrine and CNS. Arch. Ophthalmol. 1984; 102:62-67.

Sommer A. Nutritional blindness. Xerophthalmia and kerato-malacia. New York, Oxford Unicersity Press. 1982.

Sternberg J. Radiation and pregnancy. Can.Med.Ass.J. 1973;109:51-57.

Strömland K. Eyeground malformations in the fetal alcohol syndrome. In: Huber A.,Klein D. eds. Neurogenetics and Neuro-ophthalmology. Amsterdam, Elsevier-North-Holland Biomedical Press. 1981;281-284.

Terry T.L. Extreme prematurity and fibroplastic overgrowth of persistant vascular sheath behind each crystalline lens. I.Preliminary report. Am.J.Ophthalmol. 1942;25:203-204.

Wolff S.M. The ocular manifestations of congenital rubella. J.Ped. Ophthalmol. 1973;10:101-141.

THE CHANHING AETIOLOGY OF VISUAL IMPAIRMENT IN EARLY CHILDHOOL IN GREECE

KAVANOZI A., TSIKOULAS I.

FROM THE DEPARTMENTS OF OPHTHALMOLOGY AND PAEDIATRICS,
UNIVERSITY OF THESSALONIKI, GREECE

I N T R O D U C T I O N

After years of work and study on the problems of the blind children at
the "School for the Blind of Northern Greece" (S.B.N.G.) we decided to examine the causes of blindness in children who were blinded before the age of
the 6th year of their life and the possible variance of these causes as time proceeds. We believe that this experience will contribute to the prevention and the best possible management of poor vision in early childhood.
Many authors in different countries have made studies related to the causes
of blindness (Hansen 1975, Hatfield 1975, Haustrate-Gosset 1975, Lindstedt
1975, Schappert-Kimmijser et al 1975, Skydsgaard 1975, Kofinas 1977).

M A T E R I A L   A N D   M E T H O D S

We studied the cases of 284 individuals (157 boys and 127 girls) aged
6 to 25 years, students of the S.B.N.G. who were blinded before the age of
6 and have a visual acuity < 2/10. Because in Greece legally blind are considered the individuals with visual acuity < 1/20, those of our material are
divided to legally blind (252(88.7 %)) with visual acuity $\leq$1/20 and to partially sighted (32(11.3 %)) with visual acuity from 2/10 to 1/20.
   The whole study was based on the files of the S.B.N.G. and the complete clinical and opthalmological examination of all the children made by the
Ophtalmological Clinic of the University of Thessaloniki in cooperation
with A' and B' Paediatric Clinics of the University of Thessaloniki.
   The study of the socioeconomic condition of the students was based on
the reports of the social workers.
   The material of our study was divided into three decades according to
the time the students enrolled at the S.B.N.G. (1950 -59, 1960 -69, 1970 -
79), after it the cases of each decade were studied separately and then the
findings of all the decades were compared to each other.

R E S U L T S

Out of the 284 children of our material 133 (70 boys, 63 girls) enrolled at the S.B.N.G. during the decade of 1950 -59, 84(44 boys, 40 girls)
during the decade of 1960 -69 and 67(43 boys, 24 girls) during the decade
of 1970 -79. The factors which were studied and compared in this study are
the following: The number and the sex of the children, the time of blindness, the main ophthalmological lesions and their causes and finally the
origin and the socioeconomic status of the children.

Table I shows the number and the sex of the children as well as the
time of blindness.

TABLE I

Number, sex and time of blindness

	Boys	Girls	Total
Born blind			
1950 - 1959	50	51	101
1960 - 1969	37	28	65
1970 - 1979	29	19	48
Blinded later			
1950 - 1959	20	12	32
1960 - 1969	7	12	19
1970 - 1979	14	5	19
Born blind and blinded later			
1950 - 1959	70	63	133
1960 - 1969	44	40	84
1970 - 1979	43	24	67
T o t a l	157	127	284

A progressive decrease of the children who attended the S.B.N.G., as
time proceeds from 1950 to 1979, is observed (Table I). The number of the
boys is bigger than that of the girls in all three decades with a significant statistical difference ($p < 0.01$). Also the number of the children who
were born blind is bigger than the number of the children who were blinded
at a later time in all three decades.

Table II shows the main ophthalmological lesions of the children of
our material.

The congenital malformations (Table II) are at the top of the list of
ophthalmological lesions mainly during the decade of 1950 -59 (31.5 %).
During the next two decades this number decreases (1960 -69 (23.8 %), 1970-
79 (14.9 %)) with a significant statistical difference ($p < 0.01$). Another
main cause of ophthalmological lesions during the decade of 1950 -59 is the
multiple acquired lesions of the eyball (12.8 %) which gradually decreases
and reaches the percentage of 4.8 % in the 1960 -69 decade with a significant statistical difference ($p < 0.01$). During the 1950 -59 decade there is
a quite high percentage (11.3 %) of congenital glaucoma while it is gradually reduced in the next decades (1960 -69 (4.8 %), 1970 -79 (1.5 %)) with a
significant statistical difference ($p < 0.01$). During the 1960 -69 and 1970-
79 decades there is an increased number of children with tapetoretinal dystrophies compared to the previous decade (1950 -59 (11.3 %), 1960 -69

TABLE II

Main ophthalmological lesions

	1950 – 1959 No %		1960 – 1969 No %		1970 – 1979 No %	
Congenital malformations	42	31.5	20	23.8	10	14.9
Congenital cataract	22	16.5	19	22.6	13	19.4
Tapetoretinal dystrophies	15	11.3	18	21.4	16	23.8
Optic nerve atrophy. (Congenital or acquired)	19	14.3	13	15.7	11	16.4
Glioma	-	-	-	-	3	4.5
Congenital glaucoma	15	11.3	4	4.8	1	1.5
Generalized albinism	-	-	2	2.4	3	4.5
High myopia	1	0.7	2	2.4	-	-
Multiple acquired lesions of the eyeball	17	12.8	4	4.8	-	-
Retrolental fibroplasia	-	-	-	-	6	9.0
Chorioretinitis	-	-	-	-	2	3
Miscellaneous	2	1.6	2	2.4	2	3
T o t a l	133	100	84	100	67	100

(21.4 %), 1970 – 79 (23.8 %)) with significant statistical difference
(p < 0.01). There is not a case of glioma and chorioretinitis during the
1950 – 59 and 1960 – 69 decades while there are a few such cases during the
1970 – 79 decade. Also the retrolental fibroplasia appears during the 1970-
79 decade for first time. The percentages of congenital cataract and optic
nerve atrophy are steady in all the three decades.
     Table III shows the causes of the main ophthalmological lesions.
     We notice that in all three decades the main causes of blindess are
pre and perinatal factors (1950 – 59 (81.2 %), 1960 – 69 (88.1 %), 1970 – 79
(94 %)) and that at the top of the list are the inherited diseases (1950 –
59 (49 %), 1960 – 69 (64.3 %), 1970 – 79 (52.2 %)). The statistical study
with a two ways analysis of variance by which the decades, the pre and perinatal as well as the postnatal causes were studied shows that the number
of the pre and perinatal causes is statistically much bigger than the number
of the postnatal ones. This difference is steady for the three decades. No
chromosomal abnormalities have been noticed. There is no significant statistical difference in the percentages of the congenital infections among the
three decades. During 1970 – 79 8.9 % of the cases of blindness were due
to retrolental fibroplasia caused by anoxia and prematurity. No such cases
have been noticed during the two previous decades. Unknown factors hold
quite a big percentage (1950 – 59 (26.3 %), 1960 – 69 (19 %), 1970 – 79 (15 %))
of the causes for blindness; however there is a decrease of the unknown factors in the last decade, with a significant statistical difference (p
< 0.01). The percentage of postnatal causes has gradually decreased during
the three decades (1950 – 59 (18.8 %), 1960 – 69 (11.9 %), 1970 – 79 (6 %)).
The difference between the first and the third decade is statistically significant. Among the postnatal causes ocular infections occupy a 3.7 % percentage in the 1950 – 59 decade, 1.2 % in the 1960 – 69 and nil in the 1970 –

TABLE III

Causes of the ophthalmological lesions

	1950 – 1959		1960 – 1969		1970 – 1979	
	No	%	No	%	No	%
A. Pre and perinatal causes						
Inherited diseases	65	49	54	64.3	35	52.2
Chromosomal abnormalities	–	–	–	–	–	–
Congenital infections	6	4.5	3	3.6	6	8.9
Prematurity – anoxia	–	–	–	–	6	8.9
Dystocia	–	–	1	1.2	2	3
Cerebral palsy	–	–	–	–	2	3
Congenital hydrocephalus	1	0.7	–	–	2	3
Unknown	35	26.3	16	19	10	15
Undiagnosed due to the lack of evidence	1	0.7	–	–	–	–
Total (pre and perinatal)	108	812	74	88.1	63	94
B. Postnatal causes						
Ocular infections	5	3.7	1	1.2	–	–
CNS infections	13	9.8	5	5.9	2	3
Accidents	6	4.5	2	2.4	2	3
Brain tumors	–	–	1	1.2	–	–
Avitaminosis A	1	0.7	–	–	–	–
Generalized diseases of CNS	–	–	1	1.2	–	–
Total (postnatal)	25	18.8	10	11.9	4	6
T o t a l	133	100	84	100	67	100

79 decade. The number of cases due to accidents does not have a significant statistical difference in the three decades.

Table IV shows the relation between the main ophthalmological lesions and their causes.

Tables V and VI show the origin and the socio-economic status of the children in our study.

The majority of the children (table V) come from villages. However, during the last decade, there is a dicrease in the number of children who come from the villages while there is an increase in the number of children who come from the towns but, as proven by a two ways analysis of variance this is not statistically significant.

The socioeconomic status of the blind children (table VI) is low in general in all three decades. The two ways analysis of variance in the three decades in relation to the socioeconomic status, shows that there are no significant statistical changes at the socioeconomic condition during the three decades.

TABLE IV

Relation between the main ophthalmological lesions and their causes

Main opthalmological lesions

Causes	Congen. malform. (72)	Congen. Cataract (54)	Optic n. atrophy (43)	Tapetoret. dystrophies (49)	Mult.acq. lesions (21)	Congen. glaucoma (20)	High myopia (3)	Glioma (3)	Albinism (5)	Chorio-retinitis (2)	Retrol. fibroplasia (6)
Pre and Perinatal											
Inherited diseases	33	23	17	48		19	3	3	5		
Congenital infections	7	2	1	1		1				2	
Prematurity -O$_2$			2								6
Dystocia			1								
Cerebral palsy			2								
Congenital hydrocephalus			3								
Unknown	32	29	2								
Postnatal											
Infections (ocular - CNS)			11		14						
Accidents			1		7						
Brain tumors			1								
Avitaminosis A			1								
Generalized dis - CNS			1								

TABLE V

Origin of children

	Towns		Villages		Total	
	No	%	No	%	No	%
1950 - 1959	36	27.1	97	72.9	133	100
1960 - 1969	11	13.1	73	86.9	84	100
1970 - 1979	24	35.8	43	64.2	67	100

TABLE VI

Socio-economic status of the children

	Low		Medium		High		Total	
	No	%	No	%	No	%	No	%
1950 - 1959	108	81.2	21	15.8	4	3	133	100
1960 - 1969	71	84.5	13	15.5	-	-	84	100
1970 - 1979	32	47.7	25	37.3	10	15	67	100

DISCUSSION - CONCLUSIONS

This study investigates the causes of blindness and their variance of 284 individuals aged from 6-25 years who have attended the S.B.N.G. during the period 1950-79, and who were blinded before the age of 6 years. Quite a number of cases of young individuals have been studied, as the S.B.N.G. is the only institution in Northern Greece that is available for the education of blind people.

The study of the number of blind children per decade shows that there is a gradual decrease of the number of students which is statistically significant. The possible factors for this decrease might be the following: 1) The gradual decrease of individuals with congenital malformations (31.5 % in the 1950-59 decade, 14.9 % in the 1970-79 decade). The congenital malformations might be due to marriages among relatives or to congenital infections that were not diagnosed. The moving of the people from the small society of the villages to the towns has decreased the number of marriages among relatives, while the improving living conditions in this country, the broader use of inoculations and the interruption of pregnancy in cases of pregnant women suffering from rubella might be the main reasons for the decrease of congenital malformations. 2) The gradual decrease of cases with congenital glaucoma (11.3 % in the 1950-59 decade and 1.5 % in the 1970-79 decade). 3) The decrease of cases with ocular infections (endopthalmitis) or C.N.S. infections (meningitis). In the 1950-59 decade the percentage of infections was 13.5 % while in the 1970-79 decade only 3 % of all the cases was due to infections. In the 1970-79 decade there was no case of blindness due to ocular infection.

The number of boys is bigger than the number of girls. This statistically significant difference can be found in all three decades. Our findings coincide with those of other studies regarding young people with poor vision (Schappert-kimmijser et al 1975, Hansen 1975, Lindstedt 1975).

The main ophthalmological lesions of our cases were the congenital malformations (25.3 %), the tapetoretinal dystrophies (17.2 %), the congenital cataract (19 %) and the congenital or acquired optic nerve atrophy (15.1 %). These percentages are similar to those of other more developed countries such as Denmark (Skydsgaard 1975), Belgium (Haustrate -Gosset 1975), Sweden (Lindstedt 1975), Holland (Schappert -Kimmijser et al 1975), except for the percentage of congenital malformations which is higher in our study. However, it is worth mentioning that there is a continuous decrease in the percentage of congenital malformations and the 14.9 % percentage of the 1970 -79 decade is about the same with that of the above mentioned countries.

Retrolental fibroplasia appears for the first time in the 1970 -79 decade with a percentage 9 % which is about the same with other countries such as Sweden (7 %) and Holland 8 % (Linstedt 1975, Schappert -Kimmijser et al 1975) while in the 1950 -59 period the percentage in England and Wales was 29.5 % (Fine 1968).

The number of children with multiple acquired lesions of the eyeball was significantly decreased during the 1970 -79 decade. This is due to the decrease of both the ocular and C.N.S. infections with significant statistical difference.

The main causes of the ophthalmological lesions of our material are pre and perinatal in all three decades (up to 94 % during the 1970 -79 decade). The difference between the pre and perinatal causes and the postnatal ones which is statistically significant and refers to the three decades, agrees with the results of other authors regarding young people with poor vision (Nakajima 1961, Hansen 1975, Hatfield 1975, Lindsted 1975, Schappert -Kimmijser 1975). Among the prenatal causes the inherited ones are at the top of the list in all the three decades. Other authors present the same findings too.

Congenital infections vary from 4.5 % (decade of 1950 -59) to 8.9 % (decade of 1970 -79). In the U.S.A. the percentage is 2.8 % (Hatfield 1975), while in Sweden it is 8 % (Lindstedt 1975). We believe that the increase in the percentage of congenital infections of our material is not absolutely actual, but it is mainly due to a more accurate diagnosis of these cases made possible by improved medical methods used lately.

The percentage of unknown causes fluctuates from 26.3 % in the first decade to 15 % in the last one and a significant statistical decrease of the percentage is being noticed. This might be due to a better study of certain cases and most probable to better conditions during pregnancy and delivery. Our findings coincide with those of studies made in Belgium (20 %) (Haustrate -Gosset 1975), in Holland (15 %) (Schappert -Kimmijser 1975) and in Denmark (23 %) (Skydsgaard 1975). According to other authors, the percentage of causes due to unknown factors reaches the 36 -38 % (Hatfield 1975, Lindstedt 1975). This might be to the fact that the study of genetic ophthalmological diseases is not yet complete and thus many inherited diseases are put under the category of causes due to unknown factors.

The percentage of postnatal causes decreases from 18.8 % in the first decade to 6 % in the third one and thus approaches the percentage of other countries such as Sweden (6 %) (Lindstedt 1975). This gradual decrease is due mainly to the decrease of infections (ocular and of the C.N.S.). Ocular infections completely disappear as a cause of blindness during the last decade although isolated (single) cases of panophthalmia due to pseudomonas in newborn babies are being reported (Peonidis and Papayiannis 1972, Andreou et al 1982).

The percentage of accidents (4.5 % in the first decade and 3 % in the third one) is higher than of other countries e.g. Belgium (1 %) (Haustrate-Gosset 1975) and Sweden (1 %) (Lindstedt 1975). The increased percentage during the first decade was due mainly to war after effects (mines, hand grenades e.t.c.) and appeared mainly in country boys.

The study of the children's origin showed that the majority come from agricultural districts. This is valid for all the three decades and has been statistically proven. The socioeconomic status of the children is low which is also true for the three decades and has been statistically proven.

The knowledge of the causes of blindness in early childhood and its variance through the years helps us to realize the importance of prevention. The cooperation of ophthalmologists, paediatricians, genetists, neurologists, social workers, psychologists and statisticians (for the epidemiological study of blindness) is the basic prerequisite for its prevention. The early diagnosis and treatment, the genetic guidance, the study of possible carrier, the close and systematic opthalmological follow up of premature babies and the proper education of the medical and paramedical people and the public could considerably lead to a decrease of individuals with poor vision (Falls 1968, WHO 1972, Kofinas 1977).

S U M M A R Y

The main causes of blindess in 284 students of the "School for blind children of the Northern Greece" (S.B.N.G.) from 1950 to 1979, who lost their vision until the 6th year of their life, have been studied. The material of the study was divided into decades during which the children enrolled at the S.B.N.G. and then the findings of the decades were compared to each other. The majority of the children originated from villages and their socioeconomic status was low. In all the three decades pre and perinatal lesions was the main cause of blindness and among them inherited diseases was the first one. The percentage of postnatal causes had a significant gradual reduction. Congenital malformations, optic nerve atrophy, tapetoretinal dystrophies and congenital cataract were the commonest ophthalmological lesions. There was a significant gradual reduction over the decades in the congenital malformations of the eyes, the multiple acquired lesions of the eyeball, the congenital glaucoma and the infections of the eye and the C.N.S. (as a cause of blindness). Blindness due to retrolental fibroplasia has been observed only since 1970. There was also an increase over the decades in the tapetoretinal dystrophies. We believe that the knowledge of the changing aetiology of blindness contributes to the prevention and the early management of poor vision in early childhood.

R E F E R E N C E S

Andreou A, Parisis P, Iliadelis E, Kasimos C. A case of panophthalmia due to pseudomonas in a premature infant. Paediatrica Chronica 1982; 11(1):36 - 38.

Dimolitsas A. Legislative and administrative measures for the blind. Athens: 1980.

Falls FH. Significance of genetics in the daily practice of the opthalmologist. Symposium on surgical and medical management of congenital anomalies of the eye. St. Louis: Morsby Company, 1968, 1 - 13.

Fine S. Blind and partially - sighted children. Department of Education and Science. London: H.M.S.O. 1968.

Hansen E. Causes of severe visual impairment in children and their prevention in Norway. Doc. Ophthalmology, 1975; 381(39):263 -270.

Hatfield EM. Why are they blind? Sight saving Rev. 1975; 45:2 -22.

Haustrate -Gosset MF. Causes of severe visual impairment in children and their prevention in Belgium. Doc. Ophthalmol. 1975; 381(39): 249 -262.

Kofinas I. Preventive Ophthalmology and ways to be applied. Arch. of Hygiene 1977; 27(5 -8):141 -171.

Lindstedt E. Causes of severe visual impairment in children and their prevention in Sweden. Doc. Ophthalmol. 1975; 381(39):287 -297.

Nakajima A. Congenital and hereditary blindness in Japan. Japan Soc. Ophthalmol. 1961; 30:9.

Peonidis A, Papayiannis J. Panophthalmia due to pseudomonas in a premature infant. Elliniki Iatriki 1972; 41 (suppl.):40.

Schappert -Kimmijser J, Copper Ac, Dunster CB, Delleman JW, Franken S, Hamburg A, Van den Heuvel -Aghina JWM, Höefnagels KLJ, Loewer -Sieger DH, Van Veelen AWC, Verdvin PC, Volmer C. Causes of severe visual impairment in children in Netherland and their prevention. Doc. Ophthalmol. 1975; 381(39):224 -248.

Skydsgaard H. Causes of severe visual impairment in children and their prevention in Denmark. Doc. Ophthalmol. 1975; 381(39):271 -283.

WHO. Prevention de la cecité. Rapport d'un groupe d'etude de l'OMS. Genéve, 1972. 1973:518.

DISCUSSION

Jay: There are certain aspects of the physiology of vision that can keep us here for a week or two, but I am not sure whether this is the appropriate moment to discuss this topic. But the discussion is in your hands and if anyone would like particulary to mention any area or anything discussed for which collaboration might be considered then this is the moment to start.

Harcourt: Just to start the ball rolling, could you and Warburg give us any information as to how far you have got with setting up a European Ophthalmic Genetics Register. Not only national but international, in order to give us an idea of the incidence of genetic diseases.

Jay: This is a very interesting idea, and it is becoming increasingly important, with the advent of recombinant DNA technology, to have available appreciable numbers of correctly diagnosed families, including affected members with each of these inherited diseases. It is difficult in any one country to find a handful of some of these conditions and certainly a case can be made for such a register. I think this is one of the aspects we ought to be thinking about.

Warburg: In the EEC several attempts have been made to produce a European Survey of prevalences, and that has been found to be extremely difficult. The audiologist have found it so. There are studies on congenital malformations, but the money has to come from the national boards, and the end result can only be presented when everybody has delivered their report. For these reasons EEC prevalence studies are quite difficult to do. Yes, it would be very worthwhile to be together around a project concerning special disorders, and every one of us in the field knows who has described the families, so we can always get in touch. Recently, for instance, we have finished a project on Norrie's disease for which we collected families in the Netherlands and in Denmark and had them analysed in Freiburg, Germany. You could also establish a network between, for instance, the Dutch Genetic Register and the British one but there are few other countries that keep such registers.

van Hof-van Duin: You talk about the Dutch register, but even in a small country like the Netherlands it does not cover the whole country.

van Lith: It is spreading, but it is not the whole country.

Warburg: There is another question that Harcourt might have asked. Would it be possible within the EEC to establish a DNA bank of well-known families or would it be possible within the EEC to establish a mutant cell directory such as they have in North America? That is costly because one has to know the families, it requires a secretariat that keeps track of the families, and you have to monitor the bank.

Jay: I wonder how important total ascertainment is? Does it really matter whether the prevalence of some uncommon disease is one in 10,000 or one in 15,000 or one in 25,000, unless it is a condition like retinoblastoma where it has been argued that the mutation rate is increasing. The Dutch are doing this and for this to be valuable you must get total ascertainment.

Campos: I would like to propose another type of interaction, between physiologists, basic scientists and ophthalmologists in the field of amblyopia. Experimental amblyopia is a condition which is well known but no one really knows whether it matches what happens in humans. We are aware of one brain with anisometropic amblyopia which was examined, but there is no evidence of what happens in strabismic amblyopia. This may be a macabre type of co-operation but it may be very useful to have people interacting to examine the lateral geniculate bodies of humans.

Vital-Durand: What we call amblyopia in monkeys is only one specific type of amblyopia caused by pattern-deprivation of the retina. It would be very interesting to get this cooperation, but getting brains from amblyopic patients is not easy.

Campos: I think the problem is trying to get a register of all available brains.

Atkinson: Another area where I would like to see some international co-operation is in looking at visual function in children with retinopathy of prematurity. There now seems to be quite good agreement on the pathology in different stages of this retinopathy. Given that the prevalence of this illness is on the increase again as improved neonatal care leads to survival of even more premature babies, it would be nice to have some international cooperation in looking at what happens to these children in terms of vision. I see and hear a great deal about ophthalmologists looking at the various stages of the disease, but it may be more important to know what effect this has on later visual development.

Campos: It is important to analyse visual function, although one has to realise that there is not much one can really do to benefit the patient without knowing better whether the retina is potentially functional; this can be done with ophthalmoscopy. What is really important is to prevent the condition.

Warburg: I don't think that ophthalmology is all about surgery.

Campos: I agree.

Warburg: I don't see why we shouldn't know the visual acuity of children with an optical disorder.

Campos: At a given moment it is important, and I see it is to the advantage of the patient.

Atkinson: I have heard that of the children that have retinopathy of prematurity only about 10% will actually end up with a significant visual deficit. If this is the case then it is very important to know whether or not they have a visual problem, because otherwise there will be a lot of time wasted by ophthalmologists looking at cases where there is no visual problem. So I would argue very strongly that visual function has to be looked at alongside pathology and that they don't have to be done by two separate groups.

DEVELOPMENT OF VISION IN VISUALLY IMPAIRED CHILDREN

Lea Hyvärinen

City of Helsinki, Department of Health

Vision is a learned function in the normally sighted individuals and in the visually impaired children as well. A visually impaired infant must build his visual concepts based on defective visual information. He must learn to perform smooth tracking movements, saccadic movements and to accommodate and to converge. All these motor functions are needed to achieve the clearest possible image on the retina and to permit fusion in the brain of the images on both retinas.

A normally sighted infant learns these different motor functions by trial and error and is rewarded by seeing a clear image. A visually impaired infant will not see a clear image how much he may try to focus and look. Thus accommodation and coordination of the ocular muscles cannot develop as exact as those of a normally sighted child. The infant then not only has visual sensory impairment but imperfect motor functions, too.

A visually impaired infant may not become aware of his vision if the quality of the visual image is very poor. When an infant does not react to anything else but bright light, we can help him learning to see by using flash lights on which we stick different simple geometrical figures. A visual stimulus that is turned on and off is very effective. When the child has learned to react to the flash lights with adequate eye movements we can show him simple pictures and objects with very good contrast. The time of stimulation is kept long to permit the child to study the object well enough.

The human face is the most effective visual stimulus during the early weeks of life and it should be used to stimulate the infant's vision. At the same time the close bodily contact and the vocal contact with the adult help the infant to develop his communication and effectively activate the infant.

In normal infants vision is the most effective activator of the reticular formation and through it the activator of cortical functions. Many visually impaired infants are far less active in their motor functions and in observing their surroundings than their sighted peers. The quiet, seemingly content infant is not learning at optimal level and therefore activation through vision should be increased and supported by all other modalities. If we can awaken normal drive in the visually handicapped infant he will learn to see better and his whole development will improve (Sonksen et al 1984).

As soon as the infant can hold ball and other large playthings between his hands these are used to make the child aware of his hands and to bring them into the midline. Hands are the most effective playthings to train vision and to teach the child to explore. The playthings drop and the infant is unable to locate them and to try to reach. Thus an adult is needed near the infant almost constantly during the early months.

In the beginning the visual sphere of a visually impaired infant is very limited. It is difficult to entice him to look at something at a distance. The most interesting objects are the family members and, if the infant is bottle fed, the bottle. The bottle can be made better visible by painting it or by using striped bottle warmers. The family members are easier to recognize if they wear something clearly visible and, when approaching, talk to the infant to signal him their presence. Because the auditory orientation is imperfect the infant may try to locate by sight.

Orientation may be trained by constructing the surroundings of the infant so that their visual and tactile details coincide (Hyvärinen L 1983). Thus tactile information facilitates the use of vision and does not compete with it in the associative brain functions (Hyvärinen J et al 1981).

Severely impaired infants may get so little reward of looking that they do not lift their head to look around. It was quite common to see infants develop poor head lift and weak shoulders and arms when early stimulation was not routinely started. Use of colourful or illuminated playthings, and auditory stimulation up in front of the infant, and early physiotherapy result in better control of the neck, shoulders, and arms. This is a prerequisite for learning of orientation in the room and for moving.

The time between 2 months and 9 months of age should be used for effective stimulation, not to "wait and see". Today we do not know enough of playthings suitable for this age group of visually impaired infants. Many of them have other handicaps and often their capacity to use visual information is inferior to that of a normal child. Their stimulation should therefore be very well structured, long lasting and emotionally motivating. Playthings that the child could activate with easy hand movements would develop eye-hand-coordination and give the child the experience of making decisions. Development of playthings and play situations for effective stimulation in this important age is a challenge for everybody taking care of visually impaired infants.

Some infants develop the bad habbit of eye poking. It deforms the face and disturbs the child's social contacts later, and should therefore be prevented. When the infant starts to press his eyes, even gently, we use protective spectacles and make sure that the infant has enough to do with his hands so there is no time to be bored and no need of self stimulation. Good spectacle frames for infants are hard to get, quite often they have to be hand made to fit the little nose. However, it is worth the trouble to prevent eye poking immediately. It prevents the child from using his vision and it effectively cuts the contact between the child and his surroundings. The child withdraws into his own world. If eye poking has become a habbit it is nearly impossible to stop the child from practising it.

Optical correction of refractive errors is important. Because the visually impaired infants hold objects very close to their eyes in order to see them better, it is advisable to make the first spectacles as reading spectacles to decrease the amount of accommodation needed and to prevent inward squint. Those infants who have not learned to accommodate will see a much clearer image through their reading spectacles. When the visual sphere of the child enlarges his spectacles are made as bifocals with a large lower segment.

Absorptive spectacles should be used much more than they are used today.
In order to know whether the infant or child will profit from use of absorptive spectacles the vision should be examined at low luminance levels, at regular room illumination level and in bright light. Infants with achromatopsia may be so dazzled that they function like blind in "good illumination". Some children with aniridia or lens opacities will also see much better when using absorptive spectacles. If the child does not need optical correction, the use of absorptive spectacles can be reduced by adjusting the illumination in the room and by playing outside in shade or late in the evening.

On the other hand, children who need unusually high luminance levels in order to see better should get their special desks which resemble an X-ray viewing box. On them the children can see their play things and can start learning basic geometrical forms and letters and numbers. Even if they will be braille readers they will benefit from visual information. These severely impaired children have difficulties to see the structure of the rooms and to estimate distances using vision. It is important to use focal illumination in the corners of the rooms, close to the doors and edges which should be avoided to teach the child the structure of the rooms. Tactile exploration of the rooms is a necessary adjunct in learning.

Optical aids, like magnifiers, close circuit TV, and telescopes should be used earlier than they are used today, to improve the quality of visual image and to widen the world of a visually impaired child. Because he often has very short working distance he should get an easel or levated desk to prevent the development of a bad posture which can occur if he constantly leans near a usual table or desk.

Visual training and training to use different visual aids requires specialized teachers for the visually impaired children during the preschool years. At the present time there are too few of them and thus the ophthalmologist must improvise different play situations to suit the daily program of the child and must give relevant information about vision to the persons who take care of the child.

Visual training is an integral part of early habilitation and should have an athmosphere of games. It should never be experienced by the child as formal training. The different play situations should train visual fixation and pursuit at different distances, judgement of distances, direction, speed, form, etc, and to combine visual information with information from the other senses. At the same time it is important to help the child to develop his abilities to use the compensating modalities optimally.

Parents and special educators need up-to-date information on vision every second or third week during the first months and once a month when the development reaches the level of a 10 month old healthy infant. There are individual needs if the visual functions are changing rapidly, especially if vision is progressively lost.

Assessment of vision for development is a demanding task. It requires thorough understanding of the development of normal infants and that of the visually impaired infants with different visual capabilities. In most hospitals neither the ophthalmologist nor the paediatric neurologist has the experience needed and thus the evaluation may be best performed in close collaboration between the two specialists.

In conclusion, development of vision of a visually impaired child and his general development can be greatly influenced by early habilitation. If we want to help the child to develop to his maximal potential we should:

                   -diagnose the impairment as early as only possible,
                   -start early habilitation immediately,
                   -start visual stimulation as a part of habilitation,
                   -assess vision for development regularly,
                   -develop methods of stimulation, and
                   -develop our understanding of the problems related to visual
impairment of a child, in the child himself, in his family, in the day care personnel, in the hospital, because all these different problem areas have their influence on the final outcome of habilitation.

Today we ophthalmologists are blamed - with reason - for our attitude of "wait and see" during the important months of early development. We should take better care of vision of visually impaired children. Vision, although defective, is an important tool in learning and should thus be given all the special support for development that we as specialists can give.

REFERENCES

Hyvärinen J, Hyvärinen L, Carlson S. Effect of binocular deprivation on parietal association cortex in young monkeys. In: Maffei L, ed. Doc Ophthal Proc Ser 30. The Hague: Dr.W.Junk Publishers, 1981: 177-185.

Hyvärinen L. Early stimulation of visually impaired infants. Ophthalmic Paed Genet 1983;2:129-133.

Sonksen PM, Levitt S, Kitzinger M. Identification of constraints acting on motor development in young visually disabled children and principles of remediation. Child: care, health and development 1984;10:273-286.

DEFINITIONS OF VISUAL IMPAIRMENTS AND THEIR CONSEQUENCES IN
INFANTS AND SMALL CHILDREN.

Eva Lindstedt

Consequences of disease according to the ICIDH

In 1980 the World Health Organization published its
"International Classification of Impairments, Disabilities and
Handicaps - A manual of classification relating to the consequen-
ces of disease", ICIDH.

The intention was to define, describe and classify a wide range
of effects of disease, thus making it possible to evaluate health
care procedures.

"If health care processes are to be evaluated, they must be goal-
oriented, because the appraisal is concerned with the extent to
which goals are attained." (ICIDH, p.8)

The scope of the medical model of illness:

etiology -- pathology -- manifestation

was found less suitable when it came to describing the innumerab-
le individual and social consequences of disease. Another
sequence of illness-related phenomena could be presented in the
following dimensions of classification:

disease -- impairment -- disability -- handicap

The three last mentioned concepts are those of the ICIDH. The
first dimension of classification (impairment) refers to the
effects of disease on an organ or part of the body, e.g.
eye/visual system, ear, muscles etc. The second dimension (disability) refers to consequences for the individual experienced as
restriction of his ability to perform specific activities/tasks,
e.g. reading, hearing, speech, walking etc. The third dimension
of classification (handicap) refers to consequences for the
individual as related to the environment/society, e.g. physical
independence, social integration and economic self-sufficiency.

The classification scheme thus makes it possible to describe
consequences of disease from many different angles. There is,
however, one aspect which is not readily described by this classification: the developmental consequences to the young child of
prenatal, congenital or early acquired disease are not specifically mentioned.

Diseases leading to sensory impairments will deprive the infant of experience, thus constraining development.

Disability and developmental capacity

Visual impairments constrain the infant´s development in many respects. The type and degree of the constraints may depend on the type and degree of visual impairment, the age of the child and the presence of other impairments (multiply impaired children).

From the very first week of life, in the sighted child, vision takes on a leading role in general development. Vision is a trigger of motor development, an instrument for developing mental abilities, a constructor of spatial conceptions, a tool when acquiring verbal language, a means of developing emotional relationships. Vision also steers its own development; the child develops vision by using it, learns to see by seeing.

Thus in the infant and young child, the primary function of vision is connected with developmental achievements. Disabilities following visual impairments are to be defined with reference to the developmental constraints imposed, viz on visual and general development.

We know a great deal about the early visual development of the normal child - the initial capacity of the visual system, the progress of development and the duration of "sensitive periods" of development of the various visual functions. Little is known, however, about these sequences of events in the visually impaired or mupltiply impaired infant. Also, our knowledge is limited concerning the consequences of visual impairments expressed/defined as constraints on development (Sonksen et al., 1984).

At a certain developmental stage we may identify critical levels of visual function below which deprivation of experience and constraint of development will follow. Thus we might be able to define and classify disabilities of developmental capacity.

At present we do not know the exact "minima" below which specific visual functions cannot fulfil their developmental mission. This holds true both regarding critical levels below which a visual function is unable to develop and may deteriorate further, and regarding critical levels below which vision cannot pursue its developmental task.

Research is very much needed in this field. A necessary prerequisite of successful research is the further development and adjustment for clinical use of methods of assessing and measuring visual functions in preverbal children.

"Categories of vision"

Table 1 (ICIDH, p. 80)

WHO category of vision	Degree of impairment	Visual acuity (with best possible correction)	Synonyms and alternative definitions
NORMAL VISION	None	0.8 or better	range of normal vision
	Slight	less than 0.8	near-normal vision
LOW VISION	Moderate	less than 0.3	moderate low vision
	Severe	less than 0.12	severe low vision - legal blindness in some countries
BLINDNESS	Profound	less than 0.05	profound low vision or moderate blindness
	Near-total	less than 0.02	severe or near-total blindness
	Total	no light perception	total blindness

The WHO "categories of vision" (ICIDH, p.80) are evidently intended for use only in individuals having a fully developed visual system. It is inadequate in infants and young children. When attempting to outline corresponding categories of "normal vision", "low vision" and "blindness" for application in infants, we have to consider a number of facts derived from our developmental aspect of visual impairments and their consequences in young children.

- We had better be very careful when deciding which degree of a specific type of visual impairment may be considered insignificant. A minor visual impairment may have deprivational consequences of one kind or another.

- On the other hand, the developmental influence of vision during early life is so potent that even very rudimentary residual vision may be capable of developing and of promoting general development to some extent, if utilized optimally. We are best advised to postpone the diagnosis of "blindness" in an infant until we are convinced that no residual vision whatsoever is present. The use of the term "blindness" by the WHO as also referring to individuals with various degrees of residual vision is open to criticism even when applied to adults.

Early detection of visual impairment in infants

The importance of the early detection and measurement of visual impairments in infants and young children lies in the fact that there is a possibility of preventing, minimizing and/or compensating for the developmental constraints which, if nothing is done, will follow the visual impairment. remediation measures having this effect include stimulation of visual functions and different active habilitation procedures to combat disability/handicap in the child, such as retarded motor and mental development.

A complete programme of stimulation/habilitation taking into account research findings would involve co-operation between several professionals, e.g. pediatric ophthalmologist, pediatrician, psychologist, special teacher, physiotherapist, working together with the child's family.

The earlier remediation measures are applied, the more effective they will be. In other words, the earlier we are able to detect and correctly diagnose the type and degree of visual impairment, the better prospect there will be of applying the most convenient and effective measures of habilitation. Visual functions need to be re-assessed during the habilitation process, so that the procedures can be evaluated and readjusted as development progresses.

Once again, the importance of valid assessment methods is evident.

The responsibility of the pediatric ophthalmologist

Where preverbal children are concerned, the responsibility of the ophthalmologist is manifold. In addition to the diagnostic procedures and treatment of eye diseases/disorders, including refractive errors and oculomotor dysfunctions, there is the task of preventing more or less serious consequences of visual impairments.

This task implies:

- The early detection and measurement of visual impairments.

- The application of specific measures to achieve optimal visual development and utilization of vision.

- Clear information and distinct instructions, given in co-operation with other professionals, to the family and to the authorities concerning the relevant arrangements/services needed for the child, e.g. physiotherapy, family support, aids, special training, special education. It is the responsibility of the community/society to ensure that such arrangements/services are made available to the child and the child's family when a visual impairment is detected.

References

World Health Organization: International Classification of
Impairments, Disabilities and Handicaps. Geneva, 1980.

Sonksen PM, Levitt S, Kitzinger M. Identification of constraints
acting on motor development in young visually disabled children and
principles of remediation. In: Child Care, Health and Development
1984;10:273-286.

DISCUSSION

Fielder: Visual stimulation may well be important, especially in mentally retarded and mentally handicapped children. I would like to ask Hyvarinen how you distinguish in a controlled fashion between the results of stimulation and the natural course of the disease? How do you assess the effect of treatment?

Hyvarinen: There is no possibility for double blind trials in the very young. A child passes through a particular stage of development only once. The 'normal' development of a visually impaired infant and child with its variations is well known; there are enough examples of what will happen if nothing special is done. Teachers report notable improvement in the abilities of children at the age of 6 today, compared with what they were 10 years ago. We can help many visually impaired children to have almost normal motor development and to learn to use residual vision effectively. In some cases the changes have been recorded very carefully, and remarkable development is possible in the teens and even in those over 20 years of age (Carlson and Hyvarinen, Acta Ophthalmol 1983; 61: 701). If we can improve visual function at the age of 14, or even 23, it is likely that it is possible in infancy. Whenever an infant is not reaching his milestones, we try to find out why this is occurring, and we try to help him learn to master the function.

Fielder: I am interested in your observations because there are groups making a great deal of money from visual stimulation, encouraging parents to spend vast sums on this type of thing. It is a very important issue.

Hyvarinen: Our usual material for visual stimulation seldom costs more than £20 at the most. The majority of the materials used in play situations are available in every home.

Harcourt: I think that Fielder has a good point and the problem is that it is extremely important that one should be able to identify the groups carefully. One can't talk about the child whose vision is so low that he amuses himself by eye rubbing and then change from that to another child wearing a reading correction because it improves near vision or putting a dot in the field of vision so that he can follow the line properly. Within the group of which you are generally talking there are quite separate levels of vision and whether you call it blindness or slight impairment doesn't matter, but it is no good generalising when there are in fact a number of quite different groups. It is very important that this is dealt with scientifically and I agree that it is important to do matched studies in children, but part of the difficulty in doing it is that the people who are doing this are evangelical in their attitude and they by an act of faith believe that what they are doing is right. It tends to lead on to exactly the same problems that were found, for example, with the CAM stimulator for amblyopia. It is very easy for a group of people to recommend a certain method of treatment but it is difficult for other groups to conclude that their view is based on a placebo effect rather than on a scientific principle. I have also been involved with young adults in Africa who have been taught to be farmers who were blind, certainly early enough during infancy to have roving eye movements. Although it is not possible to prove they were blind from birth, they were so from early infancy but their locomotion and their hand coordination and their ability to do weaving, their ability to plant seeds and weed in a garden and to have an independent existence was excellent, so it is very difficult to talk from an anecdotal point of view about these things. We are bedevilled in Western Europe by these concepts and it is exactly the same concept that all children are born with the same intelligence and that those in the lower socio-economic order, because there are no books at home and they don't have any stimulation, then by the time they get to primary school their ability to learn has dropped away. All these have tended to become based on evangelical views rather than on good scientific sense. I agree with a lot of what was said, but I think that there should be a true scientific study.

Apkarian: I would disagree. I should like to make two points. The first is that anyone who has observed a large group of blind adults realises immediately that there are those normally adjusted to their environment to the point where they function quite well even in professions previously assumed to require vision, eg electrical engineering, or professors of politics. On the other hand, one might also observe within this group, blind individuals who are totally incapacitated and can barely dress themselves or function independently in any fashion. It is hard to believe that something like this needs scientific quantification. The early environment seems to be very important and if one is taught to be self-sufficient one tends to become just that. Early sensory stimulation is an important initial phase to normal development. As such, I would now like to bring up the second point. In terms of enriching the sensory environment of children with low vision, do you think that it is practical to use tactile stimulation to provide spatial information to the skin surface? I am referring to Bach-y-Rita's so-called "vision substitution system" whereby a camera scans a high contrast object. The image is then commutated to the skin surface via an array of vibrators. This approach has been used rather successfully with blind individuals in providing them with spatial information, concepts, and percepts otherwise unattainable. Do you think such an approach might be useful in your training programme?

Hyvarinen: No, we have not used it but we will be discussing it next month, because there is further work going on in that field. When building our stimulation programme we have the greatest difficulty in making it scientific. Every single child is so different and even if you find two children very much the same with the same diagnosis at the same age, then the families are bound to be different. You have to start with what you have, you can't ask the families for more than they can afford or can do, and you can then build around the child. Anything as complicated as a camera or a stimulator would be between the child and the parents. I would be afraid to do that early but I would be very interested in trying to do it with a child of 2 or 3 years, when the child already has some concept of space to use it for a few months, and try to find out whether children are more interested in learning to use the tactile stimulator than are adults. As you know blind people are not interested.

Arden: Can I just say one thing. I don't want to sound too censorious but one of the problems in this work is the language you use. You said the child never gets a clear image. You have no real evidence that when vision is slightly improved the child does not get the reward of a clearer image even if it isn't 100% and I think the sort of conclusions that you are drawing are bound to be less valuable than if they were more precisely formulated.

Hyvarinen: What I meant was that when the child focuses, the image will be about the same within a larger range of accommodation than in a normal child. A normal child develops much more accurate accommodation at a certain distance because he sees the difference related to the changes in accommodation. The visually impaired child will of course get a clearer image but his accommodation is not developing normally.

Arden: Is there any reason why that shouldn't be equally gratifying to the child?

Hyvarinen: I never said that, I only said that his visual functions are not as exact as those in the normal child.

Taylor: I agree with you that it is impossible to plan a scientific study of early treatment in visually handicapped children. You cannot do this because you are dealing with parents. You can't get two lots up and say "we are going to give you advice" to one only and then say "see you in two years' time." One lot will come back and another won't. We tried to do a matched control over the last 18 months and it is running into great difficulties getting the patients to come. On a practical level, if you don't have any proof about it, so what? If you use Hyvarinen's techniques or those of other people, the cost is about 10 minutes of the ophthalmologist's time if that is the least you want to do, and the amount of extra cost to the parents is zero. Let's just divorce ourselves from the scientific side for a moment. We are trying to think about treating small babies who are blind and hoping that they will see better in the long run. The scientific side of it is completely different; you don't have to have scientific evidence before you start treatment, even if people do abuse it.

Spekreijse: Is that not a strange attitude? You said you don't need scientific evidence before you start treatment.

Taylor: No, because there is no risk to the treatment.

Spekreijse: But is it doing any good to the child? It might be so slight that parents give it up, while if you would persevere it might improve in the long run.

Taylor: But if you scientifically proved it the parents are still going to give it up if they don't find it of use at all. The amazing thing is that the parents want it, they are looking for something to do and I am not just talking about keeping them busy and keeping them happy, I am talking about giving them something really positive so that they can help the child themselves and get everybody else to help and feel they are helping. Even that is of some value, assuming that it doesn't work. If it works, and again I have no evidence that it does work, one knows of a lot of patients that have been very pleased by it.

Harcourt: Of course I believe as Taylor does that these parents are in
great distress and in a terrible situation. The more that one can do to
keep them busy and happy with the feeling that they are doing something to
help their child, clearly the better. But where the danger lies is in the
exaggerated claims of some groups that this does have a scientific basis.
Of course I am in favour of doing what one can to help parents and their
children, but while I do and it is common sense to do it, I wouldn't want
to claim that it has any proven scientific basis.

Dubowitz: I would like to make a comment as a paediatrician. I think
there is a scientific basis that sensory stimulation will have an effect on
the developing nervous system in the young infant and we can see that in
other aspects of handicap. I don't think vision will be an exception and
maybe one should also draw a difference in the aetiology of visual defect.
Your best results might be in those of neurological and cortical origin as
opposed to those where there is destruction in the visual apparatus. I
think there is continual disagreement on this between ophthalmologists and
paediatricians and I must say on the whole, ophthalmologists tend to be
more pessimistic than paediatricians are, and maybe we should meet
somewhere half way.

Hyvarinen: About 15 years ago we started to study monkeys because we
wondered why some older nearly blind children do so well and some so poorly
when they were apparently about the same in the beginning. We also
wondered why some children who had reasonably good vision were far more
tactile than they needed to be. We showed that if the baby monkey does not
use vision early, tactile information will take over those cells which
should combine information from vision with other information, and once
that has happened and the critical period is over nothing will change that.
If we can use vision early, even poor vision, and make the child aware of
it, it will help the child in his development.

Loewer-Sieger: One of the important aspects of the training is the
psychological one, the learning of the parents and the child to have a
positive attitude to a task, especially the school task when the child must
read at the age of 6 years. There are scientific data on children with
slight visual impairment. Reading ability can be expressed as a reading
speed, and in one school for visually impaired children the speed of
reading was much quicker than the speed of reading of children at a normal
school, not because of training of visual acuity but because of training
and having a positive attitude to the task. I think you can discuss that
scientifically.

Harcourt: That is a different problem altogether. In any group of
children, whether visually handicapped or not, you can raise the reading
ability by training. What we are talking about is very severely visually
impaired children at a very early stage in their lives. Can the co-
ordination of their residual vision or other locomotive functions and their
other functions be so improved that in the end it is going to be raised to
a level that could not be achieved by subsequent training?

Dubowitz: If you do not have a positive attitude then you will not register these children as partially sighted. Are you going to register a child who might still recover? I would suggest that you do, so that it will get that sort of attention and you can make something of the residual visual activity.

Atkinson: Can I support Harcourt and put in a plea for scientific assessment of the implications of visual impairment. I agree that everything should be done to help these children and their families. These children are growing up all the time and we do not know what visual requirements are necessary for particular visual tasks that they are doing at different stages. Unless research is done on that aspect, and we have some idea of what constitutes blindness from a functional point of view from birth to 5 years, we won't be able to make very specific recommendations. I am in favour of helping these families much more than is done at the moment, but I am also in favour of more detailed research on the visual requirements for particular tasks that children are doing at different ages, taking into account their other disabilities, because many of these partially sighted children are also physically and mentally handicapped to some extent.

Hyvarinen: Thank you very much, I wanted to hear something like that. When we measure vision in these children we are doing it in a silly way. There is need for better assessment of vision for development, something that is very complicated.

Campos: The measurement of visual function is based mainly on visual acuity. This is probably not enough because visual acuity informs us of the threshold of potential function of the system but there are people with equal visual acuity who function differently. Contrast sensitivity could possibly inform us in a more detailed way of the capability of the subject.

Spekreijse: I think we are moving in a dangerous direction. It is not necessary to have a sound scientific basis. It is not so important to know clinical parameters like acuity or contrast sensitivity because each is completely different. Of course there are different kinds of tasks and different performance levels but still you need a simple test that you can measure data like acuity, to collect the information to know what the minimum requirements are, and how the subject is performing. That is a different matter but you know what the result is.

Arden: I would like to say that the important thing that was touched on is that there are various types of various defects. Ophthalmologists are looking at the proximal part of the visual system and they see one type of defect, whereas the paediatrician sees children who are neurologically damaged and who have much more favourable experiences. It is this sort of classification of a child's defect, not simply the measures of threshold or contrast sensitivity but the analysis of the way in which the sight and the visual system is functioning. The other thing is that every time we have looked at the plasticity of the function of the visual system, admittedly in amblyopic children without such severe difficulty, we have been able to show that the visual system of quite old children is still plastic. I don't see why we should be discouraged or limit our treatment to the first

3 or 4 years of life because 9 or 10 year old children have shown quite conclusively that they have been modified by their visual experience and I think that in children who have multiple handicaps and slow development this will be even more true. This is even more reason for pushing treatment very hard even in those children in whom you haven't begun in the first couple of years of life.

Hyvarinen: May I try to combine these two arguments. We do need the threshold measurement for diagnosis, but we shouldn't be too much surprised to find out that the threshold measurements have not changed when the vision of the child improves.

Vital-Durand: One of the slides I showed this morning was from an experiment with cats (Hein, Vital-Durand, Salinger and Diamond. Science 1979; 204: 1321). Kittens were raised in the dark until their third or fourth week. Then one eye was immobilised by intracranial surgical section of the 3 oculomotor nerves and the other eye was sutured closed. Animals were then allowed to run around freely in the light for weeks. When tested on their ability to cross a gap by stepping on a support sitting in the middle of the gap, they could not visually guide their paw to hit the support. There is evidence that the object was seen, but they could not localise it and make use of this visual information.

If the same test is performed by an adult cat deprived of eye movement, impairment will not last more than a day or two. The adult cat has acquired during infancy a representation of visual space that he can use even if the equipment needed to be built is now removed. If a young kitten has not had the device available at the appropriate time, he will never develop proper spacial coordinates. There is a sensitive period for calibrating visual space with eye movements, restricted to the first few months of life, but its precise extent is not known. From other sensitive periods in the visual system we can infer that in man it could be short or long among individuals, which could explain why some children only make use of visual information quite late.

Warburg: This discussion is not only a discussion among ophthalmologists, it is a classical discussion of how to assess the early intervention studies that paediatricians go for, early intervention for mental retardation, early intervention of children with auditory deficiencies, early intervention of the visually impaired. It goes on in all circles and there are those who stand up and say "I know what to do," and there are others who say "how on earth can you do that." The answer to this is that today we simply do not have methods of measuring or evaluating early intervention in special children. We need a new form of thinking, a new method for evaluating longitudinal intervention studies where case controls are unavailable. So somebody will have to sit and think of a method that can be used, otherwise we will go on this way for the next ten years.

THEORETICAL ASPECTS OF THE PATTERN ERG

Henk Spekreijse

The Netherlands Ophthalmic Research Institute and the Laboratory of Medical Physics, University of Amsterdam, P.O. Box 12141, Amsterdam

There have been many reports that pattern and luminance ERGs may differ widely in clinical conditions. The most obvious reason for such a difference would be that the flash ERG is in essence a mass response of the entire retina. Even when photopic Ganz-field stimulation is attempted, scotopic components can frequently be observed in the response. The pattern reversal stimulus, on the other hand, eliminates basically stray light contributions to the ERG and allows the recording of a local, and preferably macular, response. Pattern reversal with many spatial elements yields no net luminance modulation and hence also the straylight in the peripheral retina is not modulated. It is this property of the pattern reversal stimulus that prompted Riggs et al (1964) to the introduction of the moving-bar pattern stimulus. Of course some straylight effects remain present near the edge of the stimulus field, which become more important the courser the spatial elements. Therefore the pattern stimulus should always be presented with a surround field of at least the same (but preferably much higher) luminance as the patterned field.

With all precautions for straylight taken, there remains the question whether the ERG to pattern and luminance stimulation reflects electrical activity of the same retinal layers. This question is not so surprising since a) the pattern ERG cannot easily be related to the conventional components of the luminance ERG and b) the two stimulus forms have been shown to generate essentially different responses from the back of the head. Pattern EPs contain contrast specific components that are not present in the luminance EPs (Spekreijse 1966). To test for the existence of contrast-specific components in the ERG, we compared the ERG responses evoked by pattern reversal to those obtained by averaging both on and off responses to luminance flicker (Spekreijse et al 1973). This "double-trigger" procedure is necessary since the true period of the reversal stimulus is half that of the individual sets of spatial elements, e.g. checks because they are modulated temporally 180 degrees out of phase. If the modulation frequency of an individual set of checks is f, then the response to that set of checks will yield the fundamental component (f) and (if present) all higher harmonics 2f, 3f, 4f, ... The response to both sets of checks are summated by the electrode, and thus, since the two sets of checks are exactly 180 degree out of phase, the fundamental f and the higher odd harmonics 3f, 5f, ... of the two sets will be 180 degree out of phase and hence cancel. On the other hand, the second 2f and higher order even harmonics 4f, 6f, ... will be in phase, and form the response. Also possible contrast specific components in the response will have the same frequencies 2f, 4f, 6f, etc since the contrast reverses at a rate 2f. Therefore the double triggered luminance response, baptized by Arden (1982) as the focal ERG, should be compared to the pattern reversal ERG. Some of the results of the 1973 study are represented in Fig. 1.

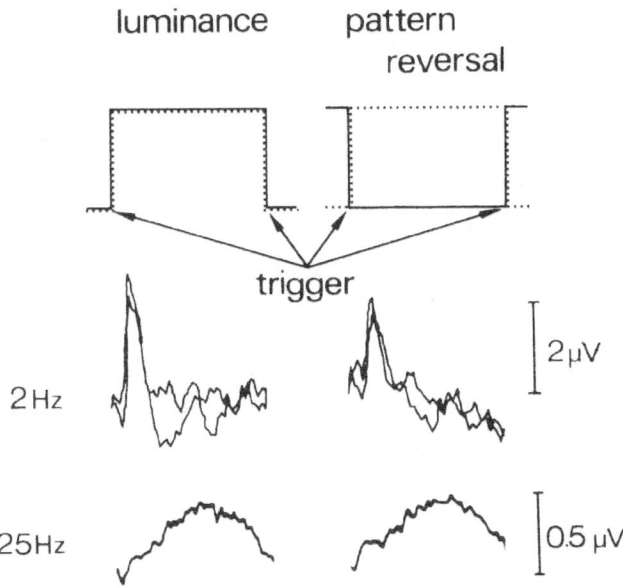

Fig. 1. ERGs to luminance modulation and pattern reversal. The averager is
triggered twice per period. Identical responses are obtained
irrespective of stimulus frequency. Mean luminance is 3000 asb;
modulation depth is 90%; checksize 60'. The stimulus field extends
8° and is surrounded by a steady field of equal luminance to
minimize straylight.

ERG responses evoked by pattern reversal rates of 2 Hz and 25 Hz are
compared to the double triggered responses to a square-wave modulated field
with the same radius (4°) as the patterned field.

A low and high temporal frequency was chosen for comparison since the
flicker fusion and temporal contrast sensitivity functions cross over at
intermediate frequency (Van der Tweel and Spekreijse 1973). So a contrast
specific component in the ERG may show up more clearly at one than at the
other frequency. Since, however, for both temporal frequencies quite
similar responses were found we concluded that the pattern reversal ERGs
seem to be determined by local luminance modulation and that the pattern
ERG does not give extra information.

THE PATTERN ERG ISSUE REOPENED

In 1981 Maffei and Fiorentini published their startling ERG findings
in cat that were obtained before and after chronic section of the optic
nerve to cause retrograde degeneration of the ganglion cells. They showed
that in the 8 adult cats in which the right optic nerve was sectioned at
the level of the chiasm, the ERGs to light flashes and flicker remained
normal and had comparable amplitude in both eyes throughout the 4-month
period following surgery. However, the pattern reversal ERG to sine wave
gratings started to decrease for the right eye as early as 18 days after
the operation. The reduction in amplitude was most outspoken for low
spatial frequencies, and progressed over time to higher spatial frequencies

till 4 months after the surgery no pattern reversal ERG could be recorded
from the right eye at all. Since the disappearance of the pattern ERG was
correlated with ganglion cell degeneration, Maffei and Fiorentini concluded
that activity of ganglion cells is the main source for the pattern reversal
ERG. So with the luminance ERG reflecting predominantly activity of the
outermost retinal layers, the pattern ERG would thus seem to be a probe for
the inner layers of the retina. This conclusion has so far reaching
consequences for clinical use that we decided to go back to the bench and
to repeat our 1973 experiments under conditions that are expected to yield
optimal contrast responses. By employing a d.t.l. electrode (Dawson et al
1979), ERGs could be recorded without interference with the optics of the
eye, allowing for the use of small checks. An example taken from this
series of experiments (Riemslag et al 1985) is depicted in Fig. 2. This
particular experiment was so designed that responses with a luminance

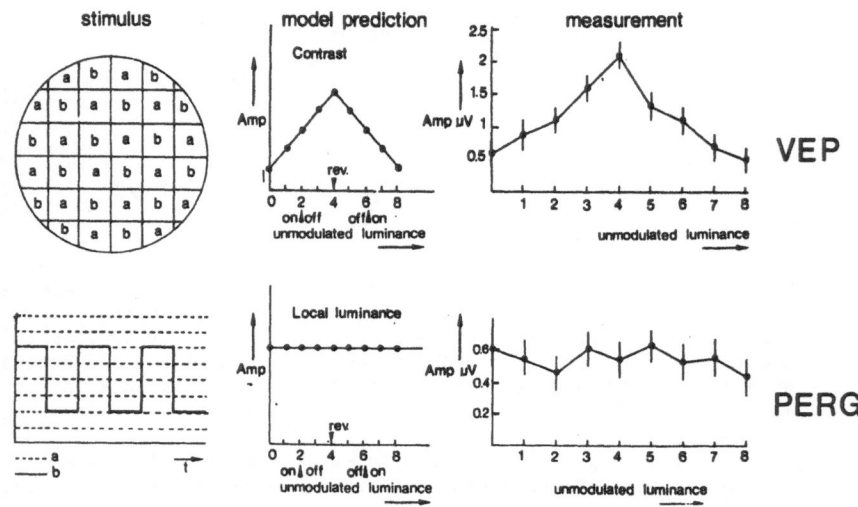

Fig. 2. One set of checks (b) was (square-wave) modulated at a frequency of
8 Hz, modulation depth 50% (continuous line). The other set (a) was
kept constant at different levels (dashed lines) for each trial.
Check size was 15 arc min, and the field size was 30 deg. The
luminance levels were as indicated: 0 = darkness; 8 = maximal, i.e.
856 cd/m^2. The luminance of the surround was ten times as bright
as the mean luminance of the modulated checks. The second-harmonic
amplitudes of the simultaneously recorded ERG and VEP are plotted
in the right column. The bars indicate standard deviation values.

origin are expected to remain constant and responses with a contrast origin
to vary. This was achieved by square-wave modulating only one set of checks
and keeping the other at a constant luminance level either lower, equal or
higher than that of the modulated checks (left column, Fig. 2). Since the
local luminance modulation is constant irrespective of the luminance of the
unmodulated checks, a response with a luminance origin should remain
constant too. On the other hand, a contrast response may be expected to
yield an optimum when the mean luminances of the two sets of checks are
about equal. In that condition the pattern reverses twice per period (mid
column, Fig. 2). The actual data, the second harmonic of the ERG and of the
simultaneously recorded VEP, are given in the right hand column of Fig. 2.

It can be concluded that local luminance dominates the pattern ERG whereas contrast plays a major role for the pattern EP! So the pattern ERGs in man and cat seem to behave differently. To verify this point, we replicated the Fig. 2 experiment also in cat (Ringo et al 1984). The results of two of such experiments are shown in Fig. 3.

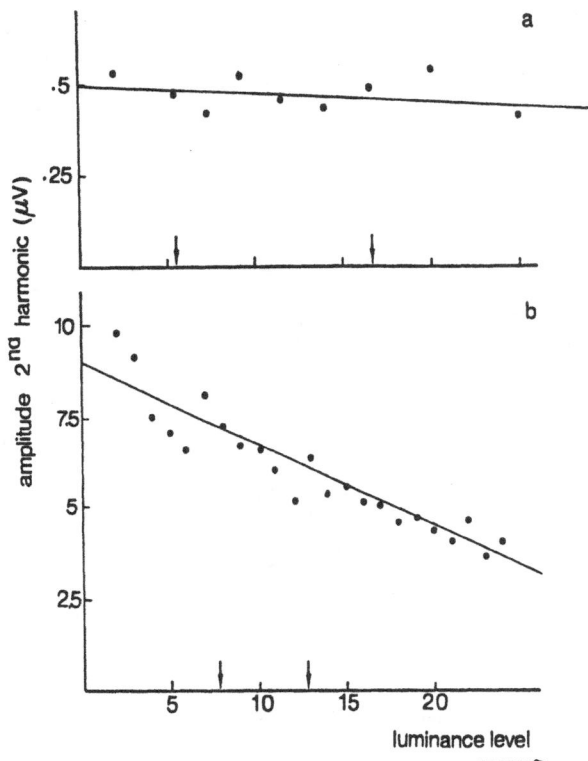

Fig. 3. Second harmonic response amplitudes as a function of the luminance level of the unmodulated set of checks. The stimulus is a 10° field surrounded by a white 10° i.d. 30° o.d. annulus. A diffuse background illuminates the entire retina. Data from 2 cats are shown. The luminance level of the unmodulated set of checks is plotted on a linear scale. 10 on this scale corresponds to 1.55×10^{10} phot.sec^{-1}.deg^{-2}. In (a) stimulation was 73% square-wave modulation, 8 Hz with 2° checks, in (b) 33% square-wave modulation, 3 Hz with 1° checks. The arrows represent the top and bottom luminance levels of the modulated set of checks. In (a) a strong background was used to suppress straylight effects. In (b) a weaker background was used. In this case strong straylight effects monotonically decrease the amplitude of the ERG for increasing luminance of the unmodulated set of checks.

The conclusion is clear: the data follow the trend determined from local luminance consideration alone. Since also in cat no maximum is found when the second harmonic pattern stimulation is maximal, any pattern driven ERG response is fully hidden in the variance of the nonlinear local luminance response.

82

No direct arguments can, however, be inferred from the data of Fig. 2
and 3 about the origin of the nonlinear luminance components. Therefore,
one of my colleagues recorded the responses to patterned and unpatterned
stimuli with a bipolar micro-electrode in the retina of an intact eye of a
macaque monkey. The responses were analysed in terms of harmonic components
(as above) and the voltage-depth profiles of these components were
assessed. The depth profiles of the second harmonic components of luminance
and pattern reversal responses were found to be the same (Riemslag and
Heynen 1984) and to resemble the b-wave depth profile (Heynen and Van
Norren 1985). So again: the recording of the pattern ERG does not provide
additional information to the classically recorded luminance ERG. Nor could
any evidence be gathered for the pattern ERG to reflect ganglion cell
activity.

THE PATTERN ERG IN GLAUCOMA

So far our search for contrast involvement and contribution of
ganglion cell activity to the pattern ERG has been negative. However, in
all our experiments healthy subjects participated, whereas the most
convincing data in literature about contrast and/or ganglion cell
involvement are from pathological conditions like the optic nerve section
in cat by Maffei and Fiorentini. Therefore, we decided to study the effect
of glaucoma on the pattern ERG (Van den Berg et al 1986). Glaucoma patients
were selected of which the two eyes also with respect to optical factors
were similar except that in the glaucomatous eye more than half of the
central 28° diameter area tested had a sensitivity loss of more than 0.6
log unit. The luminance and pattern reversal ERGs of the affected and
"healthy" fellow eyes of 5 of such strongly asymmetric glaucoma cases are
presented in Fig. 4. For neither of the 4 conditions tested the ERGs of the
two eyes differ!The same conclusion was reached for the ERGs derived from
the better and worse half fields of 7 glaucomatous eyes. In the latter
situation for certain no difference in optical quality could influence the
data.

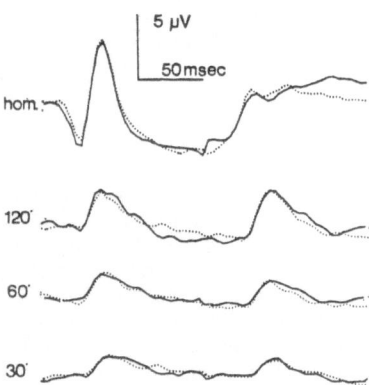

Fig. 4. Mean ERGs of 5 glaucoma subjects for luminance (top) and pattern
reversal (120', 60' and 30' checks). The continuous curves are from
the glaucomatous eyes; the dashed curves from the "healthy" fellow
eyes. The stimulus field of 28° diameter had a luminance of 200
cd/m^2. The surround was twice as bright. The two sets of checks
were 4 Hz square-wave modulated at 99% modulation depth (from Van
den Berg 1986).

CONCLUSION

Contrary to quite some number of reports in literature we were not successful in demonstrating that the ERG to pattern stimulation yields information about visual processing that cannot be obtained from the luminance ERG. The pattern ERGs can be fully described on the basis of nonlinear luminance responses, and the same retinal sources are responsible for both response types. If, however, stimulation of restricted retinal areas is wanted a pattern reversal stimulus is superior.

REFERENCES

Arden GB, Vaegan, Hogg CR. Clinical and experimental evidence that the pattern e.r.g. (P.e.r.g.) is generated in more proximal retinal layers than the focal electroretinogram (F.e.r.g.). Ann NY Acad Sci 1982;388: 580-601.

Van den Berg TJTP, De Vos GWGA, Verduyn Lunel HFE. The pattern ERG in asymmetric glaucoma interpreted as a luminance response. Doc Ophthalmol Proc Series. In press. 1986.

Dawson WW, Trick GL, Litzkow CA. Improved electrode for electroretinography. Invest Ophthalmol Vis Sci 1979;18:988-991.

Heynen H, Van Norren D. Origin of the electroretinogram in the intact macaque eye. - I. Principal component analysis. Vision Res 1985;25:697-707.

Heynen H, Van Norren D. Origin of the electroretinogram in the intact macaque eye. - II. Current source-density analysis. Vision Res 1985;25: 709-715.

Maffei L, Fiorentini A. Electroretinographic responses to alternating gratings before and after section of the optic nerve. Science 1981;211: 953-955.

Riemslag FCC, Heynen HGM. Depth profile of pattern local electroretinograms in macaque. Doc Ophthalmol Proc Series 1984;40:143-148.

Riemslag FCC, Ringo JL, Spekreijse H, Verduyn Lunel HF. The luminance origin of the pattern electroretinogram in man. J Physiol 1985;363:191-209.

Riggs LA, Johnson EP, Schick AML. Electrical responses of the human eye to moving stimulus patterns. Science 1964;144:567.

Ringo JL, Van Dijk B, Spekreijse H. Pattern ERG of the cat. Vision Res 1984;24:859-865.

Spekreijse H. Analysis of EEG responses in man, evoked by sine wave modulated light. Thesis. The Hague: Junk Publishers. 1966.

Spekreijse H, Estevez O, Van der Tweel LH. Luminance responses to pattern reversal. Doc Ophthalmol Proc Series 1973;10:205-211.

Van der Tweel, LH, Spekreijse H. Psychophysics and electrophysiology of a rod-achromat. Doc Ophthalmol 1973;2:163-173.

IDENTIFICATION OF FIRST AND SECOND ORDER VOLTERRA KERNELS FOR THE HUMAN ELECTRORETINOGRAM

Conor Minogue

Royal Victoria Eye and Ear Hospital,
Research Foundation, Dublin

INTRODUCTION

The electroretinogram (ERG) is a measurement of the massed response of the retina to stimulation by light. The ERG is most often obtained in response to an impulse-like flash of light, using a corneal surface contact electrode. This technique is deficient for a number of reasons. The Xenon flash tubes, which are widely used as stimulus sources, are very unstable in their luminous output. Usually the flash is a poor imitation of an impulse and the actual ERG recorded is dependent on the frequency content of the actual flash used. In simply recording the output of a system to an impulse one is quite defenceless against extraneous additive noise and the only recourse is in highly inefficient averaging. So multiple flashes must be presented at each flash intensity of interest with the result that the clinical procedure can become quite lenghty and uncomfortable for the patient. The state of retinal adaption is altered with each flash, (Berson et al. 1969) and further delays must be incorporated into the test procedure to maintain stationarity of retinal adaption.

The flash response ERG of itself gives no information about the nonlinear performance of the ERG mechanism. In fact, very little attention is given to nonlinear behaviour in clinical electroretinography. Nonlinear behaviour is exhibited in a number of ways, for example the b-wave amplitude of the flash ERG varies in a sigmoid fashion as a function of log stimulus intensity. The response to a pair of flashes is not simply the sum of the individual response complexes, instead the response to the second impulse is modified, depending on the interval between the flashes, which is characteristic of a nonlinear system with memory. Studies of the ERG response to sinusoidal stimulation (Troelstra & Garcia 1975), have shown signifiant second order harmonics in the response to low frequency stimuli.

The potential importance of nonlinear assessment can be seen from the results of Levy (Levy 1978), who showed that the response of a normal subject to a pair of flashes separated by 70 ms is such that the response to the second flash is suppressed. However this inhibition effect was shown to vanish early in the developement of certain inherited retinal degenerations, long before there was any subjective visual loss or other clinical signs.

Since the ERG is the bulk response of millions of current generators distributed across the retina, a reduced or altered component of the flash ERG could be the result of some of these current generators malfunctioning, or all of them malfunctioning to a lesser degree, or indeed the structures across which the ERG voltage is developed, having themselves broken down. It is hypothesized that since an assessment of nonlinear performance might reflect more closely the contribution of individual cell types, and the interactions between them, that these conditions might be better differentiated. Single flash full field electroretinography can provide little information about horizontal processes within the retina, since the ERG is a measurement of nett radial current flow. Since nonlinear effects in the ERG are quite likely due in part to mechanisms of excitation and inhibition in the horizontal direction within the retina, it is felt that nonlinear systems analysis techniques could ultimately provide useful information about this level of retinal function. It can be argued that since the ERG process is of such vast complexity that any model derived from such an approach would be of little value. However the flash ERG is itself a macroscopic measurement on this same complex system yet it has been possible over the years to identify components of the flash ERG with the response profiles of individual cell types recorded at the microscopic level. It is reasonable to expect that a similar correlation exercise would prove equally fruitful with respect to nonlinear function.

It has been the object of this work to provide a simple procedure to allow the assessment of nonlinear function in the ERG mechanism and to provide a graphical means to represent this information.

THEORETICAL BACKGROUND

The relationship between the the system output y(t) and the system input x(t) for a wide class of nonlinear systems can be expressed in terms of the Volterra functional series.

$$y(t) = \int_{-\infty}^{\infty} h_1(\tau_1) x(t-\tau_1) d\tau_1 + \iint_{-\infty}^{\infty} h_2(\tau_1,\tau_2) x(t-\tau_1) x(t-\tau_2) d\tau_1 d\tau_2 \\ + \iint \cdots \int h_n(\tau_1,\tau_2 \ldots \tau_n) \prod_{m=1}^{n} x(t-\tau_m) d\tau_m \tag{1}$$

where $h(\tau_1,\tau_2, \ldots, \tau_n)$ is the nth order Volterra kernel. In this application it is assumed that the series can be truncated after n=2, an assumption which is based on the results of Troelstra and Garcia who, in their work with sinusoidal stimulii could find no significant harmonics higher than the second. Eq (1) therefore reduces to

$$y(t) = \int_{-\infty}^{\infty} h_1(\tau_1) x(t-\tau_2) d\tau + \iint_{-\infty}^{\infty} h_2(\tau_1,\tau_2) x(t-\tau_1) x(t-\tau_2) d\tau_1 d\tau_2 \tag{2}$$

The first term corresponds to the familiar convolution integral of linear systems theory, wherein the output y(t) at any instant is expessed in terms of the immediate history of the input, with the contribution of the input at each instant τ into that history weighted according to the impulse response function $h_1(\tau)$. To this is added the second order term which expresses the dependence of y(t) at any instant on the values of the input τ_1 and τ_2 seconds into the history of the input.

An isolated nth order kernel can be measured directly by evaluating the nth order cross correlation function between input and output, if the input is derived from a Gaussian white noise source. For an isolated first order kernel, or more generally, for a system containing no nonzero kernels of odd order higher than the second then $h_1(t)$ can be measured as follows,

$$h_1(\tau) = 1/A \; \overline{y(t)x(t-\tau)} \tag{3}$$

provided the first order autocorrelation function (ACF) of the test signal is given by

$$R_{2x}(\tau) = \overline{x(t)x(t-\tau)} = A\delta(t) \tag{4}$$

where, A is the power level of the noise proces and $\delta(t)$ is the Dirac delta function.

For an isolated second order kernel, or more generally, for a system containing no nonzero kernels of even order higher than the second, $h_2(\tau_1,\tau_2)$ can be measured as follows,

$$h_2(\tau_1,\tau_2) = 1/2A^2 \; \overline{y(t)x(t-\tau_1)x(t-\tau_2)} \tag{5}$$

provided the fourth order autocorrelation function of the test signal is given by,

$$R_{4x}(\tau_1,\tau_2) = 2A^2 [\delta(t-\tau_1)\delta(t-\tau_2)] \quad , \; \tau_1 \neq \tau_2 \tag{6}$$

Some difficulties arise in the direct application of the white noise method, particularly in this application. In practice white noise is difficult to handle in the laboratory. The inevitable band-limiting means that special spectrum shaping measures must be adopted to restore the approximate Gaussian statistics, and the input output record needs to be excessively long, an unacceptable limitation in retinal electrophysiology. The method has been applied to the ERG, (Koblasz et al. 1980), using an input output record of two minutes. The method has also been applied extensively to retinal electrophysiology at the microscopic level, (Marmareliz P.Z. and Naka K.I. 1972, 1973a 1973b 1973c).

Test signals based on pseudo
random sequences suggest themselves as an attractive
alternative in that they are simple to generate and process,
yet have in principle less of the redundancy associated with
true white noise. Early attempts to apply ternary level
signals to the identification of nonlinear systems, (Hooper
and Gyftopoulos 1969), met with difficulty since the fourth
order ACF of such signals just did not have the ideal form
of eq.2. Instead there were several additional spikes
distributed across the delay space of the ACF, with the
result that the kernel estimates were corrupted by
contributions from parts of the kernel other than those
targetted for in the simple cross correlatiom measurement.
Since then, these autocorrelation difficulties have been
explained as being due to the existence of linear
deterministic relationships between elements of the pseudo
random sequences. (Barker and Pradhistayon 1970).
Eventually these very deterministic properties were
ingeniously exploited to provide a highly efficient method
for estimating the kernels of certain second order Volterra
kernels. (Barker and Davy 1978). The system described here
was designed on the basis of this latter proposal.

The Method of Barker and Davy.
The test signal in this case
is a pseudo random ternary signal with values -a, 0, +a,
clock interval T and period $(3^n-1)T$, where n is the order of
the generating polynomial of the pseudo random sequence. The
input and output are synchronously sampled to give input and
ouput sequences x_i, y_i, respectively. From this
input-output record, second order cross correlation
measurements e $(IT,<I+J>T)$ can be obtained as follows,

$$e_2(IT,<I+J>T)= 1/(8 \times 3^{n-2} \ T^2 a^4) \sum_{i=0}^{P-1} y_i \ x_{i-I} \ x_{i-I-J} \quad (7)$$
$$\text{where } P=3^n-1.$$

By taking a set of measurements with I=0, 1, 2,..etc. for
J=1, 2, 3,...etc., cross-correlation measurements are
obtained along the diagonal of the τ_1, τ_2 plane and along lines
parallel to it. It can be shown that each of the diagonal
measurements, i.e. those with J=0, in the range 0 to
(P-1)/2, can be expressed in terms of sets of kernel values
$h_2(IT,<I+J>T)$, contributing to them. Furthermore, with
certain restrictions on the domain of the kernel for a given
pseudo random sequence, these expressions can be inverted to
give all the off-diagonal kernel values simply in terms of
diagonal cross correlation measurements. In this way the
kernel estimates can be obtained by a shift-and-add
procedure on the input output record, thus relieving the
computational burden associated with conventional
correlation methods.

The method provides for the unbiased estimation of kernel values over an area of $R_m x R_m$ in the τ_1, τ_2 plane, where R_m is an index of performance for the particular pseudo random sequence used. For example the order 6 sequence, with generating polynomial $f(D)=1+D^2-D^3+D^5$ $-D^6$, has a period P = 728, with R_m= 21. The results of Koblasz et al., on the closely related Wiener kernels, indicated that the second order kernel could be considered zero outside an area of 140 x 140 ms. and within that area to have no high frequency components such that a sampling array of 21 x 21, with a unit delay of 7 ms could not adequately describe the kernel. Thus the minimum identification time in this case is 728 x 7ms.= 5.1 seconds.

IMPLEMENTATION

The system was designed around a Research Machines 380Z microcomputer having 56k RAM, twin mini-floppy disk drives with CP/M. The stimulus unit is constructed from six light bar modules (Hewlett Packard HLMP 2550) each of which comprises four high efficiency green light emitting diodes embedded in a diffusing medium, providing an approximate Lambertian radiation pattern. These devices have a peak radiation wavelength of 572 nm with a dominant wavelength of 565 nm. The diodes are multiplexed in four rows of six, refresh rate per diode 25 khz, with pulse width modulation being used to contol luminous output. The ERG signals are recovered from both eyes using gold foil corneal contact electrodes and after filtering, are multiplexed into a fast edge enabled sample and hold device and an eight bit successive approximation analogue to digital converter. Only one eye is stimulated at a time, the signal from the other being used, after severe low pass filtering, to compensate for eye movement by subtracting it from the response of the stimulated eye. This technique has proved useful with subjects who find it hard to fixate and also performs well against blink artefacts. Sampling is performed at the same rate as the stimulus sequence clock, with the sampling instant set to the midpoint of the clock cycle. The stimulus sequence can be repeated, and the ERG summed in a 16-bit wide averaging store, if required. The input output record is then passed to the cross correlation program which computes the first order cross correlation and appropriate diagonal second order cross correlation values. This process takes about two minutes for an order six sequence. The diagonal measurements are then operated on by the sets of matrices appropriate to the sequence used and finally kernel estimates are plotted on the computer display.

PROCEDURE

The subject is allowed to dark adapt for thirty minutes, mydriatic drops having being applied to block pupillary reaction. A drop of topical anaesthetic is applied to each eye and the electrodes inserted. The LED array, mounted inside a pair of goggles approximately 2 cm from the cornea is set to a luminance of 10 cd/m² and the subject is allowed to adapt to this for five minutes. The stimulus/acquisition program is activated and the LED array is modulated according to an order 6 pseudo random ternary sequence, with a clock rate of 140 hz, depth of modulation 85% and mean luminance 10 cd/m². The recovered ERG is bandpass filtered with corner frequencies 0.1 and 40 hz and mid range gain of 2.5×10^5. The mean luminance is changed to 100 cd/m² and the subject is allowed to adapt to this level for five minutes wherupon the stimulus sequence is repeated.

PRELIMINARY RESULTS

Tests were performed on ten subjects, three of whom were patients referred to the Eye and Ear Hospital Research Foundation clinic. These latter three were all members of the same family, one of whom had been diagnosed as Retinitis Pigmentosa. Typical first order Volterra kernels for the two mean stimulus levels are shown in fig 1.

(a)

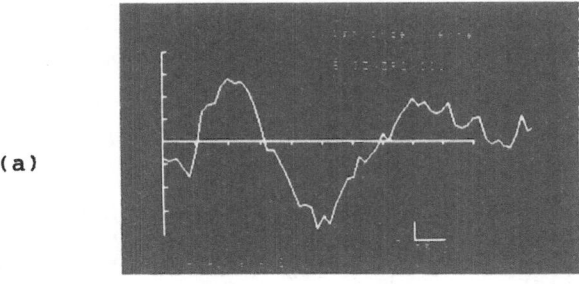

(b)

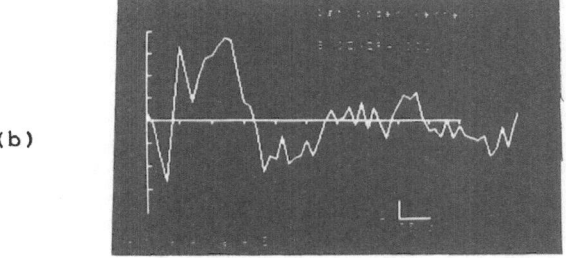

Fig. 1.   First order Volterra kernels for a normal subject with mean stimulus level of (a) 10 cd/m², and (b) 100 cd/m². Amplitude units arbitrary.

The first order kernel for the low mean luminance level closely resembles a flash ERG, having a negative going a-wave followed by a positive going b-wave and a later positive component analogous to the c-wave. The a and b-wave latentcies are respectively 30 and 70 milliseconds. With the higher mean luminance stimulus the b-wave splits into two distinct components, presumably due to the faster cone contribution at this mean level. Similar splitting of the b-wave peak is seen in flash response electroretinography, but the separation is not as distinct as has been seen here. It is worth noting that the relative amplitudes of the kernels at each luminance level are approximately the same indicating a lower system gain at higher adaption levels. The corresponding second order kernels are shown in fig 2.

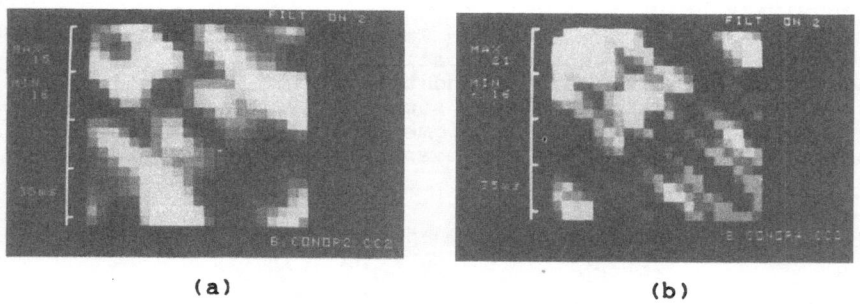

(a)   (b)

Fig. 2. Second order Volterra kernels for a normal subject at (a) 10 cd/m^2 and (b) 100 cd/m^2.

In general the kernels, viewed in this way, have ridges and valleys running paralell to the $\tau_1 = \tau_2$ diagonal. In terms of the two dimensional impulse response we would interpret a 'valley' beginning at τ seconds as representing nonlinear suppression between two impulse presented with a separating interval of τ seconds. Fig 3 shows a low mean luminance kernel with a profile drawn for the diagonal beginning at τ = 56 ms.

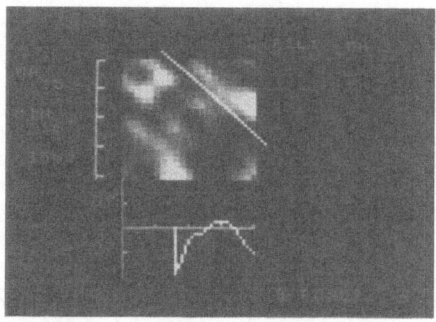

Fig 3. Profile through the kernel of Fig 2(a) at τ =56 ms.

We would interpret this as meaning that if two impulses were presented with a separating interval of 56 ms, that the response to the second one would be modified the the addition of this component of the second order kernel. In mathematical terms such an input is represented by,

$$x(t) = \delta(t) + \delta(t-\tau) \qquad (8)$$

The response to such an input for a generalised second order system is

$$y(t) = h_1(t) + h_1(t-\tau) + h_2(t, t-\tau) \qquad (9)$$

Since $h_1(\tau_1)$ and $h(\tau_1, \tau_2)$ are zero for all $\tau_1, \tau_2, < 0$, then as t increases from zero we get, first of all, the contribution of $h_1(t)$ alone. Then as t reaches τ the contributions of the second and third terms in eq. 9 come into play. If, as is the case in fig. 3, the second order kernel is negative along such a diagonal then the h_1 response will be opposed by the h_2 response. Similarly a ridge running diagonally would mean that the second order kernel contribution would add constructively to the first order component.

                Fig. 4 shows the first and second order kernels, at low mean luminance level, of a young man with Retinitis Pigmentosa. His flash response ERG was grossly diminished and his vision was very poor. The first order kernel is virtually zero, however the second order kernel retains much of the characteristic diagonal structure, except along the diagonal which is strikingly different. Fig. 5 shows profiles drawn through this and the 'normal'kernel. It would appear therefore, that while the linear component of his response has been diminished, that the second order component is intact. A single flash ERG analysis could give a zero response if the h (t) response was opposed by the diagonal h (t,t) component. The interesting possibility is raised whereby a zero response is obtained in a single flash experiment whereas a nonzero response occurs at the second of a pair of flashes. It could be speculatd that since this type of nonlinearity with memory is related in part to horizontal activity within the retinal layers, that the transmission of signals radially within the retina has been selectively affected by this disease.

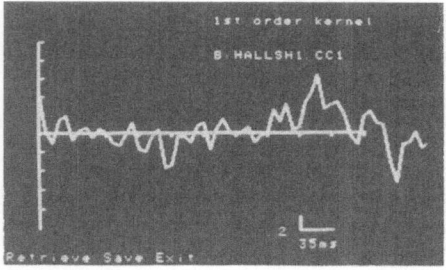 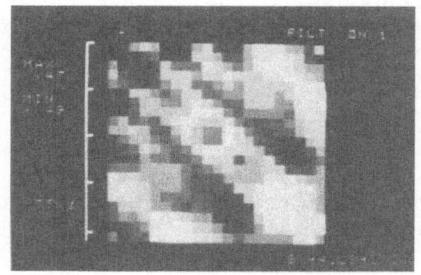

Fig. 4   First and second order kernels at the 10 cd/m   level
for patient S.H.

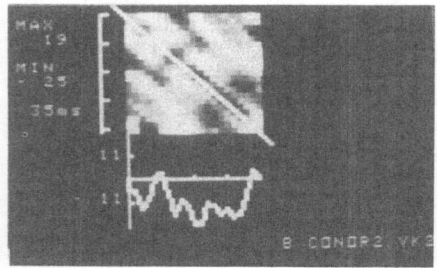 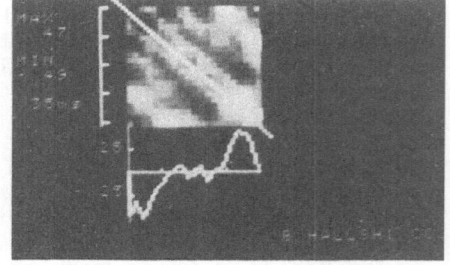

Fig. 5   Profiles drawn through diagonal of the second order
         kernel for (a), a normal subject and (b), patient
         S.H.

                              Figs. 7 and 8 show the
results of the nonlinear analysis for his brother who is two
years younger. His flash ERG studies were normal and he had
no subjective loss of vision or other clinical signs of
retinal disease. Tests were also performed on their younger
sister however she was quite agitated and it was impossible
to obtain a blink free recording, indicating that the
procedure as presently constituted requires a measure of
co-operation which could not be expected of all patients.

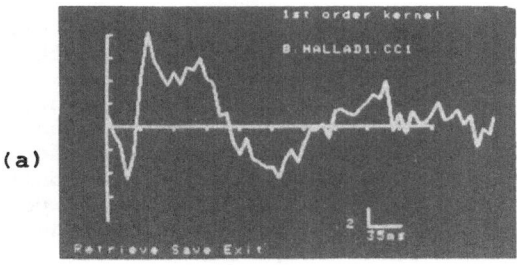

(a)

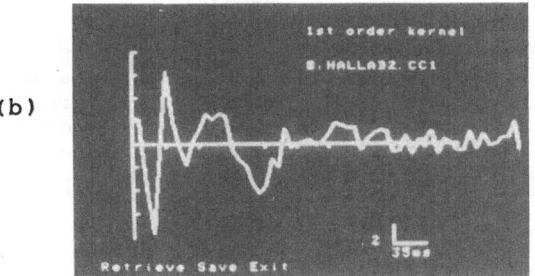

(b)

Fig.7   First order kernels for patient A.H.

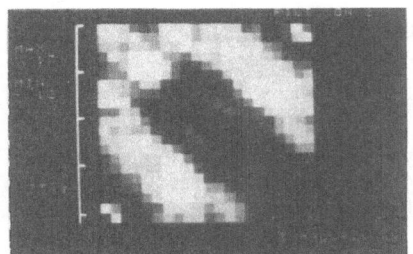
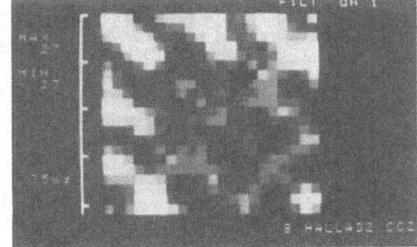

Fig.8   Second order kernels for patient A.H

CONCLUSIONS

The technique of input-output cross correlation has been used to obtain estimates of the first and second order Volterra kernels of the human ERG, with the stimulus derived from a pseudo random ternary sequence. The superior noise reduction offered by the cross correlation process is of significant advantage in the noisy envirinement of ERG recording, where speed of data acquisition is of such importance. By exploiting the deterministic properties of the pseudo random sequence used as the basis for the luminous stimulus, the second order kernel estimates can be made from a set of first order correlation measurements alone. The correlation process reduces to a shift and add algorithm on the input output record and can therefore be readily implemented within the instruction set of a standard 8 bit microprocessor.

The first order Volterra kernel has been found to closely resemble in form the conventional flash ERG. The actual response to an ideal impulse can be calculated from the first order kernel and the diagonal of the second order kernel. The second order kernel can be interpreted in terms of the interaction between paired flashes and therefore describes a nonlinear memory effect within the ERG mechanism. It is not possible, at present, to interpret the form of the second order kernel in terms of known retinal electrophysiology and as such the model provided by this type of signal analysis can only be of empirical value. Nevertheless, some interesting questions are raised even from the results of this preliminary study. It can be shown that it is mathematically possible for a system represented as a generalised second order nonlinear system to have a zero response to a single impulse, and yet have a nonzero response to the second of a pair of impulses, however it is not immediately apparent how this effect could occur in the case of the ERG system, as has been found here.

REFERENCES

[1]   E.L. Berson, P. Gouras and M. Hoff, (1969), "Temporal effects of the ERG." Arch. Opth. Vol. 1, No. 6, pp. 784-786, Dec 1969.

[2]   N. Troelstra and C.A. Garcia. (1975), "The electrical response of the human eye to sinusoidal light stimulation.", IEEE trans. Vol. BME-22, No.5, Sept. 1975

[3]   N. Levy. (1978), "Early diagnosis and evolution of dominant retinitis pigmentosa.", Am. J. Opth. Vol.86 pp 552-556. Oct. 1978

[4]   A. Koblasz, J.L. Rae and J.C. Manning. (1980), "Wiener kernels and frequency respose functions for the human retina.", IEEE trans. Vol. BME-27 No. 2, pp 68-75, Feb. 1980

[5]   P.Z. Marmarelis and K.I. Naka, (1972), "White noise analysis of a neuron chain. An application of the Wiener theory", Science, Vol. 175, pp 1276-8.

[6]   P.Z. Marmareliz and K.I. Naka (1973a, b, c), "Nonlinear analysis and synthesis of receptive field responses in the catfish retina, Parts I, II, and III", J. Neurophysiol., Vol. 36, pp 605-548.

[7]   H.A. Barker and T. Pradisthayon, (1970), "Higher order autocorrelation functions of pseudorandom signals based on m-sequences.", Proc. IEE, Vol. 117, No. 9, Sept. 1970

[8]   H.A. Barker and R.W. Davy. (1978), "Measurement
          of second order Volterra kernels usong pseudo
          random test signals.", Int. J. Control, Vol. 27,
          No. 2 pp 277-291, Feb. 1978.

DISCUSSION

Campos: I want to make a point concerning Spekreijse's paper. I have no way of judging whether the pattern ERG is an expression of genuine contrast sensitivity. I have results from patients in which there was a discrepancy between the pattern ERG and the flash ERG. Typically, patients with optic nerve injury who have not yet developed optic atrophy show pattern ERG changes, but no flash ERG changes. I have also seen a severely glaucomatous patient who did show the same discrepancy, and I have seen this discrepancy in severely amblyopic patients with a visual acuity of less than 0.2.

Spekreijse: In all those the pattern ERG was changing in which direction, moving down?

Campos: Yes, moving down.

Spekreijse: My problem is that nothing is changing in the retina but stray light becomes more and more important. The response will go down. The pattern ERG is rather dangerous because you really need control to be certain that in two situations comparing responses the subject really fixated and accommodated in exactly the same way. My patient was given a cycloplegic and corrected optically before the tests.

Fiorentini: Under certain conditions you can influence the ERG response to a pattern, while the response to diffuse light remains unchanged. This cannot be an artefact. Certainly this is true in the animal situation. With some kinds of stimuli, for instance with very large checks of high contrast, the local luminance response in a sense prevails on the response to contrast modulation. This is one possibility, but I don't think it is the only one.

Spekreijse: It was one of the weaknesses of our initial experiments and was the reason for the new interpretation. We decided to review the problem and use stimulus conditions at their optimum level for hitting the contract mechanism. We were able to show that there was a very good correlation between the distortion in the ERG and the pattern ERG. There is no need to choose a separate mechanism.

Fiorentini: We never used a 90% contrast. We used a much lower contrast, thus reducing the effects of stray light. I think that as far as the clinical application is concerned, the main point is that you can differentiate the two responses. Thus the pattern ERG is a diagnostic tool. I agree that the problem of the origin of the two responses is still open.

Arden: The techniques that we have used to avoid stray light artefacts are to use very large checks, which we believe produce luminance responses, and rather smaller ones than the 60' size which you use. What we and others have found is that the response to the smaller checks is actually larger than that to the big ones, so that there is a bell-shaped curve, as there is for example with other visual functions which depend upon the size of the units in the retina which produce the response. I think Spekreijse's demonstration that there is a luminance-generated response is absolutely undeniable, but I don't see why we would get this differentiation, this large increased amplitutude response to smaller checks, unless the generating units had receptive fields. This increase is the thing that vanishes in retinal disease. This is in exactly the wrong sense for changes due to scattered light or changes due to abnormalities in refraction, but this occurs in cases as different as diabetic retinopathy, amblyopia or maculopathy. We see that the response to the large checks stays high but the augmented response to the smaller checks declines, and I agree with Fiorentini that this is extremely useful clinically. It would even be useful without this because the pattern reversal stimulus enables one to know what part of the retina the response is coming from and for us that is very important.

Spekreijse: I agree with you that this is important for localising ERG recordings to certain areas of the retina but not the suggestion that it is also hitting a completely different mechanism. One of the arguments for this is the bell-shaped curve that you have used, and even if you start to think about stray light to explain it, this brings about the two neighbouring bars again, both are moving up and down. So it is a homogenous field and this bar will affect stray light and this one will reduce the effect of modulation of this stimulus and will be less than the affected modulation of this stimulus because when this is fairly bright this is fairly dim. There is a little line leading from here to there and so the net modulation is larger. So the response will come from a homogenous field through large checks to the smaller checks because the stray light drops off too as a function of distance and therefore the latitude that lies first goes up first to the smaller checks and then of course has to drop again because there you get other kinds of things.

Van Lith: I would like to ask Spekreijse - I have heard him often and today I listened very carefully in the discussion to what he said and he said there was no necessity to assume another mechanism. I would like to ask him whether clinically we have completely the same results as other clinicians in that the pattern ERG is disturbed in glaucoma patients. This is completely different from the Amsterdam results. I would like to ask you how sure are your experiments in excluding the contrast component? You said that it was not necessary to be sure but can you exclude it?

Spekreijse: You never can prove something is not there, but the best you can say is if it is there it is of the same order as the variablity.

van Hof-van Duin: I was under the impression that Fiorentini used pattern ERGs in order to get thresholds for acuity whether it is in monkeys or in humans. If there is no difference between flash ERG and pattern ERG how is it possible that apparently the amplitude of the pattern ERG decreases when the size of the gratings becomes smaller and smaller.

Arden: The point is that there is no effective change in retinal luminance when the bars become small, but I think this does not mean that what one is seeing is the same thing as contrast sensitivity which depends on something quite different.

van Hof-van Duin: But it isn't true, Fiorentini, that if one keeps the contrast constant and uses smaller and smaller gratings, one can obtain an acuity value for the pattern ERG.

Fiorentini: It is certain that the amplitude of the ERG decreases when the spatial frequency of the grating increases above certain values in man and monkey and it is possible to evaluate an ERG acuity, as the highest spatial frequency at which an ERG can be recorded.

Apkarian: My question is a matter of whether or not you are looking at different mechanisms. Can you find comparable changes between the pattern and flash ERG when looking at different aspects of the flash response, for example, the second harmonic? Will this higher harmonic luminance response be more closely related to the changes found in the pattern ERG? That is, the fundamental response of the uniform field ERG may be normal but the second harmonic may, for example, attenuate in a fashion similar to the pattern evoked response, also a second harmonic measure.

Spekreijse: We believe that there are different mechanisms and we know that contrast is correlated at threshold levels to our contrast sensitivity curve so that you can use it as a substitute. Then have a look at the functional fields and for the ERG again in the luminance condition and the contrast condition you can compare in the same way.

PATTERN VEPs IN VERY YOUNG INFANTS

Vittorio Porciatti

Divisione Oculistica USL 13 57100 Livorno Italy

INTRODUCTION

Studies of the development of spatial vision by means of pattern-visually evoked potentials (VEPs) have dealt mainly with the development of acuity and contrast sensitivity (see Dobson & Teller 1978, Banks & Salapatek 1981, Atkinson 1984 for review). These studies have shown that both acuity and contrast sensitivity improve rapidly during the first six months and then more slowly, approaching adult levels at about one year of age. However, the rate of development seems slower in the early post-natal period (Atkinson et al 1979, Porciatti et al 1982, Porciatti 1984).

Relatively few studies have been devoted to the temporal properties of the pattern VEPs in infants (Sokol & Jones 1979, Moskowitz & Sokol 1980, 1983) and newborns (Porciatti et al 1982, Porciatti 1984). The present study attempts to elucidate some characteristics of the VEP amplitude and latency (temporal phase) in response to a phase-alternated checkerboard of various temporal and spatial frequencies in newborns. In addition, the changes of such properties during the first two months of age were followed to evaluate their potential clinical use as an index of neurological development.

METHODS

Twenty-eight normal term-infants of both sexes were examined: their chronological age ranged between 3 and 50 days. In particular 12 infants were 3 days old and for two of them we had the opportunity to carry out a longitudinal study. The other 16 infants were of different ages under 2 months. The visual stimulus consisted of a checkerboard pattern electronically generated on a TV screen in which the dark and light elements spatially alternated at constant mean luminance. The alternation frequency ranged from 1 rev/s to 16.6 rev/s. The angular dimensions of the single checks ranged from 15 to 240 min. The mean luminance was 72 cd/sqm, the contrast was about 84% and the field was circular with a diameter of 29 cm. The subjects fixated its centre binocularly from 45 cm distance. The cortical responses were conventionally recorded from the scalp by using a midline electrode placement Oz-Cz (2 cm anterior to the inion-vertex). The ground electrode was placed on the forehead. The signal was amplified with a frequency band-pass of 1.5-33 Hz (-3 dB/oct) and stored on a magnetic tape. The signal processing was done off-line by averaging and Fourier analysis of the averaged waveform.

All infants were examined with the following procedure: 30 min. before the feeding time the electrodes were located in place. The subjects were then held in a seated position on the lap of a nurse with their head reclined on the nurse's breast. The room was the darkened, the only source of light available being that of the photostimulator. After the infants were prepared we waited until them woke up naturally, which generally occurred after a few minutes. When they were awake and behaviourally alert the infants gazed at the stimulator intermittently, for a time varying usually between 5 and 15 min.. During this period an observer, watching the infants from behind the stimulator, controlled the trigger signal, and switched it off whenever they did not gaze at the center of the screen.

RESULTS AND DISCUSSION

Representative VEP responses of one 3 day-old infant and one adult at different reversal rates are shown in fig. 1A and B. At low reversal rates, both the neonatal and adult responses show a major positive wave which appears with a peak latency of about 265 msec and 110 msec respectively. At increasing temporal frequencies, the responses show a sinusoide-like waveform. Further increases in alternation rate cause a progressive reduction in the response amplitude. Figure 1D shows the amplitude of the fundamental harmonic of the responses as a function of the reversal rate. Both the neonatal and the adult VEPs show a temporal tuning. In the neonate the maximal amplitude occurs at lower frequencies (around 4 rev/s) than in the adult (around 8 rev/sec). Moreover, the amplitude fall-off in the high range of frequencies is steeper in the newborn than in the adult. Figure 1C shows the phase shift of the fundamental harmonic of the responses as a function of the reversal rate. The phase shift increases approximately linearly over the range of temporal frequencies both in the neonate and in the adult. Therefore, the VEP latency independent of temporal frequency can be evaluated from the slope of the phase vs frequency function (apparent latency). The slope of the function gives in the adult an apparent latency of about 110 msec, which is similar to the peak latency of the transient response. A close correspondence between the peak latency of the transient-reversal response and the apparent latency evaluated by the phase plot of the steady-state reversal response has been previously reported for normal adults (Porciatti & von Berger 1981, Riemslag et al 1982). The slope of the phase characteristic is in the neonate much steeper than in the adult and its apparent latency is around 265 msec. This value is of the same order as the peak latency of the transient response. Comparable results were obtained in three other infants of the same age.

Thus, the difference in peak latency between the neonatal and adult transient responses seems to represent a real difference in response latency. Therefore, shifts in peak latency of the major positive deflection of transient responses could be considered indicative of age-related changes of the visual system. This view is supported by the finding that this component is consistently present at all ages (Sokol & Jones 1979, Moskowitz & Sokol 1980, 1983, Porciatti et al 1982, Porciatti 1984) and its peak latency shifts smoothly from neonatal to adult values.

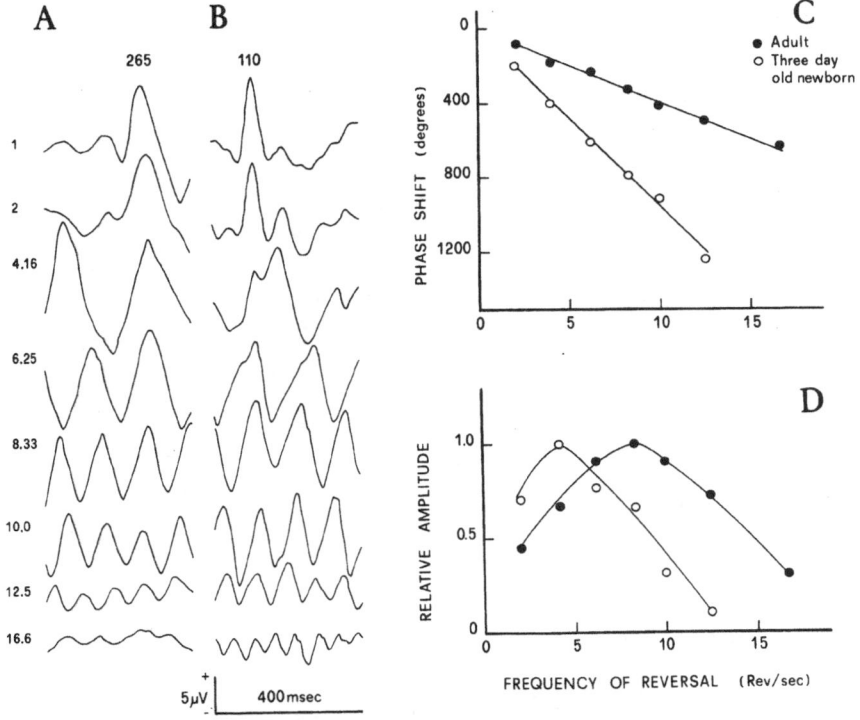

Fig. 1. Representative VEP responses of a 3 day-old infant (A) and an adult (B) to a checkerboard (60 min. checks, 84% contrast, 36 deg. field) presented with different reversal rates. Phase shift (C) and relative amplitude (D) of the fundamental harmonic of the responses as a function of the reversal rate (open circles: neonate; filled circles: adult). (from Porciatti 1984)

All the above-reported differences in the temporal parameters between the neonatal and adult responses might be used in the evaluation of the infants' developmental changes. However, the brief period of alertness of very young infants precluded in most cases the determination of amplitude and phase characteristics over a full range of temporal frequencies. Therefore, only the peak latencies of transient-reversal VEPs could be studied systematically.

In infants 3- to 50 days of age, transient VEPs to large checks (60 min.) have been recorded. As shown in fig. 2, the peak latency as a function of post-menstrual age decreases rapidly from about 266 msec at 40-41 weeks (mean value: S.D.=7) to about 221 msec at 47-48 weeks (mean value: S.D.=7). The longitudinal recordings of the two different infants

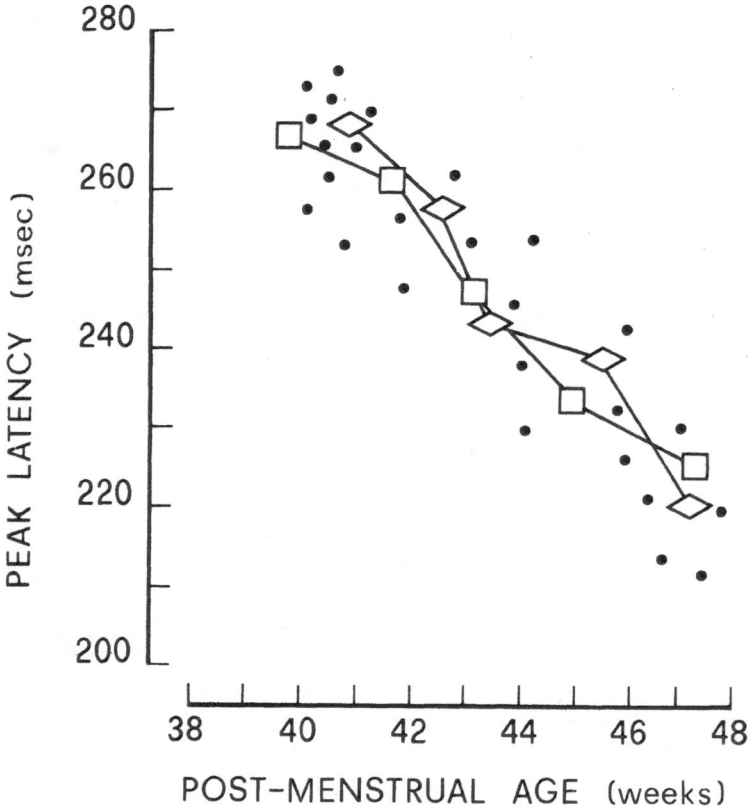

Fig. 2. Peak latencies of transient reversal VEPs (60 min. checks, 84% contrast, 36 deg. field, 1 rev/s) as a function of post-menstrual age. The filled circles represent single infants. The open symbols joined by lines represent two different infants tested at various ages. (from Porciatti 1984)

show latency variations of the same order. The recorded latencies of the older infants agree well with previous measurements obtained in infants of the same age under similar experimental conditions (Sokol & Jones 1979, Moskowitz & Sokol 1980, 1983).

Figure 3 shows the amplitude of the fundamental harmonic of the neonatal VEPs to an optimal reversal rate of 4.1 rev/s as a function of check size. Data were obtained from two different neonates. It can be noticed that in both subjects the VEP amplitude is maximal for checks ranging from 240 min. to 60 min.. At 30-min. checks there is a sharp drop in amplitude, and at 15-min. checks responses are at noise level. The VEPs recorded from the same infants at 1 month of age still show the same behaviour as a function of check size.

Thus, the actual threshold (VEP acuity) of neonates and 1 month-old

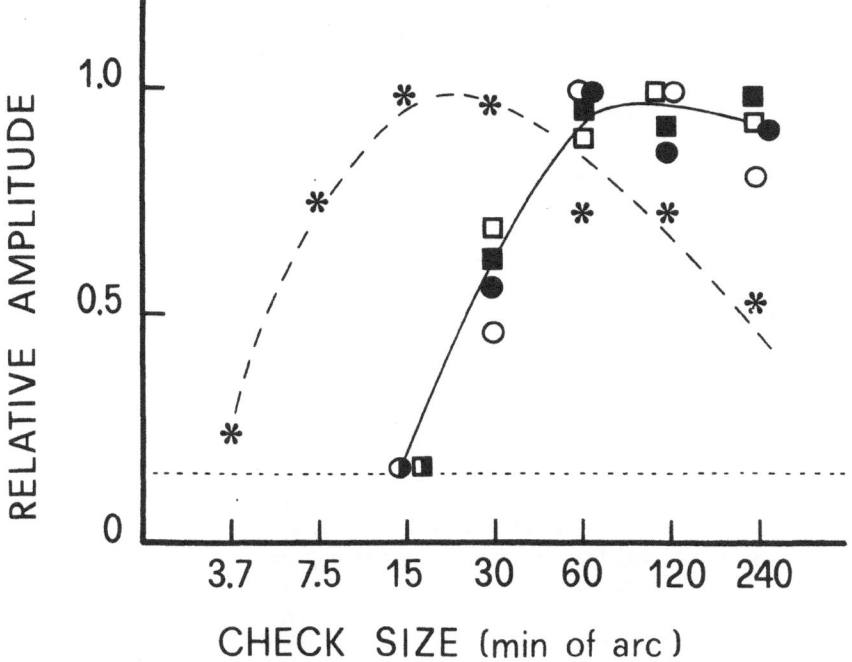

Fig. 3. Relative amplitude of the VEP response (fundamental harmonic) as a function of check size (84% contrast, 36 deg. field, 4.16 rev/s). The open circles and squares represent two different 3 day-old infants. The filled circles and squares represent the same infants at 1 month of age. Asterisks: normal adult. Dashed line: noise level. (from Porciatti 1984)

infants lies at a point between 30 min. and 15 min.. This value of acuity is in the range of previously reported VEP acuities in infants of the same age (Marg et al 1976, Atkinson et al 1979, Sokol & Jones 1979, Baraldi et al 1891, Porciatti et al 1982, Porciatti 1984). The present results suggest that a possible improvement of VEP acuity during the first month would be limited to within one octave range.

Figure 3 shows in addition that, under comparable experimental conditions, the adult VEP is spatially tuned, with a clear peak at around 15–30 min. checks.

CONCLUSIONS

Detecting developmental or sensory ipmairment by means of objective criteria is particularly important in the early post-natal period. In this limited age range the parameters which show the highest rate of maturation should have the best potential for clinical use.

The present study shows that several parameters of the pattern-reversal VEPs differ considerably between young infants and adults. In comparison with the adult the neonatal spatial tuning function is shifted towards lower spatial frequencies and does not show an optimal check size. This function does not seem to change appreciably during the first month. In addition, the temporal tuning function in the neonate is shifted towards lower temporal frequencies in comparison with the adult. However, previous measurements obtained under very similar experimental conditions (Moskowitz & Sokol 1980) show that the temporal tuning functions of 2-month-old infants are comparable to those we found in newborns. Therefore, it seems reasonable to suppose that the temporal tuning does not vary substantially over the first 2 months of life.

The neonatal pattern-reversal VEP in comparison with the adult is much delayed. The peak latency of the major positive component shortens rapidly during the first two months with a slope of around 1 msec/day. Previous studies in which comparable experimental conditions have been used (Sokol & Jones 1979, Moskowitz & Sokol 1983) show that the peak latency decreases rapidly beyond two months approaching adult levels by 4-5 months. It is well established that sharp age-related changes in the peak latencies of VEP responses to flashes- or patterned flashes of light also occur in the first months of life (e.g. Barnet et al 1980, Blom et al 1980). However, these responses vary greatly in amplitude and latency both within and between subjects and therefore they seem unsuitable for making judgements about individual infants. Moreover the neonatal waveform is different from the adult one and hence a direct comparison between the two responses is not possible.

On the contrary, the major positive component of the transient-reversal response to 1 deg. checks is consistently present at all ages and show a low inter-subject variability in its peak latency. This last parameter, therefore, might have a useful clinical application as index of neural development in the early post-natal period when threshold measurements are not easily obtained.

It should be noted, however, that the reported data refer to a homogeneous group of normal-term-subjects. Preliminary observations (Porciatti et al unpublished) indicate that there is a negative correlation between body weight and latency in the early post-natal period.

SUMMARY

Pattern-reversal VEPs to a checkerboard presented with different reversal rates and check sizes have been recorded in infants 3- to 50 days old. It has been found that the neonatal temporal and spatial tuning functions, as compared with the adul ones, are considerably shifted towards lower temporal and spatial frequencies respectively. These functions do not seem to show marked changes in the early post-natal period. The neonatal response latency, in comparison with the adult, is delayed about 150 msec. The VEP latency shortens dramatically during the first two months with a low inter-subject variability. These findings suggest a possible clinical use of the pattern-reversal VEP latency as an index of neural development in the early post-natal period.

REFERENCES

Atkinson J. Human visual development over the first 6 months of life. A review and a hypothesis. Human Neurobiol 1984;3:61-74.

Atkinson J, Braddick O, French J. Contrast sensitivity of the human neonate measured by the visual evoked potential. Invest Ophthalmol 1979; 18:210-213.

Banks MS, Salapatek P. Infant pattern vision: a new approach based on the contrast sensitivity function. J Exp Child Psychol 1981;31:1-45.

Baraldi P, Ferrari F, Fonda S, Penne A. Vision in the neonate (full term and premature): preliminary results of the application of some testing methods. Doc Ophthalmol 1981;51:101-112.

Barnet AB, Friedman SL, Weiss IP, Ohlrich ES, Shanks B, Lodge A. VEP development in infancy and early childhood. A longitudinal study. Electroenceph Clin Neurophysiol 1980;49:476-489.

Blom JL, Barth PG, Visser SL. The visual evoked potential in the first six years of life. Electroenceph Clin Neurophysiol 1980;48:395-405.

Dobson V, Teller DY. Visual acuity in human infants: a review and comparison of behavioural and electrophysiological studies. Vision Res 1978;18:1469-1483.

Marg E, Freeman DN, Peltzman P, Goldstein PJ. Visual acuity development in human infants: evoked potentials measurements. Invest Ophthalmol 1976;15: 150-153.

Moskowitz A, Sokol S. Spatial and temporal interaction of pattern-evoked cortical potentials in human infants. Vision Res 1980;20:699-707.

Moskowitz A, Sokol S. Developmental changes in the human visual system as reflected by the latency of the pattern-reversal VEP. Electroenceph Clin Neurophysiol 1983;56:1-15.

Porciatti V. Temporal and spatial properties of the pattern-reversal VEPs in infants below 2 months of age. Human Neurobiol 1984;3:97-102.

Porciatti V, von Berger GP. Visual potentials evoked by pattern stimulation in retrobulbar neuritis. Doc Ophthalmol Proc Series 1981;27:67-76.

Porciatti V, Vizzoni L, von Berger GP. Neurological age determination by evoked potentials. In: Francois J, Maione M, eds. Paediatric Ophthalmology. John Wiley & Sons and Cortina Verona, 1982:345-348.

Riemslag FCC, Spekreijse H, van Walbeek H. Pattern evoked potential diagnosis of multiple sclerosis: a comparison of various contrast stimuli. In: Courion J, Mauguiere F, Revol M, eds. Clinical applications of evoked potentials in neurology. Raven Press, New York, 1982:417-426.

Sokol S, Jones K. Implicit time of pattern evoked potentials in infants: an index of maturation of spatial vision. Vision Res 1979;19:747-755.

V.E.R. TESTING OF CORTICAL BINOCULARITY AND PATTERN DETECTION IN INFANCY

Oliver Braddick, Janette Atkinson, John Wattam-Bell

Visual Development Unit, Department of Experimental Psychology, University of Cambridge.

INTRODUCTION

The visual evoked response (VER) is now a well established means of studying normal and abnormal visual mechanisms. Developments of this technique can take one or both of two routes. One line of development is to refine the response measures that we take, for instance by characterising the details of the waveform more closely (e.g. amplitude and latency of specific components), undertaking more sophisticated statistical analysis of the signal, or by studying the detailed topography of the response in an attempt to locate the underlying sources. A second line is to use new types of visual stimulus to elicit the VER, with the aim of isolating mechanisms within the visual system that respond to specific stimuli; a simple example would be the use of pattern-appearance rather than a simple flash, to generate a VER associated with pattern processing.

A great deal of effort has been put into the refinement of recording techniques and measures (see for example the contributions of Srebro & Wright, Lesevre, and Duffy in Bodis-Wollner, 1982). However, there is still controversy about the origins and significance of the different components in VERs recorded from adults, and the difficulties of interpretation are increased when considering infant VERs, in which the latency, topography, and relative amplitude of components might be quite different from those known in the adult. In using the VER as a tool to study visual development, we have taken the other route: that is, to use stimuli selected to be informative about the development of specific aspects of visual function. In this approach, the response measures used need not be elaborate; the question is simply whether a statistically reliable VER occurs at all in response to a particular stimulus. However, some ingenuity and care is required to design and control displays for which the VER signal can be unambiguously ascribed to a particular property of the stimulus.

We outline here two examples of this approach using VERs to test for stimulus-specific mechanisms in early infancy. The first is the use of dynamic random-dot correlograms to elicit VERs that indicate cortical binocularity. The second is a dynamic display which elicits VERs specific to orientation-selective mechanisms in visual cortex.

CHOICE OF RECORDING METHODS

With both stimulus techniques we have used relatively high stimulus frequencies (typically, 4 Hz), leading to "steady-state" rather than "transient" VER recording (Regan, 1982). The principal advantage of this for infant work is that the higher the repetition rate, the larger the number of responses that can be cumulated in the signal averaging computer in a given time. Since usable records can only be obtained from a calm and alert infant who will fixate the display, and infants (particularly newborns) only remain in this state for rather brief periods, it is important to gather data as quickly as possible. Of course, if the stimulus frequency is made too high, there is the risk of going beyond the optimal frequency for the response of the infant's visual system. However, in both the methods described here, we have carried out pilot experiments exploring a range of stimulus frequencies to verify that enhanced responses were not obtained at lower repetition rates. At "steady-state" frequencies, detailed features of the signal waveform are lost and the response appears approximately sinusoidal. While this would be a disadvantage in studies concerned with the form of the response, we are here concerned only with its presence or absence. In this case the uniform form of the response may even be an advantage since it leads to an unambiguous measure of response strength (i.e. signal amplitude at the stimulus frequency).

Similarly, we have had no reason to use complex arrays of recording electrodes. All our recordings have been bipolar, with one Ag/AgCl electrode at the inion and a second at the vertex, and an indifferent electrode on the forehead.

VER TESTING OF CORTICAL BINOCULARITY

To be assured that a VER arises specifically from binocular interaction in the infant's visual system, we must use a stimulus in which neither eye's input taken separately could generate the observed response. Such a stimulus, in which an essential feature emerges only as a result of the combination of information from the two eyes, has been called 'cyclopean' (Julesz, 1971). Our cyclopean stimulus is a dynamic random-dot correlogram (Julesz, Kropfl & Petrig, 1980; Braddick, Atkinson, Julesz, Kropfl, Bodis-Wollner & Raab, 1980). That is, the infant faces a wide-screen video display of continuously changing red and green random dots, alternating between two phases. In the 'correlated' phase, the dynamic dot patterns displayed in red and green are identical and superimposed; in the other, 'anticorrelated' phase every bright dot displayed in the red channel is superimposed on a dark dot in the green channel, and vice versa. The infant wears lightweight red-green goggles, so that each set of dots can be seen by one eye only. Since the dots are continuously changing, the alternation between the two phases is detectable only as a change in the relationship between the red and green patterns. Therefore, either eye alone sees only a 'snowstorm' of random dots and this is also what is seen with both eyes open by an individual who lacks binocular function. However, with normal binocular vision the correlated phase is fused, while the anticorrelated phase cannot be fused. This leads to a visible pulsation and to a VER time-locked to the alternation between the phases. This VER can only arise from interaction of the two eyes' signals at a binocular neural site.

Figure 1 illustrates VER records obtained from an infant subject with this technique. If negative results are to be interpretable, we must verify that they result from an absence of binocular function and not simply from the use of spatial and temporal display parameters outside the range of the particular infant's visual system. This is done by testing

the infant without the red-green goggles: the correlated phase of the
stimulus now appears as a yellow-black dot pattern and the anticorrelated
phase red-green. This contrast change elicits a clear VER from the infant
at both ages illustrated, indicating that the dot pattern was neither too
fine nor varying too fast for the infant's visual system to respond.
However, at age 60 days this infant showed no VER evidence of binocularity
when viewing the pattern through the red-green goggles. Two weeks later,
at 74 days, the binocular VER is clearly present. Statistical comparisons
with a control condition, in which there is no stimulus at the alternation
frequency, verify that there is reliable evidence of a binocular response
in the signal recorded at 74 days but not at 60 days; this may also be
verified by a test of the consistency of the signal phase in successive
blocks of the recording (Wattam-Bell, 1985).

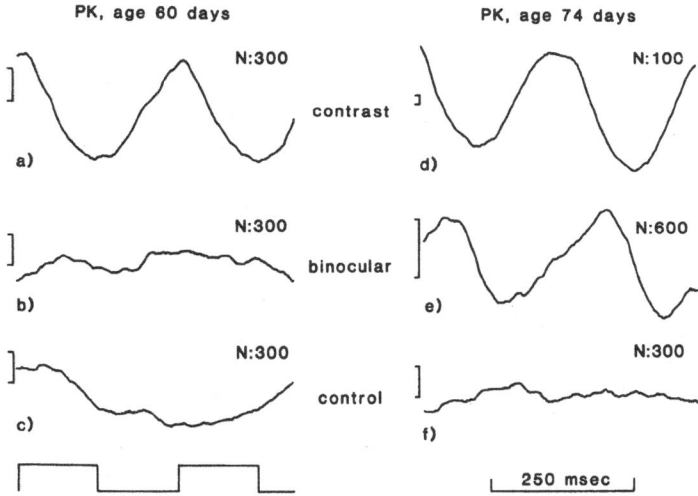

Figure 1. VER records showing the attainment of binocular response
by a particular infant between the ages of 60 days (a-c) and 74 days
(d-f). a,d: responses to contrast changes in the dot-pattern (i.e.
without goggles). b,e: responses with the infant wearing red-green
goggles; positive response in this condition is evidence of cortical
binocularity. c: control condition looking away from stimulus. f:
control condition with red and green patterns vertically misaligned
to prevent fusion. N by each record gives the number of repetitions
averaged; vertical bar indicates the scale of a 2 microvolt response
in each case. Bottom left: timing of alternations between correlated and anticorrelated phases.

In a study of a large group of newborns using this technique
(Braddick, Wattam-Bell, Day & Atkinson, 1983), we found no evidence of
functional binocularity at birth, even when VERs in the contrast condition
showed that the infants were responsive to the dynamic dot patterns.
Longitudinal measurements at approximately 2-week intervals on a group of
normal infants showed a median age of 13 weeks for the first positive
results on the VER test of binocularity. A variety of other techniques
have concurred with this result in placing the normal onset of
binocularity between 3 and 4 months of age (see review by Braddick &

Atkinson, 1983). It should be emphasised, however, that even in normal development there are marked individual variations, e.g. from 8 to over 15 weeks in this study.

Disorders of binocular function are the commonest problems facing the paediatric ophthalmologist, so the capability to assess binocularity at an early age is obviously of potential clinical interest. Following animal models (Hubel & Wiesel, 1965; Blakemore, 1978) it is widely supposed that loss of binocularity is a consequence of strabismus of oculomotor or accommodative origin, which leads to misalignment of the eyes in a sensitive period in early life. However, we should be alert to the possibility that in some cases the sensory defect might be primary: a child lacking functional binocularity beyond the normal age of its development might be expected to fail to maintain accurate eye alignment. To explore this hypothesis, we are currently following up a group of 100 infants who have a history of early strabismus or amblyopia in a primary relative. VER testing showed that compared to infants without such a history, this group showed a longer 'tail' in which development of binocularity was late or absent during the period of study (up to 5-6 months). As this group develop through the age of high risk of strabismus, it should be posible to determine whether an apparent early deficit of cortical binocularity can be a precursor of later strabismus.

5% of this group with family history of strabismus actually developed manifest strabismus during their first 6 months. Such cases must be expected to fail the VER test since misalignment of the eyes will presumably prevent them from registering the correlation of binocular images, whatever sensory mechanisms the infant may possess. It might be argued that oculomotor development is also critical in the normal onset of binocular-specific VERs, but the evidence (reviewed in Braddick & Atkinson, 1983) is against this. Clearly, however, it would be valuable both scientifically and for the strabismus surgeon to have a measure of sensory binocularity which could be applied even when the eyes were not aligned. It may prove possible to achieve this in the future, by developing the VER method to use random-dot patterns with variable alignment.

VER SPECIFIC TO CORTICAL ORIENTATION DETECTORS

In the visual pathway, the striate cortex is the earliest stage at which binocular signals converge onto single neurones. It has been suggested (see discussion by Atkinson, 1984) that the striate cortex may not play an effective role in vision in the early weeks of life, raising the question whether the lack of functional binocularity up to 3 months may just reflect a broader immaturity of cortical function. Is it possible to test cortical function in other respects, without having to make assumptions about the anatomical origin of particular components of the infant VER?

One of the best established features of striate cortical physiology in higher mammals is the predominance of neurones which respond to edges or bars in particular orientations (Hubel & Wiesel, 1962). Such neurones are absent in earlier stages of the visual pathway, so a VER which was a specific response to orientation would be strong evidence for visual cortical function. Normally, if the orientation of a pattern is changed, this will entail widespread local contrast changes. A response to these changes will occur even in neurones which are not orientation-sensitive,

e.g. in the optic radiation. How can we exclude these responses from
contributing to the VER?

In the correlogram display used to test binocularity, many individual
dots have to change in the alternation from correlated to anticorrelated.
This change could have generated a VER even monocularly. However, by
making the dot patterns dynamic, we ensured that the alternation was part
of a continual sequence of changes, distinguishable only by specific
binocular mechanisms. We have devised an analogous technique for
isolating orientation detection (Braddick, Wattam-Bell & Atkinson, 1984).
A stripe pattern is presented on a video display, with a random
displacement occurring on every TV frame, so that the stripes appear in
rapid irregular

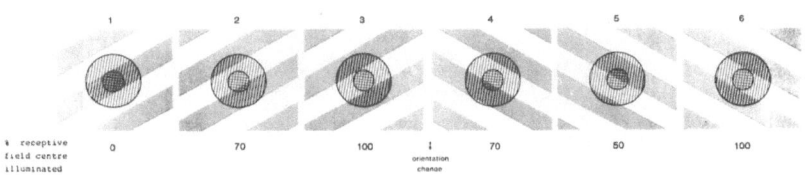

Figure 2. 1-6 illustrate the grating displayed in six successive TV
frames of the dynamic stimulus used to elicit orientation-specific
VERs. After three frames (1-3) in which random displacements of an
obliquely oriented grating occur, the orientation changes to the
opposite oblique which undergoes random displacements for three more
frames (4-6), and so on. The grating is shown falling on the
circular receptive field of a visual neurone, e.g. an l.g.n. cell
with an axon in the optic radiation. The fraction of the receptive
field centre illuminated, and hence the cell's response, varies
randomly from frame to frame; nothing about the stimulus change
between frames 3 and 4 (the orientation reversal) differentiates it
from the displacements between other frames, for such a non-
orientation-specific cell.

motion. At a lower rate (every third frame) the orientation of the
stripes is changed through 90 degrees. A visual neurone with a non-
oriented receptive field will pick up a random change in stimulation at
each displacement, and the orientation change will be another,
indistinguishable change in this series (Figure 2). Such neurones may
generate a response at the high frequency of the frame-by-frame
displacements, but will not show any distinctive response at the lower
frequency of the orientation changes. In contrast, a cortical neurone
with a specific orientation sensitivity will register the orientation
change as a much more significant transition than the intervening
displacements which leave orientation unchanged.

A large percentage of young infants are astigmatic (Howland,
Atkinson, Braddick & French, 1978; Mohindra, Held, Gwiazda & Brill, 1978).
This means that for any given amount of accommodation, edges in one

orientation will be more sharply focussed than in the orientation at right angles, and so a switch between these orientations will be accompanied by a contrast change that would be detectable by non-orientation-specific neural mechanisms. To avoid this problem, we have used alternation between oblique orientations, as illustrated in Figure 2. The great majority of astigmatic infants have astgmatic axes near the horizontal and vertical, and for those who have oblique axes, these are almost invariably mirror-image in the two eyes; alternation of obliques will therefore not produce any overall contrast change.

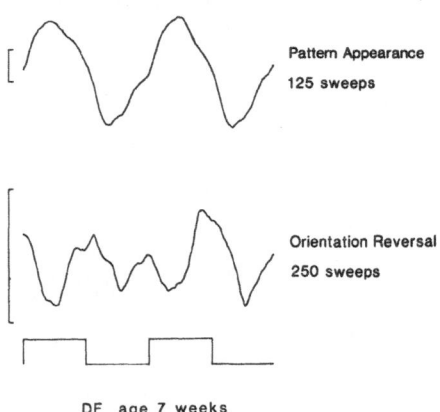

Pattern Appearance
125 sweeps

Orientation Reversal
250 sweeps

DF   age 7 weeks

Figure 3. Example of VER records obtained from a 7-week-old infant using the dynamic orientation stimulus explained in the text and Figure 2. Upper: with pattern-appearance stimulus (randomly displaced grating of constant orientation alternates with uniform field). Lower: with orientation-reversal stimulus. Bottom: stimulus trace of orientation or pattern alternations (total duration of trace, 250 msec). Note that since the two orientations are symmetrical, there is are peaks in the VER both for 45-135 degree alternations and for the reverse, i.e. double the alternation frequency. For pattern-appearance, 'on' and 'off' are not equivalent events and so the major component is at the alternation frequency. Each vertical marker corresponds to 5 microvolts at the scale of the adjoining record.

Figure 3 shows an example of the VER recorded from a 7-week infant using this stimulus. The upper record represents a control condition. It was obtained with a display where the grating underwent random displacements, as in the left-hand half of Figure 2, but these were not alternated with an opposed orientation. Instead, they were alternated with a uniform field matched in mean luminance. This is similar to a conventional pattern-appearance stimulus, except that the pattern which appears is dynamic rather than static. The occurrence of a clear VER demonstrates that the infant's visual system was responsive to the dynamic pattern, i.e. the rapid random displacements did not effectively blur out the grating for the infant.

The lower record was obtained with the dynamic orientation-reversal stimulus. The clear and statistically reliable VER must arise in orientation-specific neural mechanisms in the infant's cortex. Thus we can conclude that this particular child was showing at least one aspect of mature striate cortical function at the age of 7 weeks.

In contrast, Figure 4 shows similar recordings from a newborn infant. As with the 7-week-old, a clear and statistically reliable response was obtained with the pattern-appearance stimulus, so the infant was capable of detecting the grating despite its rapid random movements. However, no VER was apparent for the orientation-reversal stimulus, and this is confirmed by statistical testing. We conclude that this infant shows no evidence of functioning cortical orientation detectors.

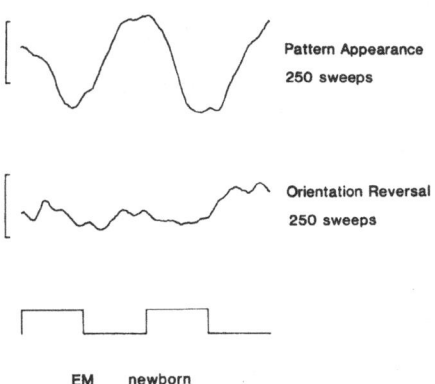

Pattern Appearance
250 sweeps

Orientation Reversal
250 sweeps

EM   newborn

Figure 4. Example of VER records obtained from a newborn infant using the dynamic orientation stimulus of Figure 2. Upper and lower records, and the stimulus trace at bottom, correspond to those shown for an older infant in Figure 3. There is no evidence of an orientation-specific response.

The results shown in Figure 4 are typical of those we found in newborn subjects. In a group of 20, selected from a larger group on the grounds that they showed a statistically reliable pattern-appearance response, we saw no case of a reponse to orientation change. In five of these we extended the recording to 500 sweeps or more to increase sensitivity, but still found no evidence for an orientation response. We conclude that if the striate cortex is functional at all in newborn infants, its receptive field properties must be very immature. One question to which we cannot yet give a definite answer is where the pattern-appearance VER observed in newborns originates. It may be a response of pre- or sub-cortical mechanisms, or it may be due to cortical neurones whose receptive fields are still very immature and non-specific.

We currently have underway a longitudinal study of a group of infants, to determine the age at which an orientation-specific response can first be detected. While this study is not complete at the time of writing, results so far suggest that 5-6 weeks is the age at which this aspect of cortical function generally emerges. This is an age around which many striking developments of visual function occur (Atkinson,

1984); however, comparison with our data on binocularity implies that the latter is a separate and specific development.

The use of orientation-specific VERs offers a possible index of specifically cortical function, which may prove to be of value in assessment of children in whom impairments of visual behaviour may be the product of cerebral damage. The technique is already in use in our programme of visual assessment (see Atkinson and Braddick, this meeting). One example is a six-month-old referred to us with spastic quadraplegia following severe birth asphyxia. She showed little behavioural evidence of visual function either in informal testing of fixation or in preferential looking, field testing, or photorefractive examination of accommodative responses. Optokinetic responses were very weak. VER testing with the pattern-appearance stimulus showed a statistically reliable response; with the orientation-specific stimulus, no consistent response was present although there may have been brief episodes of a time-locked signal. This pattern of VER response somewhat resembled a normal newborn. Our interpretation must be cautious, but it seems possible that the VER we see in this patient may depend on subcortical structures. We do not yet know the implications of this for the patient's present and future visual capabilities; the VER results will have to be related to continuing assessment of the child's visual performance.

SUMMARY

Our approach has been to record visual evoked responses using stimuli that are tailored to isolate the response of particular sensory mechanisms - in these examples, binocular interaction and orientation-selective neurones. These methods have provided valuable normative data on how central visual functions develop in early infancy. In future, VER recording with these special stimuli should prove useful tools for clinicians, as components of a fuller assessment of vision, in the diagnosis and management of binocular disorders and of cerebral impairments of vision.

ACKNOWLEDGMENTS

This work is supported by a programme grant from the Medical Research Council. We thank Jacqueline Day, Shirley Anker, Rose Anne Hall, and Carol Evans for their assistance. We are grateful to Dr N C R Roberton and the staff of the Rosie Maternity Hospital, Cambridge for their co-operation, without which our studies of newborns would not have been possible.

REFERENCES

Atkinson J. Human visual development over the first six months of life: a review and a hypothesis. Human Neurobiol 1984;3:61-74.

Blakemore C. Maturation and modification in the developing visual system. In: Held R, Leibowitz HW, Teuber HL, eds. Handbook of Sensory Physiology, vol VIII: Perception. Heidelberg: Springer-Verlag. 1978.

Braddick O, Atkinson J. Some recent findings on the development of human binocularity: a review. Behav Brain Res 1983;10:141-150.

Braddick O, Atkinson J, Julesz B, Kropfl W, Bodis-Wollner I, Raab E.

Cortical binocularity in infants. Nature 1980;288:675-677.

Braddick O, Wattam-Bell J, Atkinson J. Evoked potentials specific to orientation detectors in adults and infants. Perception 1984;13:A27.

Braddick O, Wattam-Bell J, Day J, Atkinson, J. The onset of bincoular function in human infants. Human Neurobiol 1983;2:65-69.

Bodis-Wollner I, ed. Evoked Potentials. Ann NY Acad Sci 1982;388.

Howland HC, Atkinson J, Braddick O, French J. Infant astigmatism measured by photorefraction. Science 1978;202:331-333.

Hubel DH, Wiesel TN. Binocular interaction in striate cortex of kittens reared with artificial squint. J Neurophysiol 1965;28:1041-1059.

Hubel DH, Wiesel TN. Receptive fields, binocular interaction, and functional architecture in the cat's visual cortex. J Physiol 1962;160: 106-154.

Julesz B. Foundations of Cyclopean Perception. Chicago: University of Chicago Press. 1971.

Julesz B, Kropfl W, & Petrig, B. Large evoked potentials of dynamic random-dot correlograms and stereograms permit quick determination of stereopsis. Proc nat Acad Sci USA 1980;77:2348-2351.

Mohindra I, Held R, Gwiazda J, Brill S. Astigmatism in infants. Science 1978;202:329-331.

Regan DM. Comparison of transient and steady state methods. Ann NY Acad Sci 1982;388:45-71.

Wattam-Bell J. Analysis of infant VEPs by a phase-sensitive statistic. 8th European Conference on Visual Perception, Peniscola, Spain. 1985.

DISCUSSION

Fells: Could I ask Braddick why you used the oblique orientation instead of the vertical and horizontal when you know that they give a better physiological response than the oblique ones?

Braddick: The reasons were that we were concerned that our response was genuinely a function of cortical activity and we know that a large fraction of newborn infants are astigmatic. The majority of those are in the vertical and horizontal axes so that they could have a differential blur which might induce a response even with a non-orientated neural system. Oblique astigmatism is much rarer and is also symmetrical between the two eyes, but I agree that we should go back and repeat some of these measurements with vertical or horizontal orientations on a selection of infants who have been screened for the absence of astigmatism.

Campos: When you studied binocularity, which of the binocular functions did you test?

Braddick: Operationally we are testing the ability to distinguish between the correlated and the non-correlated patterns, if you like between a fused pattern and a non-fused pattern. This does not refer directly to true stereopsis because no disparities are involved and it is conceivable that infants might have a system that was sensitive to fusion in the sense of correlation between the two eyes, but which could not distinguish between correlated but disparate images. That is a question we shall have to pursue, whether we show not only binocularity in this sense but also disparity sensivity. You may know that there are results in the literature that show stereoscopic discrimination in infants, but it is at least possible that detection of correlation is an earlier stage in the development of binocularity, and I don't think it can be resolved until we look at the same infants longitudinally that this may be an earlier stage in the development of binocularity.

Hache: How do you examine babies for electrophysiological tests and particularly for pattern ERG, because attention and results change with the posture of the baby? We do 20 examinations a week but we have not succeeded in getting a method.

Braddick: I can tell you what we do, you saw a picture of our babies in the seated posture. We are recording with silver/silver chloride electrodes that are entirely on the midline, with the indifferent electrode on the forehead and recording between electrodes on the vertex and above the inion.

Hache: Contact?

Braddick: Yes. One very important factor is that you are not going to get a visually evoked response from the baby who is not looking at the stimulus and so it is important to monitor continuously the child and only to accept signals for averaging when the child is reasonably stationary and is fixated on the screen. One point I make here is that most commercial averagers, if they have a rejection button, enable you to reject the next sweep, but the one coming in is already accepted. In our microcomputer with a program for this purpose we have a foot switch with which you can throw away the sweep that is currently coming in. I don't know how much difference that makes, but in general it is important to be able to reject data or discard data obtained when the child is not in an appropriate state.

Atkinson: We should also make the point that skin resistance is much higher in the neonatal period than even two months postnatally, so it is necessary to get skin resistance down a little more thoroughly in the newborn. We do this by rubbing them with surgical spirit to get a clean skin surface. We should say that we haven't actually managed to record VEPs from between half and two-thirds of the newborns who get as far as the testing room because of practical state problems. A very warm maternity hospital is one of our problems.

Van Lith: Even then normal babies start crying when electrodes are fixed.

Atkinson: No, not at all.

Van Lith: But they don't know the people who are doing it. How long is such a session?

Braddick: One thing you have to be very clear about is age and the question of whether the baby knows the individual. A one-month-old baby is a very different creature from a 9-month-old baby and psychologists will tell you that separation anxiety and stranger anxiety is something that emerges well after six months of age. So who is holding the baby doesn't make a lot of difference in this early age group, although it is important to have somebody holding him who is competent and experienced with babies and knows the requirements of the recording session, holding the baby straight and keeping the electrodes away from the holder's body, and so on. The other point is about the number of sweeps. You must remember that these are relatively fast, in the order of 250 msec sweeps, so that 250 sweeps would take about a minute in an uninterrupted run. Obviously they are going to take rather longer than that because of rejection problems. A recording of say 5 minutes for a particular record and 10-15 minutes for the whole session would be typical of these studies.

Taylor: I think on a very simple practical level there are methods of getting the right state, in other words awake and looking and yet not being overexcited. Get them to come to your session or your clinic when they are starved and then you gratify them with their bottle and towards the end of the feed and for a little while afterwards they are often in a very good state. What you do with breast feeding, I don't know.

van Lith: We also starve the baby before they come into the session and give them the bottle during the session but they become so sleepy.

Taylor: Yes, but isn't it quite a long time afterwards that they become sleepy rather than immediately?

Braddick: I think there is a general point to be made. If you are going to record successfully under 6 months of age, then the baby has to be setting the timetable. You will not get the results if you expect the baby to appear on appointment, you will get even less good results if you give the baby or the parents an appointment for 10 o'clock and start recording at 11.30. Particularly with newborns, the way we did the study is to rove the hospital and find those infants that are ready and we may walk round all morning and only find two. Now I think this means that if you are going to use this diagnostically in a clinic, it is going to be very different from older children and from adults.

Apkarian: One relevant issue that emerges from this discussion is that recording procedures in infants are far from standardised. Although one can make the same comment regarding VEP measures in general, the problem is further exacerbated in infant populations because of the difficulties associated with state determination; the latter influences the final measures and consequent data interpretation.

Fiorentini: In very young infants we use external electrodes that we make ourselves with silver wire, and that we stick to the lower eyelid with sticky tape. We have two equal electrodes for the two eyes so that one is the reference electrode for the other one. While recording the ERG from one eye the other eye is covered. This is done in order to minimise contamination from VEPs. These electrodes work very well and the subjects do not complain.

Hache: Do you have sufficient attention of the baby?

Fiorentini: Yes, provided it is the right time preferably soon after feeding. However, the ERG is much less successful than the evoked potential because the signal is smaller and you have to record for a longer time. I would say that about 60% of sessions are successful in young infants to get enough data for estimating an ERG acuity.

VISUAL FUNCTION IN THE NEWBORN INFANT: BEHAVIOURAL AND
ELECTROPHYSIOLOGICAL STUDIES

J. Mushin[*], L.M.S. Dubowitz[*], G.B. Arden[**]

 * Department of Paediatrics and Neonatal Medicine,
   Royal Postgraduate Medical School, London.
** Department of Clinical Ophthalmology,
   Institute of Ophthalmology, London.

Assessment of visual function forms an important part of the
neurological evaluation of the newborn infant. It provides information on
the integrity of the visual pathway and also has been claimed to be a marker
of higher cortical function and thus a reliable predictor of later intellectual
performance (Hack et al 1977).

The introduction of routine cranial ultrasonography in the neonatal
unit made possible the early diagnosis of ischaemic hypoxic lesions such as
periventricular/intraventricular haemorrhage (PVH/IVH), periventricular
leukomalacia (PVL), porencephalic cysts and ventricular dilatation (Levene
et al 1985). This allowed a better correlation of visual function with
anatomical lesions. We would like to review the present methods used to
evaluate visual function in neonates and how far the new correlative studies
still support the old hypotheses.

METHODS OF ASSESSMENT OF VISUAL FUNCTION IN THE NEWBORN

Behavioural Testing

Tracking: The infant is propped up at about 30° in the supine position
and a red woolly ball held approximately 20 to 25 cm from its face is moved
slowly horizontally and vertically. The infant's eyes should converge and
follow the target demonstrating the ability to fixate and track an object.
This test can be used in a neonatal unit, inside and outside an incubator
(Brazelton 1973, Dubowitz et al 1980).

Preferential Looking Technique: Fantz (1963) demonstrated that newborn
infants have a definite preference for patterns of different shape, size and
complexity. To test this the infant is presented with two spatially
separated stimuli which consist of patterns on a uniformly illuminated stage
and preference for one of the patterns is judged by deviation and fixation of
the eyes in the direction of the preferred pattern. The four pattern pairs
used by us are illustrated in Fig. 1. The test can be elaborated by making
the patterns gratings of various spatial frequency and presenting them
together with a uniform grey surface matched for luminance. By this means a
measure of visual acuity can be obtained (Ordy and Udelf 1962, Miranda 1970,
Vassella et al 1977, Morante et al 1982).

120

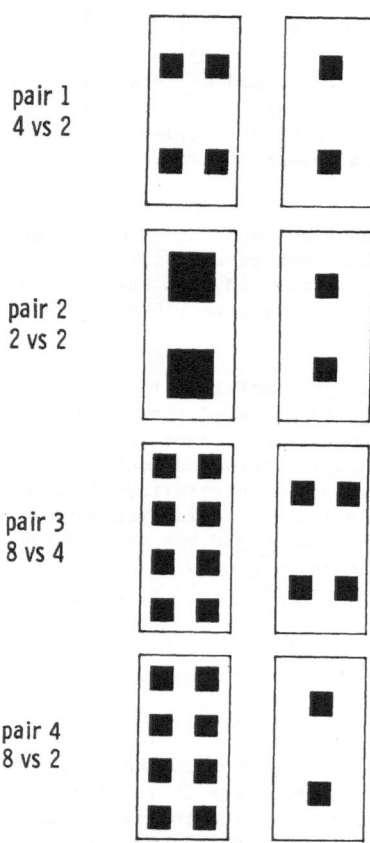

pair 1
4 vs 2

pair 2
2 vs 2

pair 3
8 vs 4

pair 4
8 vs 2

Pairs of patterns used in that order

Figure 1.   Four pairs of patterns used in testing pattern preference.

Visual Evoked Responses

The maturational changes of the visual evoked response (VER) in the preterm and full-term infant have been described by various authors using a Xenon discharge stroboscope (Ellingson 1960, Ferriss et al 1967, Umezaki and Morrell 1970, Watanabe et al 1972, Hrbek et al 1973, Barnet et al 1980, Blom et al 1980). The stroboscope has several disadvantages when used in a neonatal intensive care unit and to overcome these a photostimulator has been developed which consists of an array of light emitting diodes (LEDs). This has been shown to evoke VERs in newborn infants which are comparable in latency and waveform to those elicited by a stroboscope (Mushin et al 1984). Three or four silver chloride electrodes are attached to the infant's scalp. Single channel recordings are made with a single active electrode on the midline at the inion. Two channel recordings are made with active electrodes 2cm lateral to the inion. The reference electrode is placed on the midfrontal region and the ground electrode on the mastoid. Interelectrode resistance should be below 6kOhms. Thirty-two or 64 flashes are averaged using a medelec 'Sensor'.

THE DEVELOPMENT OF VISUAL FUNCTION IN NEUROLOGICALLY NORMAL INFANTS

Behavioural Testing

Tracking: From 32 weeks gestational age infants are able to fixate on and track an object during the first week of life. By 34 weeks postmenstrual age (PMA) over 80% of neurologically normal infants can track. When these infants reach 40 weeks PMA their ability to track is superior to that of full-term infants during the first week of life (Fig. 2).

Preferential Looking Technique: Pattern preference can be successfully tested in 60-70% of infants above 32 weeks gestation who are well enough to be taken out of the incubator. Using the four pairs of patterns shown in Fig. 1, preterm infants of 34 weeks gestation or less that can be tested are able to disciminate between pattern pairs 2 and 4, in 60-70% of tests performed under one week of age. However, very few of these infants are able to differentiate the other two pairs. Over 70% of full-term infants distinguish all four of the pattern pairs. The evolution of pattern preference with increasing gestational age is illustrated in Fig. 3.

Using vertical stripes of subtense 160', 80' and 40' arc it is found that visual acuity improves with increasing gestational age. At 32 weeks more than 90% of infants are able to distinguish between the high contrast 160' arc stripe and a blank field, but only one third are able to recognise the 80' arc stripes. The increase in visual acuity determined in this way with gestational age is shown in Fig. 4.

Visual Evoked Responses

VERs have been recorded in infants from 24 weeks gestational age (Hrbek et al 1973). The first response is a simple surface negative wave. Between 32 and 35 weeks a positive wave precedes the negativity. The peak time of the positive wave varies in normal premature infants from 200-250 msec. By 40 weeks the positivity has increased in amplitude and a preceding negativity has appeared, giving the N-P-N complex. The latencies subsequently shorten and the waveform becomes more complex, so that by 6 months there should be

Evolution of Visual Orientation in Preterm and Full Term Infants.

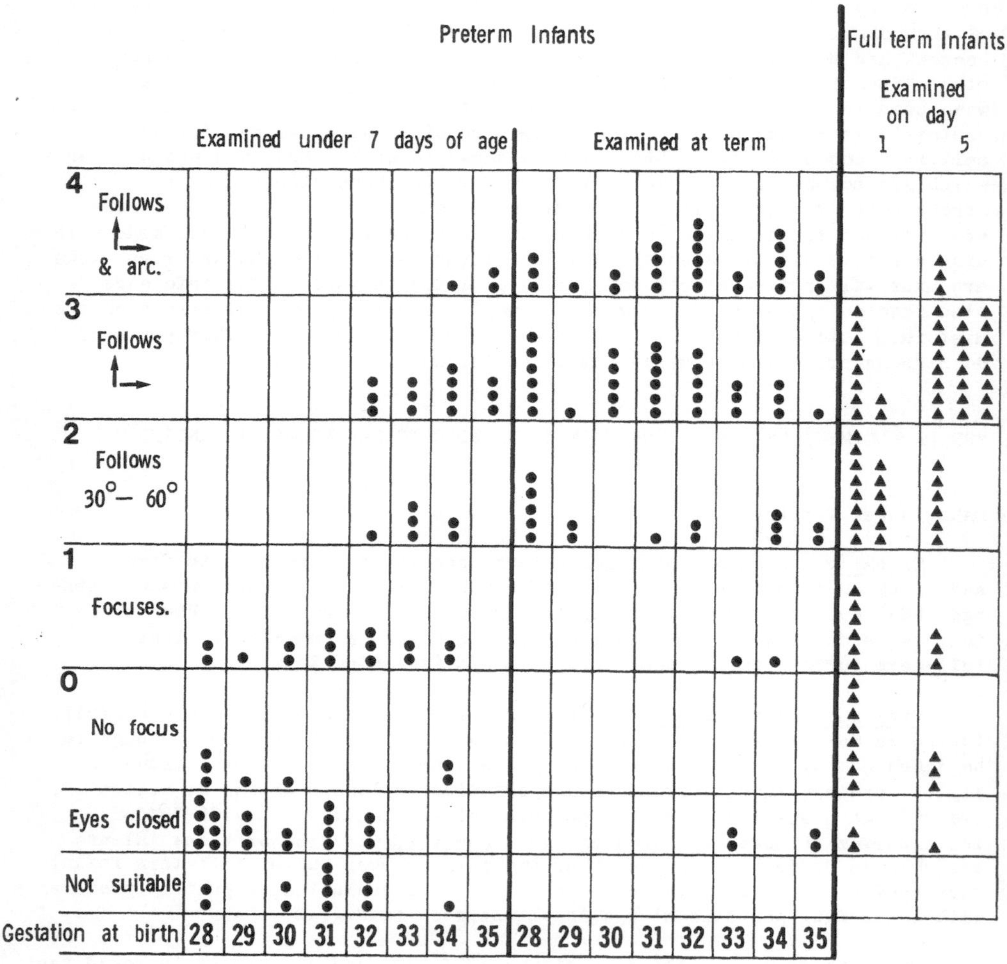

Figure 1. Evolution of visual orientation in preterm infants (gestation 29-30 weeks) assessed in the first seven days of life and at term (38-40 weeks PMA) compared with full-term infants assessed on the first and fifth day documented in the right-hand column.

Pattern preference in normal infants, preterm (≤ 36w) and term (≥38w), examined during the first week of life.

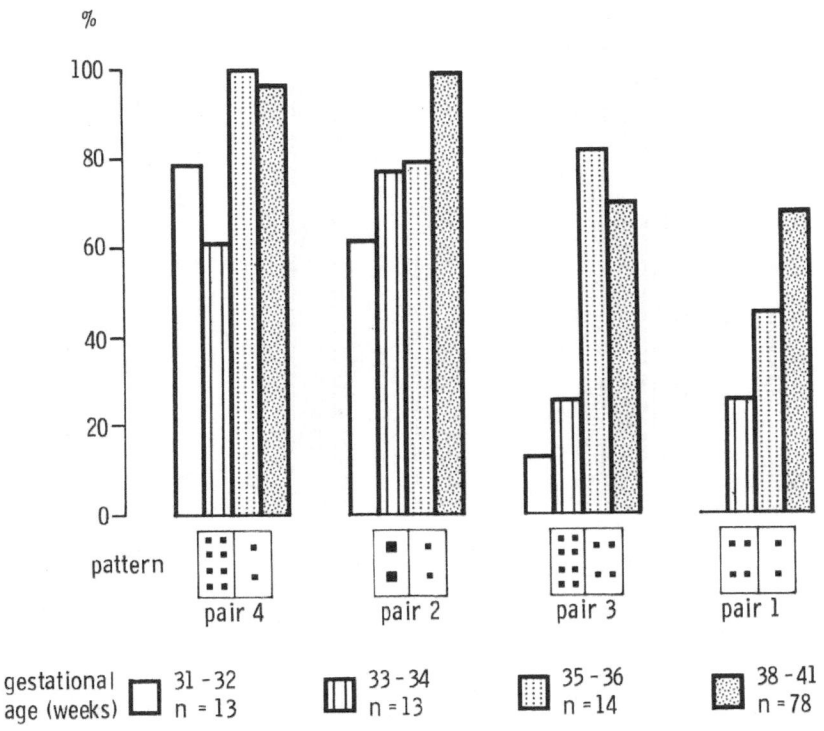

Figure 3.

124

Visual acuity in normal infants, preterm (≤ 36w) and term (≥38w), examined during the first week of life.

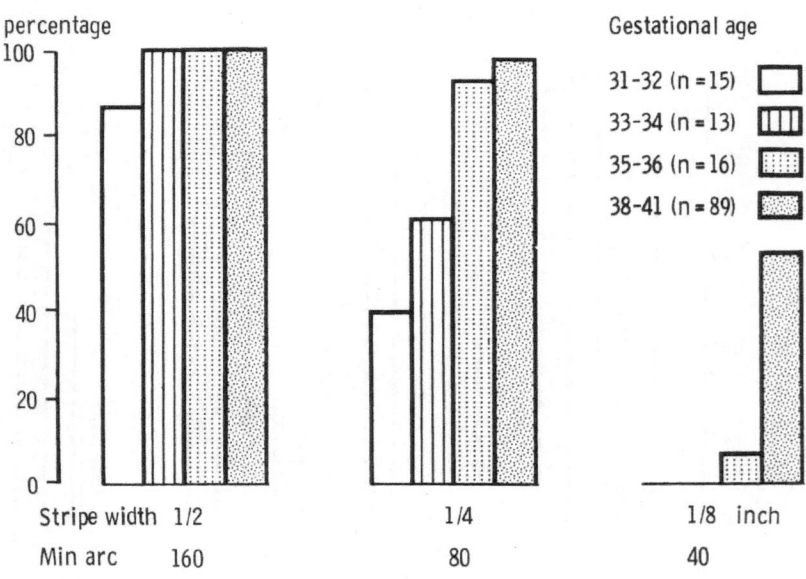

Figure 4.

a nearly adult waveform with a prominent surface positive component peaking at 100-150 msec after the flash. Ellingson (1960) has described a bimodal curve relating latency to age with a steep reduction in latency values between 1 and 2 months of age in infants born at term.

Figure 5A shows serial VERs obtained in a normal preterm infant born at 32 weeks gestational age. By 34 weeks PMA a well marked positive deflection can be seen preceding the negative peak. The positivity was present in 38% of VERs obtained from normal infants at 32 weeks PMA and in over 90% of VERs recorded at 36 weeks PMA. The sequence of development of the VER, and in particular the appearance of the positive wave, is a more reliable indicator of maturation than either latency or amplitude measurements (Watanabe et al 1972). This is especially so, as in the sick or immature infant response amplitude and latency have been shown to vary with the rate of stimulation (Table 1).

TABLE 1. Stimulus frequency and the VER for premature infants*

| Frequency Hz** | Amplitude (% of 0.2 Hz) | | | Latency (msec) | | |
| | Age range (weeks) | | | Age range (weeks) | | |
	<32	33-35	>35	<32	33-35	>35
0.2	100	100	100	284	278	250
1	76	82	83	301	302	257
2	43	63	65	320	335	312

*   Neurologically normal and abnormal children included
** No differences observable between 0.2 and 1 Hz for full-term controls

Comparison Between Changes in Visual Acuity (Preferential Looking) and the VER

In a series of preterm infants (31-39 weeks PMA) (Placzek et al 1985) it was found that in 79% of cases there was an association between the development of acuity of 80' of arc and the presence of a positivity in the VER.

THE DEVELOPMENT OF VISUAL FUNCTION IN THE NEUROLOGICALLY DEVIANT INFANT

Behavioural Testing

Tracking: The development of this function in the neonatal period is frequently delayed, particularly in those infants with periventricular and/or intraventricular haemorrhage (PVH/IVH). However the magnitude of the delay bears no relationship to the size of the haemorrhage or to the presence of ventricular dilatation. Surprisingly, infants with extensive cystic periventricular leukomalacia (PVL) often show normal fixation and tracking in the neonatal period (Dubowitz et al 1985).

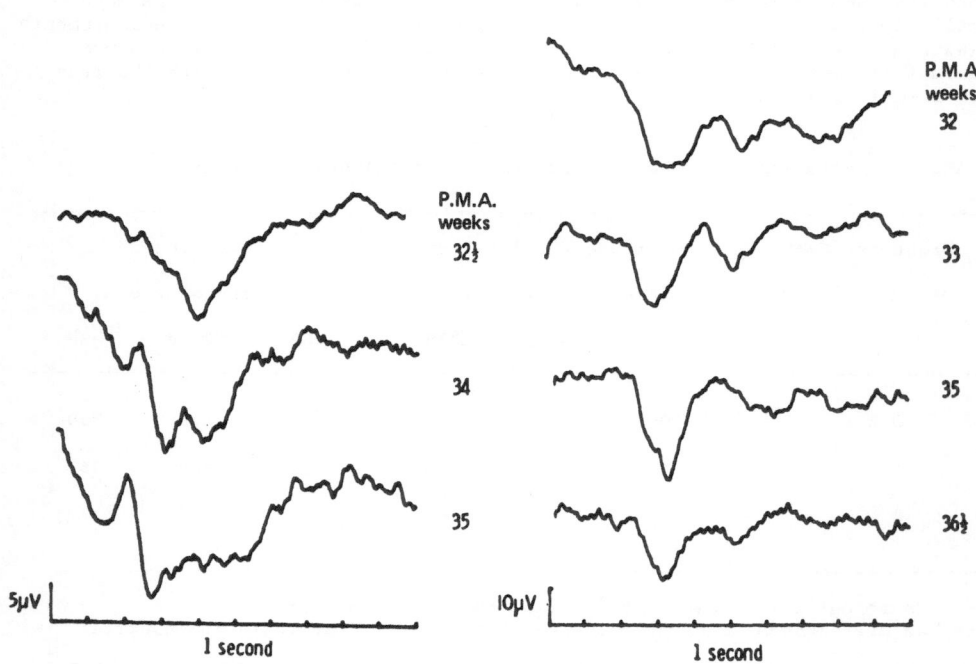

A - NORMAL   32 weeks G.A.   B - ABNORMAL 27 weeks G.A.

Figure 5.   A)   Serial VER recordings in a normal infant born at 32 weeks
                 gestation.
            B)   Serial VER recordings in an infant with an intraventricular
                 haemorrhage born at 27 weeks gestation.
            Positivity upwards.   Note delay in appearance of positive wave.

Pattern preference in neurologically normal and abnormal preterm
infants examined at 36 and 40 weeks post-menstrual age.

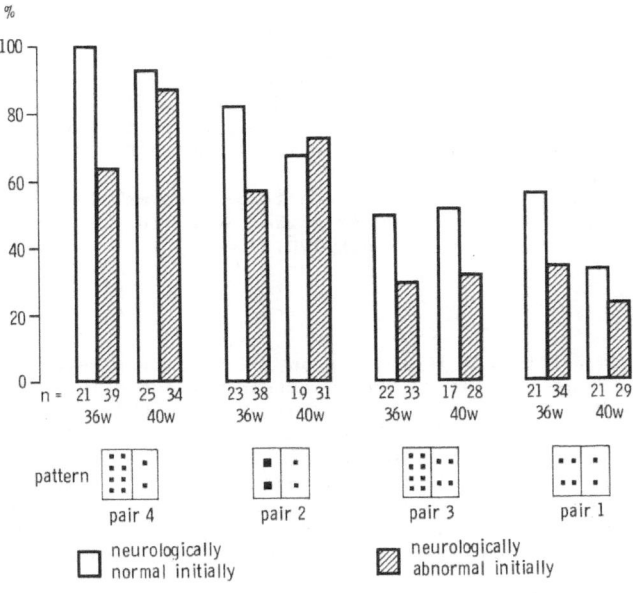

Figure 6.

Preferential Looking: Neurologically abnormal full-term infants show significantly poorer pattern preference than normal full-term infants on initial examination and show only little improvement when re-examined 4-6 weeks later.

Preterm infants with abnormal neurological findings on their initial· examination also show significantly poorer development of pattern preference compared to normal preterm infants of corresponding age (Fig. 6). There is, however, no significant difference in pattern preference in those infants who suffer a PVH/IVH and those who do not. Some pattern preference for the more striking patterns has been observed in infants with extensive PVL.

In the neonatal period, visual acuity tends to be abnormal in those infants with neurological deficits. The most marked delay in the development of visual acuity was seen in infants with PVH/IVH. (Fig.7.)

Visual Evoked Responses

Figure 5B shows the serial VER records in an infant with a severe intraventricular haemorrhage born at 27 weeks gestational age. The appearance of the positivity is delayed and occurs only after 35 weeks PMA. In a group of infants with large IVH only 38% of VERs showed a positivity by 36 weeks PMA. This compared with 54% in a group with less extensive IVH and 50% in a group with abnormal neurological signs including hypotonia but no IVH (Placzek et al 1985). An additive logistic model was fitted to the data (Fig. 8). This shows that VER maturation as measured by the appearance of the positive wave is significantly delayed in the neurologically abnormal infants (groups II, III, IV) compared with the normal (group I).

The delay in VER maturation showed no correlation with ventricular enlargement, but appeared to be more marked in infants in whom the haemorrhage extended downwards towards the thalamus. In infants with asymmetrical dilatation associated with cyst formation, bilateral VER recording demonstrated no difference in the VER waveform between the two hemispheres in infants less than 40 weeks PMA. However, later recordings in the same infant showed asymmetrical responses (Fig. 9).

It is of interest that a VER with an abnormal waveform was elicited from an infant with proven holoprosencephaly (Fig. 10). VERs recorded in patients with periventricular leukomalacia tended to be normal in cases where the cysts were mainly confined to the occipital region, but were grossly abnormal in cases with more extensive lesions.

DISCUSSION

Although fixation and tracking and some pattern preference can be demonstrated in premature infants it is quite likely that this is not cortical in origin. The evidence in support of this is that infants with widespread involvement of the occipital cortex, such as periventricular leukomalacia, are able to track and follow well in the neonatal period. On the other hand, infants with IVH/PVH and presumably hypoxic lesions in the colliculi show more marked disturbances of visual function. In one infant tested with complete absence of visual cortex, an apparent VER could be recorded initially. Further evidence of the non cortical origin of the VER comes from the observations that in three infants with asymmetrical lesions affecting the occipital cortex, symmetrical evoked responses were recorded from the two hemispheres in the neonatal period.

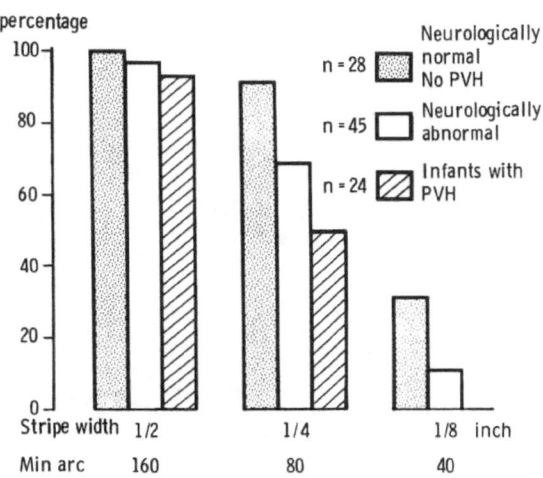

Comparison of visual acuity at 40 weeks PMA in initially neurologically normal and abnormal premature infants.

Figure 7.

130

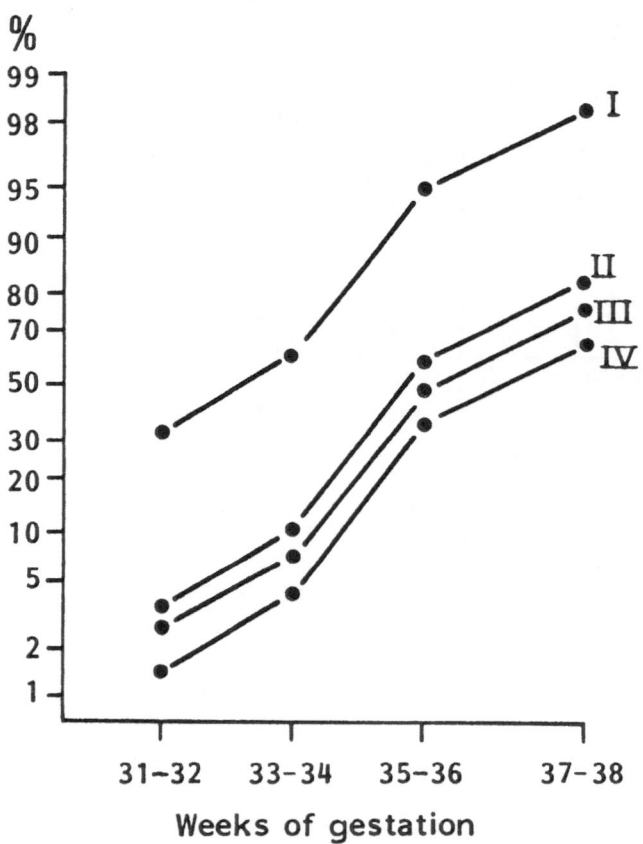

Figure 8. Graph showing percentage of VER records in which positive wave is present for normal infants (Group I) and neurologically abnormal infants (Groups II, III and IV).

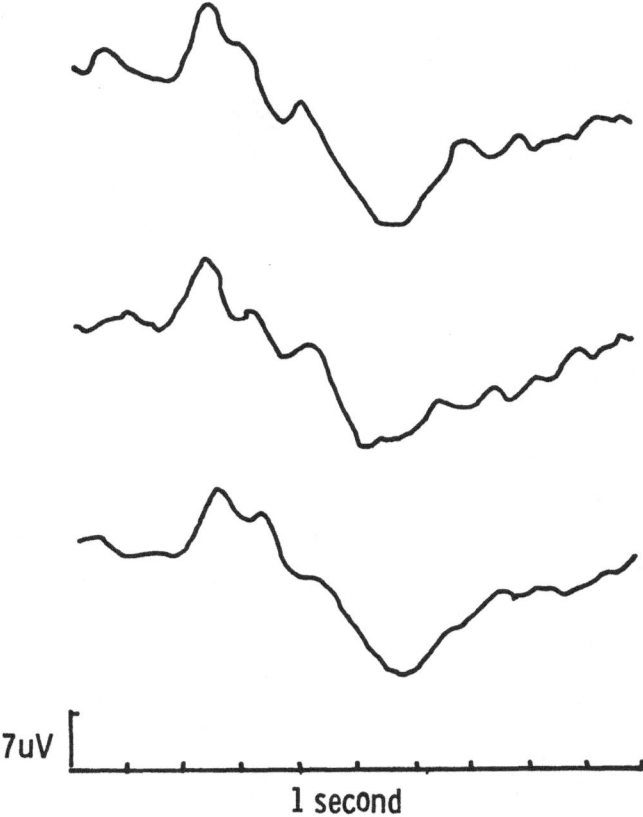

7uV

1 second

Figure 10.   VERs recorded from single electrode on inion in infant with
holoprosencephaly age 38 weeks PMA.

132

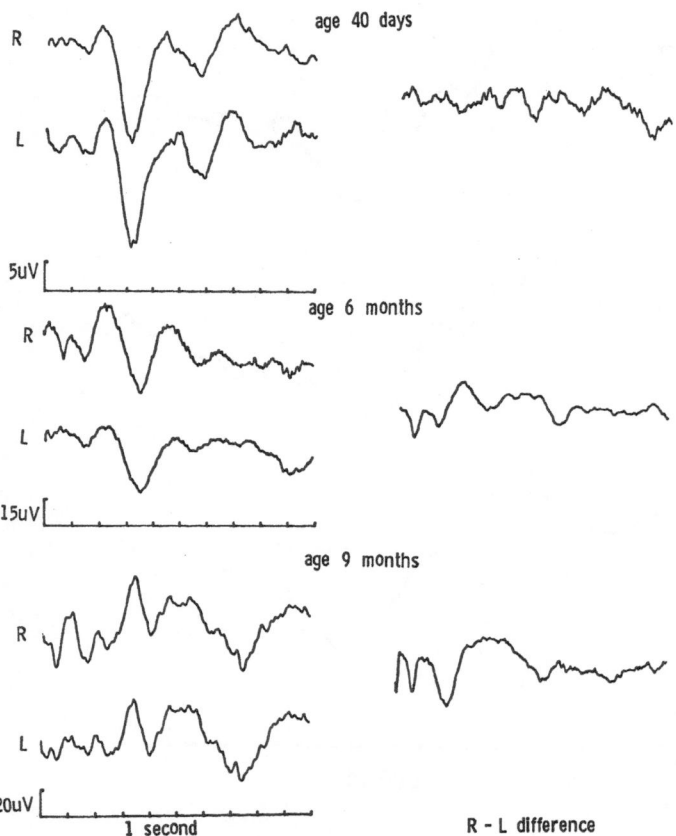

Figure 9. Bilateral VERs recorded from an infant with asymmetrical occipital dilatation as demonstrated by ultrasound scan. Initially symmetric, later asymmetric responses were recorded.

In our experience, vision appears to become cortical at around 44 to 48 weeks PMA. At this stage, infants with PVL who were able to track in the newborn period become cortically blind. The VER becomes asymmetrical in those infants with asymmetrical lesions.

Other investigators have described concurrent changes in the visual system at this time. There is a marked reduction in the latency of the flash VER between one and two months post term (Ellingson 1960); it becomes possible to elicit evidence of binocular stereopsis (Atkinson and Braddick 1985); a true pattern VER can be elicited (Marcus 1977), and acuity determined by the pattern VER begins to increase (Moskowitz and Sokol 1983).

These observations would suggest that there is a developmental shift in the physiological locus of control of infant visual function from a subcortical to a cortical locus over this age range (Hoffman 1978). This implies that the predictive value of early assessment of vision as a marker of higher neurological function is questionable.

REFERENCES

Atkinson J, Braddick O. Docum Ophthalmol Proc series. 1985, in press.

Barnet AB, Friedman SL, Weiss IP, Ohlrich ES, Shanks B, Lodge A. VEP development in infancy and early childhood: a longitudinal study. Electroenceph clin Neurophysiol 1980,49:476-489.

Blom JL, Barth PG, Visser SL. The visual evoked potential in the first six years of life. Electroenceph clin Neurophysiol 1980,48:395-405.

Brazelton TB. Neonatal Behavioural Assessment Scale. Clinics in Developmental Medicine, No.50. London: SIMP/Heinemann. Philadelphia: Lippincott. 1973.

Dubowitz LMS, Dubowitz V, Morante A, Verghote, M. Visual function in the preterm and full-term newborn infant. Develop Med Child Neurol 1980,22:465-475.

Dubowitz LMS, Bydder GM, Mushin J. Developmental sequence of periventricular leukomalacia. Arch Dis Child 1985,60:349-355.

Ellingson RJ. Cortical electrical responses to visual stimulation in the human infant. Electroenceph clin Neurophysiol 1960,12:663-677.

Fantz RL. Pattern vision in newborn infants. Science 1963,140:296-297.

Ferriss GS, Davis GD, Dorsen MM, Hackett ER. Changes in latency and form of the photically induced averaged evoked response in human infants. Electroenceph clin Neurophysiol 1967,22:305-312.

Hack M, Fantz RL, Fanaroff AA, Klaus MH. Neonatal pattern vision: a predictor of future mental performance. J Pediatr 1977,91:642-647.

Hoffman RF. Developmental changes in human infant visual evoked potentials to patterned stimuli recorded at different scalp locations. Child Develop 1978, 49:110-118.

Hrbek A, Karlberg P, Olsson T. Development of visual and somatosensory evoked responses in preterm newborn infants. Electroenceph clin Neurophysiol 1973, 34:225-232.

Levene MI, Williams JL, Fawer C-L. Ultrasound of the Infant Brain. Clinics in Developmental Medicine, No.92. Oxford: SIMP/Blackwell. Philadelphia: Lippincott. 1985.

Marcus MM. Visual evoked potentials to flash and pattern in normal and high risk infants. In: Desmedt JE, ed. Visual Evoked Potentials in Man: New Developments. Oxford: Clarendon Press, 1977:490-499.

Miranda SB. Visual abilities and pattern preferences of premature infants and full-term neonates. J Exper Child Psychol 1970,10:189-205.

Morante A, Dubowitz LMS, Levene M, Dubowitz V. The development of visual function in normal and neurologically abnormal preterm and fullterm infants. Develop Med Child Neurol 1982,24:771-784.

Moskowitz A, Sokol S. Developmental changes in the human visual system as reflected by the latency of the pattern reversal VEP. Electroenceph clin Neurophysiol 1983,56:1-15.

Mushin J, Hogg CR, Dubowitz LMS, Skouteli H, Arden GB. Visual evoked responses to LED photostimulation in newborn infants. Electroenceph clin Neurophysiol 1984,58:317-320.

Ordy JM, Udelf MS. Maturation of pattern vision in infants during the first six months. J Compar Physiol Psychol 1962,55:907-917.

Placzek M, Mushin J, Dubowitz LMS. Maturation of the visual evoked response and its correlation with visual acuity in neurologically normal and abnormal preterm infants. Develop Med Child Neurol 1985, in press.

Umezaki H, Morrell F. Development study of photic evoked responses in premature infants. Electroenceph clin Neurophysiol 1970,28:55-63.

Vassella F, Giambonine S, Heits B, Kaufman R, Kehrli P, Walti U. Development of visual discrimination (pattern preference) in normal infants. Helvet Paediat Acta 1977,32:319-329.

Watanabe K, Iwase K, Hara K. Maturation of visual evoked responses in low birthweight infants. Develop Med Child Neurol 1972,14:425-435.

DISCUSSION

Fielder: I am a little concerned. I don't want to disagree about whether the flash VEP is a cortical response or not. For example, I saw an infant with good visual function, but there appeared to be no occipital cortex on CT scan. We put the electrode anteriorly instead of the usual place and obtained a good VEP response. I am unhappy about correlating CT scan or ultrasound with visual function.

Arden: I think that is the point we are bringing out, that there are these measures of function, both psychophysical and electrophysiological, which may not correlate with the child's ultimate performance, and they don't predict whether or not the part of the brain we expect to test is even there or not.

Fielder: With respect, you use the word apparent, though in fact the child appeared to see and did see. You didn't give us pattern preference findings.

Atkinson: What do you use, when you say they are cortically blind? With those children have you tested them behaviourally, is that what you mean? Do they lose their visual response later on?

Dubowitz: Completely. They have definitely been seen by others and the diagnosis was not in fact made by us on these 3 children. They are all ophthalmological and they have been test behaviourally, up to 2 months we were able to get them to focus and then at about 6 months there was some doubt and after 6 months we got practically nothing.

Atkinson: That is very nice because it fits well with our data and is the rationale for us going over to using this orientation shift because we were very unhappy with the pattern appearance potentials being regarded as indicators of cortical vision.

Hyvarinen: Did the child not lose only cortical function or also midbrain function?

Dubowitz: Yes, apparently. After the child is 6 months old I refer to the ophthalmologists who, in the initial months, did not know the original diagnosis and this has been the diagnosis of all these children.

Mehdorn: How was the pupillary reaction in these patients? What was the state of the optic nerve?

Dubowitz: That was normal.

Mehdorn: I ask this question because many patients with porencephaly show optic atrophy.

Dubowitz: They have normal optic nerves.

Warburg: At what age please?

Dubowitz: The oldest of these is 18 months.

Harcourt: Are you wishing to use this as a general test, a prediction of
neurological function? I wonder whether you have compared the development
of the VER with the auditory evoked responses in the same children.
Auditory evoked responses are being used more as a general test. Do you
think visually evoked responses have more or less value in that sense?

Dubowitz: Our experience was mainly in premature infants. You cannot
predict neurologically what will happen to these children, whether children
who show initial delay are going to be the ones who have some abnormality
of visual function later, particular if they have difficulty in visual
scanning, difficulty with binocularity which is quite likely. These
children are not old enough to be tested for that, but that is one of the
aims of the project. But it has not predicted neurological abnormality in
gross terms. I think the same applies to the AVR because these children
with AVR get a 90% incidence of abnormal auditory evoked potentials.

Harcourt: But in your series did the results of the AVR pretty well fit in
with the results?

Dubowitz: We can't get all the results onto one collected result.

Spekreijse: They don't tell you much about the development of the visual
system. The best way is not to pay too much attention to the accuracy of
the timing, whether it is 10 seconds more or 20 seconds less, as long as
you make the recordings at the same time. With the pattern VEP, you can
have normal results at one month of age with normal peak latencies and
there you have a reflection from the primary visual cortex. It is only
later in children from the age of 3 or 4 months that you can see little
gratings riding on top of the components, the non-specific components are
evidence of the maturation of the visual system.

Dubowitz: Thank you very much for these comments, because we completely
agree with them. One of the interesting children was one who had quite a
marked difference in the negativity, but it was the early components that
were asymmetrical. It was the early components on which we noticed the
asymmetry and not on the large negative ones.

Braddick: I think we are using the word subcortical in two slightly
different senses. We may be referring to the wholly subvisual-cortical
pathway to midbrain centres or we can be talking about the earliest stages

in the geniculo-striate pathway. Presumably if we are looking at behaviour, that is being controlled by some route that doesn't actually involve the cortex. If we are looking at the evoked potential it could be contributed by geniculate neurons which are not actually getting to the cortex because the cortex is immature.

Arden: Apart from the difficulty in determing that (in children where we have made fragmentary recordings) the evidence is the way that their behaviour goes is with the evoked potentials and therefore I would suggest it likely that we are looking at something from the midbrain.

DEVELOPMENT OF SEPARATION-ABILITY OF CONTOURS DURING CHILD-
HOOD - QUANTIFICATION OF THE CROWDING PHENOMENON IN AMBLYOPIA.

Wolfgang Haase   Annemarie Hohmann

University Eyeclinic, Hamburg

The development of visual acuity in the first year of life has
been well documented (Atkinson, 1982; Dobson and Teller 1978),
likewise that over 4 years of age (Slataper, 1950; Oppel, 1964;
Frisén and Frisén 1981). The authors used either isolated symbols, such as optotypes from Snellen or Pflüger, or group presentations constructed along the Snellen principle. Gratings
are used to obtain measurements in infants. The acuities reported using these various technics do not differ much in the
normally developed visual system. Misleading good results can
be obtained in amblyopic patients when using gratings (Gstalder
and Green 1971). It was proposed by the international conference in Napels (1909) to use Landolt rings as the standard
test object. Even with the Landoltring the measured acuity can
vary, depending on the horizontal spacing between two rings.
Various authors observed a worsening of acuity when other contours were in the vacinity of a given test symbol - "crowding
phenomenon" (vom Hofe, 193 ; Irvine 1948; Müller 1951). Flom
and coworkers (1963) have quantitatively measured this contour
interaction effect.
Since then it has been demonstrated that contour interaction
also alters other visual functions, e.g. Vernier acuity (Westheimer and Hauske 1975), the orientation perception threshold
(Westheimer et al., 1976) and the stereo threshold (Butler and
Westheimer, 1978). Up till now visual acuity in cases of suspected amblyopia has been measured with single symbols or
Snellen charts. The latter is designed along the following
lines: The horizontal distance between two objects is proportional to their hight. We have found in some commercially
available near tests that the interspacing for large symbols
is over 30' of arc - which is beyond the contour interaction
zone, whereas interspacing in smaller types lies within this
zone.

METHODS
The following requirements need to be considered when developing a clinically useful "crowding"   test: The surround of
a single test type should be contour-free within 30 minutes of
arc because of the extension of the contour interaction (Flom
et al. 1963). If one wants to measure the contour interaction
or its pathologic exaggeration in amblyopia then the interspacing between two symbols has to be kept constant for all acuity values. That implies the Snellen principle cannot be applied.
The difference in acuity between single symbols and line symbols with constant interspacing is a quantitative measure of
crowding.

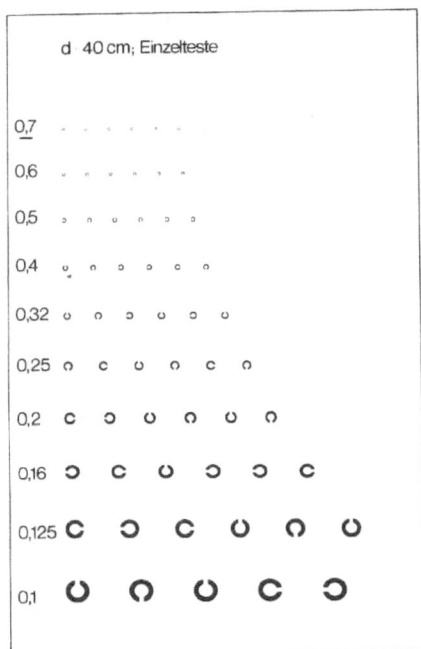

Fig. 1
C-Test - example of the
acuity values 0.7 to 0.1,
constant interspacing of
35' arc.
0.7 means an additional
value to the logarithmic
scale.

The acuity values run in decibel steps (Westheimer, 1979).
We have available testing charts for 5 meters, acuity steps
between 1.25 and 0.16. The near test (40 cm) includes steps
of acuity from 0.02 to 1,4. To not overtax children the Landoltrings are only orientated vertically or horizontally. We
presented 8 Landoltrings per line, 6 correct answers constituted the threshold. 80% of the children between 3 1/2 years
and 4 years of age were able to perform the test. The examiner points to the ring with a rod and asks: "Where is the
tyre broken? Where can a captured mouse escape from?"
The child should point its hand in the appropriate direction.
The individual symbol has to be pointed out because of the
homogenity of the chart.
The test which we have named "C-Test" is available from
OCULUS. We have examined 288 children in kindergartens and
schools. They had a complete ophthalmic examination (Retinoscopy, Ophthalmoscopy, binocular functions, Bagolini striated glasses and Titmus stereotest).
We also examined normal (n = 50) and organically determined
low vision (n = 23) adults with this test.

The amount of interspacing has to be determined. The maximal physiological contour interaction occurs when a neighbour contour appears within 2' - 3' arc (Flom et al., 1963). The contour interaction is hardly detectable for interspacing larger than 5 minutes. A test which is also capable to detect the "physiological crowding" must have line-optotypes with an interspacing of 2' - 3' arc. We used a chart with an interspacing of 2,6' arc. This interspacing is similar to that which appears in small newspaper print. The exaggerated contour interaction in amblyopia can be as great as 30' arc. We have developed another line optotype chart with an interspacing of 17,2' arc. To evaluate the extension of the individuals crowding zone. Technical reasons determined the unusual figure of 17,2' arc interspacing.

The complete test is comprised of 3 charts: a) The single Landoltring, separation approximately 35' arc. b) Line Landoltrings, separation 17,2' arc. c) Line Landoltrings, separation 2,6' arc. (Fig. 1, 2, 3).

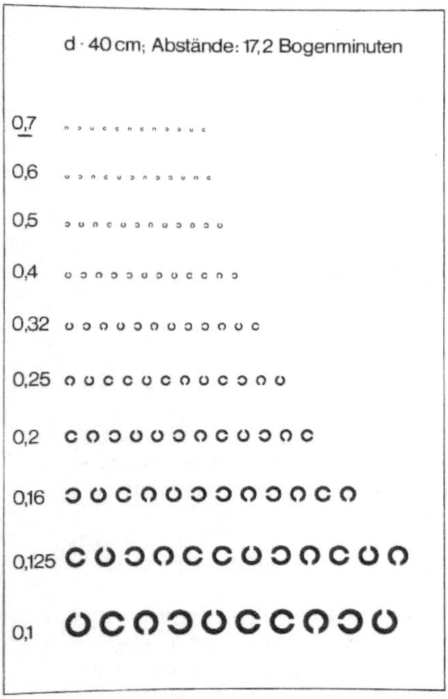

Fig. 2

C-Test - acuity values 0.7 to 0.1 with constant interspacing of 17.2' arc.

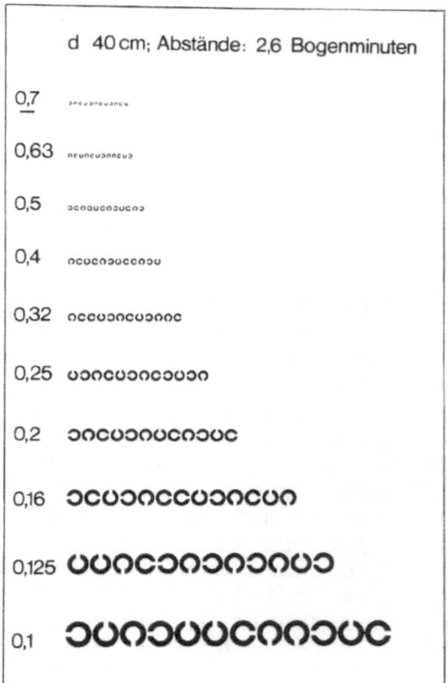

Fig. 3

C-Test - the interspacing between 2 symbols is kept constant through all values of acuity.

RESULTS

Visual acuity, as measured using isolated Landoltrings, has developed to 1.0 or better by the age of 5 years. This well known development is practically identical for line optotypes with the larger interspacing of 17.2' arc. In contrast we find acuity values in 4 years old children approximately 4 decibel levels lower when using the compacter line Landoltrings (2.6' interspacing). The acuity improves until the 11th year of life. It then resembles that of adults which, in the rule, is 1 - 2 levels below that of isolated Landoltrings (Fig.4). Even patients with organically based low vision show a difference not greater than 1 - 2 steps between isolated symbols and line symbols. Approximately 90% of amblyopes measured with the C-Test exhibit crowding. Both amblyopes with foveal fixation and those with eccentric fixation show the crowding phenomenon (Fig. 5,6). A clinical example will demonstrate the importance of a quantitative measurement of the crowding phenomenon in the course of therapy and the follow up period. (Fig. 7) A 7 year old child has beeing treated succesfully by occlusion and pleoptics. After the pleoptics period we ordered penalization and periodical occlusion. During a follow up period of 8 weeks the visual acuity with isolated symbols or Snellen charts remained on a high level of 0.8 - 0.9. The line acuity (2.6' interspacing) plunged down to 0.16.

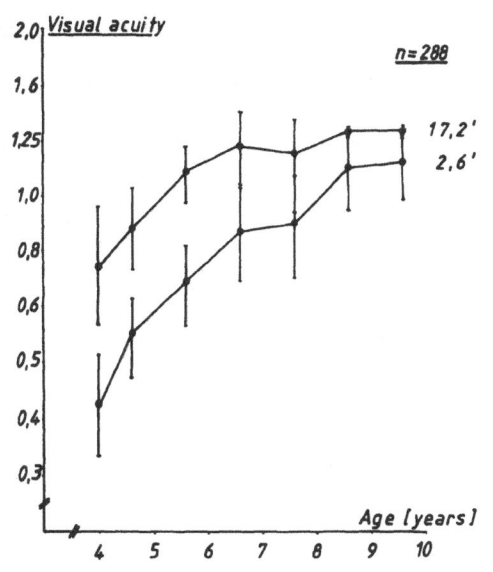

Fig.4

Normal development of visual acuity in childhood: 17.2' = C-Test measurements with symbols which are horizontally 17.2' arc (upper trace) or 2.6' arc (lower trace) apart from each other.
Each age group contains 25 children at minimum.

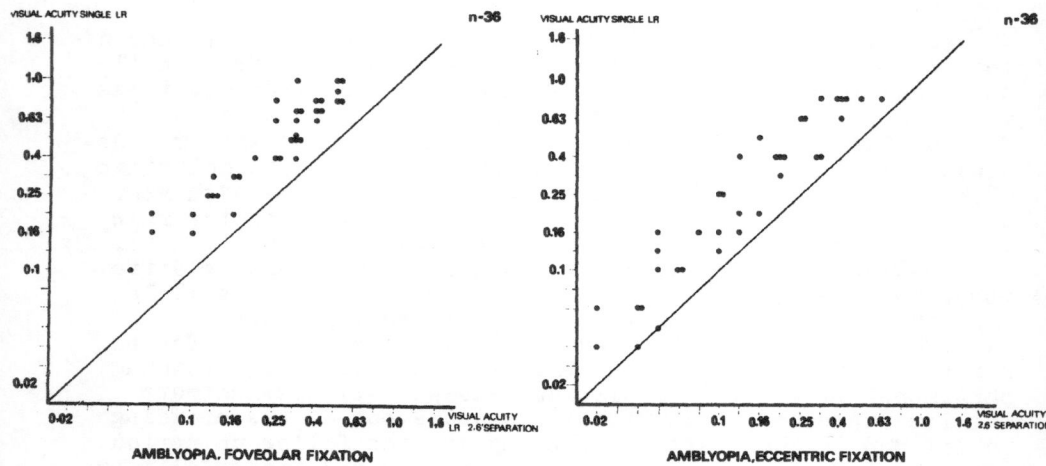

Fig. 5

visual acuity in amblyopic
patients with foveolar fixation.
C-Test: acuity values in
logarithmic steps (factor 1.2589),
abcissa: line Landolt rings
horizontally separated 2.6' of
arc, ordinate: isolated Landolt
rings. The majority (89 %) of
the patients show crowding of
more than 1 step of acuity.

Fig. 6

C-Test - visual acuity in
patients with eccentric fixation.
Abcissa and ordinate as in Fig. 5.

Fig. 7

Course of treatment in a 7 years
old child. Single Landolt ring
acuity tends to gain a too good
result. A masked crowding remain

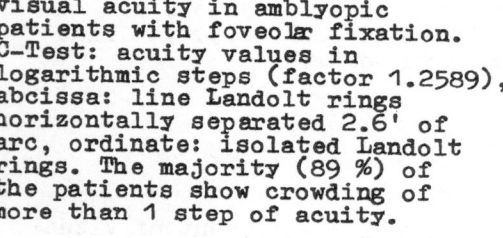

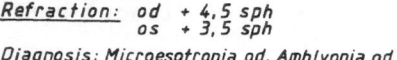

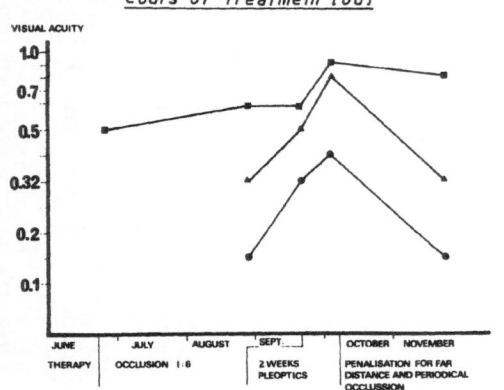

DISCUSSION

Irvine (1948) was the first author who described the crowding phenomenon in amblyopes in a more detailed way. Flom and his coworkers (1963) measured this phenomenon quantitatively, they also showed the extension of the effect up to approximately 30' arc. around a symbol. Despite the clinical importance of crowding, a practically applicable test had not been developed. The so called "C-Test" (Hohmann und Haase 1982; Haase und Hohmann 1982) is based on the findings of Flom et al. (1963): The symbol is the Landoltring. We do not want to examine higher visual functions e. g. reading ability but visual acuity. The crucial point in the C-Test is the comparison of the visual acuity with single Landoltrings with Landoltrings in a horizontal line with constant interspacing through all steps of acuity values. The difference between both acuities shows the quantity of crowding. As we found in children between 4 years and 11 years of age the ability to separate contours is not yet well developed when they enter school at the age of approximately 6 years. Some of the difficulties which many children have during their first attempts to learn to read may be based on "physiological crowding". The lower line-acuity in preschool children has to be taken into account for differentiation of normal visual status and amblyopia. The majority of amblyopic patients exhibit crowding (90%). The phenomenon seems to depend on the case history: During treatment the visual acuity with isolated symbols increases first, the line acuity follows with variable delay. Beside this treatment effect even amblyopes who have never been treated show crowding (Thomas - Decortis, 1959). We examined different etiological groups of amblyopia - squint-,ametropic-, anisometropic- and early deprivation amblyopia - all reached higher visual acuity with single optotypes than with narrow neighboured symbols. The phenomenon appears independent of the fixation pattern. The reliability of the C-Test for the detection of amblyopia seems to reach about 90%.

144

References

Atkinson J.
Braddick O.
: Assessment of Visual acuity in infancy
and early childhood
Acta Ophthalmologica (Copenhagen)
1983; Supplement 157: 18 - 26

Butler T.W.
Westheimer G.
: Interference with stereoscopic acuity:
spatial, temporal and disparity tuning.
Vision Res. 1978; 18: 1387 - 1392

Dobson V.
Teller D.Y.
: Visual acuity in human infants: A review
and comparison of behavioural and electro-
physiological studies
Vision Res. 1978; 18 : 1469 - 1483

Flom M.L.
Weymouth F.W.
Kahnemann D.
: Visual resolution and contour interaction
J. Opt. Soc. Amer. 1963; 53 : 1026 - 1032

Frisén L.
Frisén M.
: How good is normal visual acuity ?
Albrecht v. Graefes Arch. klin. exp.
Ophthalmol. 1981; 215 : 149 - 157

Gstalter R.J.
Green D.G.
: Laser interferometer acuity in amblyopia
J. Ped. Ophthalmol. 1971; 8 : 251 - 256

Haase W.
Hohmann A.
: Ein neuer Test (C-Test) zur quantita-
tiven Messung der Trennschwierigkeiten
("crowding") - Ergebnisse bei Amblyopie
und Ametropie
Klin.Mbl.Augenheilk. 1982; 180 : 210 -
215

Hohmann A.
Haase W.
: Development of visual line acuity in
humans
Ophthalmic Res. 1982; 14 : 107 - 112

vom Hofe K.
: Untersuchungen über das Sehen in Fällen
von Schielamblyopie
Klin.Mbl.Augenheilk. 1930; 85 : 79 - 80

Irvine R.A.
: Amblyopia ex anopsia
Trans.Amer.Ophthalmol.Soc. 1948; 46:
527 - 575

Müller P.
: Über das Sehen der Amblyopen
Ophthalmologica 1951; 121 : 143 - 149

Oppel O.
: Über die Entwicklung der Sehschärfe bei
Kindern in Vorschulalter
Klin.Mbl.Augenheilk. 1964; 145 : 358 -
371

Slataper F.J.   :   Age norms of refraction and vision
                           Arch.Ophthalmol. 1950; 43 : 466 -481

Thomas-Decortis G.   :   Acuité visuelle angulaire et acuité
                           visuelle morphoscopique dans l´ am-
                           blyopie ex anopsia
                           Bull.Soc.Belge Ophthalmol. 1959
                           123 : 488 - 499

Westheimer G.   :   Interference with line orientation
Shimamura K.   sensitivity
Mc. Kee S.P.   J.Opt.Soc.Amer. 1976; 66 : 332 - 338

Westheimer G.   :   Temporal and spatial interference with
Hauske G.   Vernier - acuity
                           Vision Res. 1975; 15 : 1137 - 1141

MEASUREMENT OF VISUAL ACUITY IN YOUNG
CHILDREN BY A NEW INSTRUMRNT : CASIMIR

M. LOULY - ORTHOPTIST - CLINIC OF OPHTHALMOLOGY - CHR of LILLE
S. FOSSATI, H. RAMES, N. PHANN & J.C. HACHE (LILLE)

We are all aware of the great progress that has been achieved since the application of computer techniques to our investigation methods. In conjunction and close collaboration with the Lille laboratory of vision RAMES and PHANN from Essilor International have developed an automated device for measurement of central visual acuity in kindergarten or nursery school children based on the Sheridan Gardiner matching method. 484 children have been tested by one of our orthoptists, Mrs FOSSATI, who has devoted her time to mass screening and detection of visual impairment in these children over the past few years.

Casimir is different from the usual distant acuity chart.By simply changing of floppy disk the contents can be modified.

- A wide range of exams are offered (different tests, presentation), 54 in all.
- Optotypes in a given size are selected and displayed randomly eliminating memorization.

It introduces a new form of visual acuity measurement: the fuzzy sets theory.

Casimir can be used:

- either for automated testing (in this case the child's responses determine the choice of the following tests)
- or manually as an ordinary distant visual chart, yet storing the results.

For a correct response the child is rewarded with a little music or the projection of a movie on the monitor screen.

The child's responses are processed.

In brief, Casimir saves the previous data, computes, stores and gives the results which can be displayed on request.

MATERIAL and METHODS
A - Material

Casimir is mainly a microcomputer with its peripherals, built for easy manipulation and transportation featuring 2 packages:

1° - The microcomputer : a compact machine which already includes some peripherals (2 disk storage units) a

DETAILS OF CASIMIR

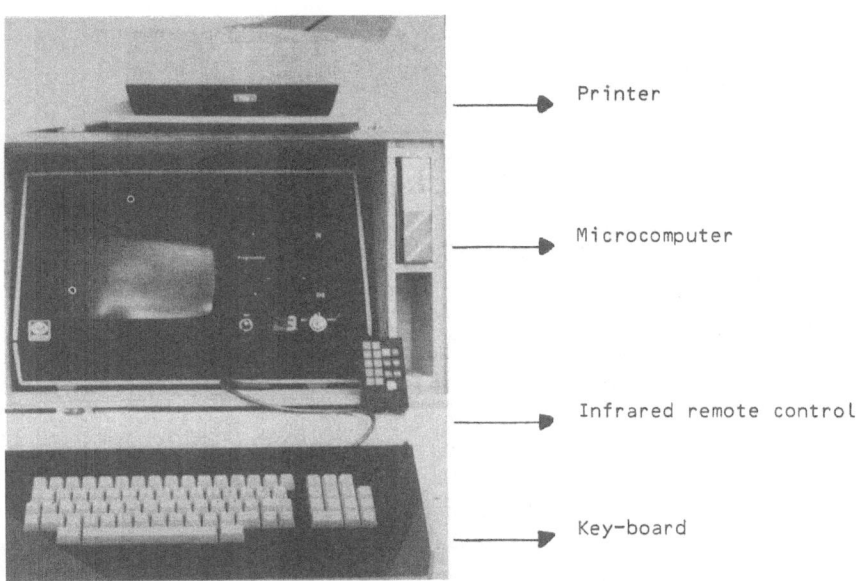

→ Printer

→ Microcomputer

→ Infrared remote control

→ Key-board

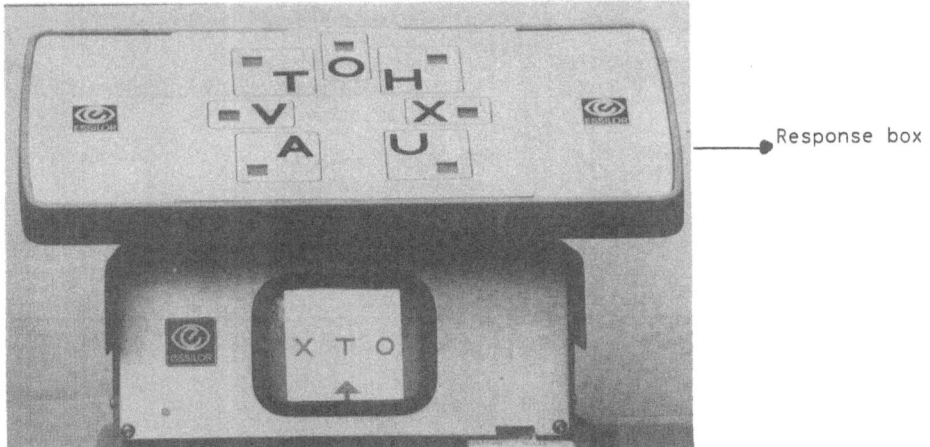

Response box

Television monitor with matching tests

TV display screen, an alpha numeric key-board & new
diskettes storage

2° - The peripherals, fixed in a second case including:

- the response-box,
- the printer,
- the television monitor to display the tests
- the infrared remote control which executes the
  orders and allows the examiner free movement.

Response box
The microcomputer displays visual acuity targets on a
television monitor situated at 2m 50 (8 feet) from the child
seated in front of the response box. The response box has 8
large buttons corresponding to the randomly projected tests.
The child matches the tests by pressing on the appropriate
button.

The response generates:

- The projection of the following test (except in the
  manual procedure or at the end of the examination).
- A reward in case of a correct response
- The result if the examination is over

B - Procedure and methods
Visual acuity targets
These can be displayed under the following conditions:

Number	Parameter	Choice
1	Contrast	1 Black targets - white background 2 White targets - Black background
2	Presentation	1 Isolated 2 Horizontally grouped targets 3 Vertically grouped targets
3	Test	1 Snellen E 2 Sheridan matching letters 3 Dor images
4	Strategy	1 Manual 2 Increasing progressively) (20/100 20/20)Auto- 3 Fussy sets theory)mated
5	Adaptation phase	1 Yes

1 target can only be displayed for low acuities (20/200 -
20/100)

3 targets up to 20/60

5 targets over 20/50

The index can be dimmed by remote control.

STRATEGY

Obviously the child will need some explanation; so it is highly recommended to begin with a pre\,miminary adaption phase (include the following parameters: targets, contrast, presentation) using a large target (20/30)

A - Manual procedure

The examiner determines the value of acuities to be presented by using a remote control. To store the results, he must calculate the responses before entering the final result.

B - Automated procedure
.Progressively increasing type

Can be initiated either at 1/10 (22/100) or at the acuity evaluated during the previous testing. If all responses are correct, the size of targets increase progressively. For an incorrect response, the same optotype is projected once again. After two mistakes, the lower size target is displayed. The following conditions stop the examination:

- no mistakes
- 2 successive correct responses, 2 incorrect responses at the superior target size
- for each target size, 3 presentations are permitted.

.Fuzzy sets theory

In this system the child's responses are not considered as absolutely accurate. The graph of probability of perception of the displayed tests is modified according to the child's responses.

A correct response increases the probability of perception of the tests having a bigger size than that presented.

An incorrect response decreases the probability of perception of the tests of smaller size than that presented.

The examination stops when there is a low incertitude on the child's visual acuity.

This technique is faster than the progressively increasing method and has, above all, the great advantage of tolerating the child's errors.

OUR FINDINGS
. Comparative Study

* 484 Children have been screened with Casimir
  148 Chiildren aged 5 years or more
  223 Children from 4 to 5 years of age
  113 Children from 3,6 to 4 years of age

* only 338 out of the 484 children tested figure in our statistical study of acceptability
* only 212 have undergone both Casimir and ROSSANO/WEISS standard symbol chart.

150

I - For CASIMIR
   - Age and acceptability

Between 2,6 and 3   years 75 %
        3   and 3,6   years 95 %
        3,6 and 4   years 97,3 %   3 exams : impossible
        4   and 4,6   years 97,8 %   3 exams : difficult
        4,6 and 5   years 100 %   Refusal = 6/338 = 1,7 %
        5   and 5,6   years 97,4 %
        5,6 and 6   years 100 %

                Acceptability = 98,3 %

   - Test acceptability

.DOR test prefered by 8 children out of 338

Between 2,6 and 3   years 50 %= 2 children
        3   and 3,6 years 20 %= 4 children   Refusal=8/338=2 %
        3,6 and 4   years 2,7 %= 1 child
        4   and 4,6 years 1,1 %= 1 child

.SNELLEN E prefered to SHERIDAN letters : 1 child

.SHERIDAN prefered to SNELLEN E

Between 4   and 4,6 years 3,3 %= 3 children
        4,6 and 5   years 1,7 %= 1 child

In brief, .SHERIDAN has been accepted by 98%
          .DOR has been prefered by   25% age ranging from
                                         to 2,6 and 3,6 years
          .SNELLEN is not accepted better

          - Presentation and acceptability
.Isolated test prefered

Between 4   and 4,6 years 5,6 %= 5 children
        4,6 and 5   years 3,5 %= 2 children
        5   and 5,6 years 1,3 %= 1 child

II - For ROSSANO/WEISS
          Standard symbol chart

          - Age and acceptability

Between 2,6 and 3   years 50 %
        3   and 3,6   years 66 %
        3,6 and 4   years 86 %   9 exams : impossible
        4   and 4,6   years 95 %   5 exams : difficult
        4,6 and 5   years 93 %
        5   and 5,6   years 96 %
        5   and 6   years 100 %

                Acceptability = 93,4 %

III - CASIMIR versus WEISS

Out of 212 children tested with both methods:

Casimir = 1 difficult exam between 4 and 4,6 years
1 difficult exam between 5 and 5,6 years
(but Weiss accepted)
1 refusal Casimir (or Weiss)

Readily accepted by all the others

Weiss = 5 difficult exams
9 refusal

Refusal
1 child refuses either method
1 child refuses Casimir but accepts Weiss
9 children refuse Weiss but accept Casimir
201 children accept either method

CONCLUSIONS

Obviously the most important thing is to detect visual impairment as early as possible; any method available is welcomed in this case.

Computerized techniques nowadays offer so much more accurate possibilities that we cannot ignore them if we want to progress in this field.

We tried to find here an attractive yet very scientific procedure to test children and children definitely appreciated "playing" with Casimir.

In practice, the average age of acceptability of the instrument can be situated around 36 months, but the use of an isolated test can sometimes allow screening of younger children.
In the future, this prototype will be reduced to a portable all built-in system not exceeding the size of the actual monitor.

Key-words : Visual screening
Children's acuity
Automated measurement
Fuzzy sets theory

DISCUSSION

Dubowitz: Can I ask you how much it costs?

Louly: It is a prototype.

Hache: We use it for testing our method, and for measuring and verifying the usefulness of responses, but it is a prototype.

Dubowitz: The accuracy compared with the Sheridan-Gardiner test is 80%. I have been using the Sheridan test for several years and it costs about £5.

Louly: I think it is only that they play much more easily and they give a response.

Hache: We have also used the Sheridan test, but in school this equipment is very useful and all results are printed immediately.

Warburg: So that you can keep them and put them into the child's case history?

Spekreijse: When we compared the acuity estimates from VEPs, there was very good correlation in children between the ages of 3 to 4.5 years and then the subjective test was slightly lower than the objective test. Don't young children have more difficulty with the task and therefore they are underestimating their own ability?

Haase: I think it is indeed so, because the results I showed in normals were first examination results in kindergartens. When we compared the results of our children in our office who we see more often, we can compare the results for the good eyes in amblyopes and the results are just the same or sometimes one line different.

Warburg: But isn't that the usual finding in visual acuity testing? Isn't it so that when testing visual acuity you cannot expect more than a 50% correlation, so that your children are actually performing better than what we usually find?

Haase: What do you mean?

Warburg: I mean if we test and retest children and get a certain visual acuity by repeated testing we may as well get one line above or one line below. The chance of getting the same result is only 50%, and you are telling us that your correlation is closer.

Haase: Yes, it is indeed, maybe one line worse on repeated examinations, but this is true for line acuity and for single type acuity. When you have a second or third examination they show a pseudo-increase of one line.

Atkinson: One way you might be able to check your data to see whether a cognitive problem of understanding or spatial confusion is coming into it, is to compare the accuracy of doing top/bottom with left/right, because there is a lot more confusion in left/right than there is with saying "it is the top or the bottom." Have you looked at your error scores to see whether there is any difference between these two? Because if there is, it would suggest that there is some spatial confusion occurring, particularly with these younger children.

Haase: Yes we did, and in addition we also examined in a vertical line where there is less crowding than in a horizontal line. What you mean is there is a difference between the vertical gap and the horizontal gap.

Atkinson: I mean that top/bottom is an easier combination than left/right for children.

Harcourt: What effect do you think using a pointer to point out the symbols makes? If you use the Sheridan-Gardiner test for instance and match linear against single optotypes, trying to show a difference between the two eyes, once you are pointing to the letter the whole confusion system breaks down and you get much better results, so that there is a difference between asking children to select symbols either vertically or horizontally out of a line without pointing to them and doing it with pointing. You are doing it all the time with pointing.

Haase: Yes, without pointing it would be impossible to remain objective and they become absolutely confused.

Harcourt: But for instance if you do projecto-type where you can take out a line of say 5 in a row either vertically or horizontally because there are not so many symbols that confuse, perceptive confusion is less. When they are faced with a whole long line of random symbols that touch each other it is extremely confusing. I just wonder what the general feeling is about what effect confusion in pointing out the symbols makes.

Mehdorn: We routinely use the Haase-test, and we often find a lot of crowding even with pointing. There may be a marked difference between visual acuity measured with single optotypes and measured with the Haase-test. So I think that pointing at the symbols does not substantially affect the results.

EVALUATION OF ELECTRODIAGNOSTIC TESTS IN CHILDREN.

G.van Lith and S.Vijfvinkel

Eye Hospital,Erasmus University,Rotterdam

In the context of this meeting, results of 6 years electrodiagnostic examination· of children in their preverbal age will be presented rather than an overview of all methods that can be used in children or of results that can be obtained in various diseases. A recent and excellent review has been written by Carr (1983) in Harley's textbook Pediatric Ophthalmology.

The children, examined by us, were referred by our own out-patients department as well as by ophthalmologists outside the hospital for 3 main reasons. These are:
- Diagnosis or confirmation of a suspected diagnosis when generalized retinal abnormalities or pale discs are seen;
- Detection of possible abnormalities and functional assessment when dense medial opacities prevent proper fundus examination; in these instances electrodiagnostics are usually combined with sonography;
- Functional assessment when an abnormality in the fundus is seen and known or when a suspected low vision cannot be explained after fundus examination.

Age	0 - 1 yrs.	1 - 4 yrs.
Diagnosis	18	54
Medial Opacity	24	15
Visual Function	64	46
Unknown	2	1
Total	108	116

Table 1: Number of children referred for electro-physiological examination, subdivided into a group below the first year and a group between 1 and 4 years. Reasons of referral were: diagnostic problems, diagnostics and functional assessment in medial opacities or functional assessment per se.

The distribution of these 3 groups is presented in table 1, subdivided into children before their first year, the babies, and those between their first and fourth year.
The babies often had severe pathology, like general retinal pigment

.dystrophies, white discs or vitreous opacities with retrolental fibroplasia. They are commonly referred at a 3-4 month age, when the parents
are in doubt whether their child can see or not.
In the older age group many mentally retarded children with normal fundi
were seen. More often the main question in this group was how much the
child could see and whether pathology of the visual pathways or at the
cortical level could be spotted.

The examinations were carried out without sedation. Before the mid-
seventies we were used to apply general anesthesia. For various reasons,
however, we changed our strategy, one of the main being that anesthetics
may cause a decrease of the evoked potentials. Nowadays we discuss after
examination without general anesthetics:
- whether examinations under general anesthesia can provide additional
  information;
- whether additional information is needed to solve the child's problem
  or that of the parents;
- whether it is compulsory to solve the problem, at that very moment,
  realizing that most abnormalities seen by us cannot be cured and
  information needed for further help or for education can gradually be
  discovered during early childhood.

Concerning these aspects, our thoughts were always shared with the parents,
who often proposed themselves to abstain from further examination. When
general anesthesia was applied, it was generally done for other reasons too,
such as sonography, careful slit-lamp or fundus examination.

The ERG-potentials were led off with skin electrodes when contact lens
electrodes were not accepted. This makes the signal to noise ratio and
consequently the detection power of the test lower, but this of course
is only a problem when no response is seen. The common place for a skin
electrode is the margin of the lower eyelid. It produces responses of
approximately 25% of the contact lens values.
In babies we often used an electrode on the nose-bridge, revealing 10%
responses. We experienced the golden foil electrode (Arden et al. 1979)
as well as the DTL electrode (Dawson et al. 1979) as less succesful in
these children.
The occipital potentials (EPs) were registered via electrodes in the
midline 2 and 4 cm above the inion referential to an electrode at the
earlobe.

Age	0 - 1 yrs.		1 - 4 yrs.	
Result	+	–	+	–
ERG	86	16	66	11
Lum.EP	96	10	75	2
Patt.EP	2	2	41	3

Table 2: Results of ERG, luminance evoked potentials
and pattern evoked potentials. A plus sign indicates
that the recordings could be measured or assessed; a
minus sign that reasonable results could not be
obtained.

Analyzing our results, the first question we were faced with was how often
reasonable recordings were obtained in our clinical setting, implying not

.more than that the recordings could be measured and assessed. From the results of table 2 it appears that this could not be done in more than 10 per cent of the luminance responses in the baby-group.
Pattern-responses were hardly performed in this group.
Better scores are seen in the luminance and pattern evoked potentials in the older age group.

Age	0 - 1 yrs.	1 - 4 yrs.
Positive	13	38
Doubtful	5	16

Table 3: Number of children with a positive or doubtful contribution of the electrical recordings to the diagnosis.

The next questions we looked for were, how often the electrophysiological results contributed to the diagnosis (table 3), were helpful for decision making in case of medial opacities (table 4) or could provide reasonable information concerning visual function (table 5).

Contribution to the diagnosis was doubtful (table 3) in more than one third of the number of children in both age groups. The negative results usually concerned 'no' visible abnormalities or possible abnormalities of the visual pathways as indicated by pallor of the optic discs. Apparently, luminance evoked potentials are not always clearly abnormal in these instances, even when visual functions are lowered. Reversely in children with a doubtful retinal disorder, electrodiagnostics could generally provide a positive contribution to the diagnosis. The reason very probably is that mostly the ERG is clearly disturbed in retinal abnormalities except for macular diseases, which however are not common in these age groups.

Age	0 - 1 yrs.	1 - 4 yrs.
Positive	21	14
Doubtful	3	1

Table 4: Number of children with a positive or doubtful contribution of the electrical recordings to the decision in medial opacities.

Better results than in the diagnostics group were seen in the medial opacity group (table 4), the results being doubtful in approximately 10 per cent of the patients.
In congenital cataract retinal and occipital eletric responses were generally good, in vitreous pathology often disturbed.

		Normal	Disturbed	Absent	Failed
ERG	0 - 1 yrs.	44	5	8	5
	1 - 4 yrs.	21	2	4	2
Lum. EP	0 - 1 yrs.	44	2	13	3
	1 - 4 yrs.	23	5	3	0
Patt. EP	0 - 1 yrs.	0	0	0	0
	1 - 4 yrs.	10	4	4	2

Table 5: Results of ERG, luminance EPs and pattern EPs in children with presumed disturbed visual functions.

An interesting group, especially in comparison with other studies at this meeting, is the group of the functional assesment (table 5). For this interest, the number of failures in obtaining reasonable results are provided for this group separately. Most remarkable in this group is the high number of normal results. Mainly it concerned seriously mentally retarded children with normal media and fundi, suspected of low vision. An explanation for the normal results very probably is that in these children abnormalities are beyond the level, where we measure the evoked potentials, for example , when defects are situated in the high visual centres or even in the memory.
At any rate luminance EPs appeared to be not refined enough to assess visual function in this group. Whether pattern EPs can provide reliable and fruitful information in these children is rather doubtful.
From examination of adults we know that in our set-up detectable luminance EPs under photopic conditions generally point to a visual acuity higher than 0.1, but that there are exceptions dependent on the diagnosis. This is even more so for pattern EPs. For example in demyelinating diseases and compressive lesions these responses are relatively more disturbed than visual acuity, whereas in atrophies and defects often the reverse is seen. Results, therefore, has to be interpreted with caution, both when they are good or non-detectable (van Lith, 1980).

The main conclusions of this evaluation are:
- Electrophysiological examinations of children in the preverbal age has to be applied and assessed with reserve;
- Results are more fruitful in diagnostic problems rather than in functional assessment;
- As yet electrodiagnostics are more profitable in retinal diasorders than in abnormalities of the visual pathways or of the visual centres;
- In combination with sonography, electrodiagnostics are helpful in medial opacities;
- Functional assessment often fails, very probably due to abnormalities situated beyond the level of the origin of the evoked potentials; this can be expected in mentally retarded children;
- Furthermore, it has to be in mind that in general dependent on the nature and the location of an abnormality, the electrophysiological potentials may be more or less disturbed compared to psychophysical results.

158

REFERENCES

G.B. Arden, R.M.Carter, C.Hogg, I.M.Siegel. A gold foil electrode:
extending the horizons for clinical electroretinography. Inv.Ophthal.
and Vis.Science. Vol 18, No.4, pp 421-426, april 1979

R.E.Carr. Electrodiagnostic tests of the retina and higher centers.
Harley's textbook: Pediatric Ophthalmology, pp 189-207, 1983

W.W.Dawson, G.L.Trick, C.A.Litzkow. Improved electrode for electroretinography. Inv. Ophthal. and Vis. Science. Vol 18, No.9,pp 988-991,
september 1979.

G.H.M. van Lith. The application of visually evoked cerebral potentials
in ophthalmological diagnosis. Clin.Neurol.Neurosurgery. Vol 82-2,
85-91, 1980.

THE PATTERN REVERSAL ERG AND ITS APPLICATION TO THE MEASUREMENT OF INFANT VISUAL ACUITY

Adriana Fiorentini and Lamberto Maffei

Istituto di Neurofisiologia del C.N.R., Pisa, Italy

The pattern reversal ERG in monkeys after section of the optic nerve.

Evidence derived from experiments in cats in which one optic nerve had been sectioned intracranially (Maffei & Fiorentini 1981, 1982; Holländer et al 1984) showed that the steady-state pattern ERG (ERG in response to gratings reversed in phase at 8Hz, 16 rev/sec) is severely affected and eventually disappears following retrograde ganglion cell degeneration, while the ERG in response to flashes of diffuse light is unaffected. This finding indicating that in the cat integrity of ganglion cells is necessary for generating a normal ERG response to gratings has important implications for humans: the pattern ERG may become an important diagnostic tool to signal ganglion cell dysfunctions.

Recently this findings has been extended to the monkey (Maffei et al, in press). The right optic nerve was sectioned intracranially in 3 adult monkeys (Macaca nemestrina) and ERG responses were recorded from the anaesthetized (Ketamine) and paralyzed animals (Pancuronium bromide) at various times after surgery. The experimental procedure was the same as previously used in the cat (Maffei & Fiorentini 1981, 1982). The stimuli were sinusoidal gratings of various spatial frequencies, (contrast 55%, mean luminance 100 cd/m^2). The stimulus subtended 30° X 20° or 15° X 10° to the eye.

The ERG responses to alternating gratings in the monkey, as in man and cat, have an approximately sinusoidal waveform with a temporal frequency corresponding to the second harmonic of the stimulus. For a fixed contrast of the grating the response amplitude is a function of the spatial frequency, with a peak around 3-4 c/deg, similarly to what has been reported for humans (Hess & Baker 1984).

The results obtained in monkeys with intracranial section of the optic nerve show that the ERG response to phase reversal gratings is considerably reduced in amplitude already 10 days after the section. Three weeks after the section, a response can be obtained only at intermediate spatial frequencies, but its amplitude is much smaller in comparison with the normal eye response. Five weeks after optic-nerve

160

section the ERG in response to gratings is down to noise
level. The ERG responses to diffuse retinal illumination are
unaltered: their amplitude is comparable in the two eyes (Fig
1).

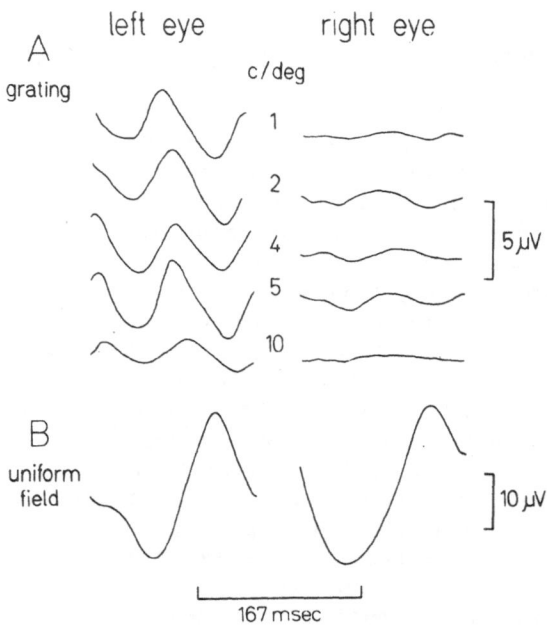

Fig 1,A - ERG responses to sinusoidal gratings of various
spatial frequencies reversal in phase at 6 Hz (12 rev/sec)
recorded from the two eyes of a monkey the right optic nerve
of which had been transected intracranially 3 weeks before the
recording session. Records averaged over 300 to 600 stimulus
sweeps. Grating contrast 55%, mean luminance 100 cd/m^2. B: ERG
responses to uniform field sinusoidal modulation (6Hz) of the
same display used in A. Records averaged over 20 stimulus
periods.

Histological examination of whole mounted retinas of two
monkeys sacrificed 6 and 8 weeks respectively, after right
optic nerve section showed in the right retina a severe
degeneration, ganglion cells loss and glial reaction. The
degeneration was present in the whole retina, but particularly
pronounced in the temporal hemiretina.
These findings are in line with those previously obtained

in the cat, in that they show that ganglion cell degeneration is accompanied by the impairment of the steady-state ERG response to phase-reversal gratings. Since circular disturbances can be excluded in our preparation, the reduction in grating ERG responses has to be interpreted as a consequence of ganglion cell degeneration or dysfunction.

The results on the monkey are particularly important in view of the application to humans, because of the similarity between the human and monkey retina.

In particular it is of interest that in the monkey the impairment of the pattern ERG is observable much earlier after transection of the optic nerve than in the cat. One would expect that the amplitude of the ERG in response to phase-reversal grating may be altered quite early in human patients following traumatic or inflammatory alterations of the optic nerve. Cases supporting this expectation have recently been reported.

Retinal acuity in infants evaluated with the pattern ERG

Although the exact location of the retinal sources of the pattern ERG is still unknown, the activity of retinal cells with center surround organization is likely to play a role in the generation of the pattern ERG. And indeed, the amplitude of the steady-state ERG respose to phase-reversal gratings of moderate contrast decreases at spatial frequencies below 2-4 c/d.

An interesting question is whether this retinal response reflects the limits of spatial resolution of the retina. In the adult, the amplitude of the steady-state (6Hz) ERG in response to gratings of high contrast decreases progressively with increasing spatial frequency and falls to noise level for spatial frequencies around 20-25 c/deg. The subjective acuity is around 30-35 c/deg at this temporal frequency of reversal. The acuity extrapolated from cortical visual evoked potentials (VEP) is close to the subjective acuity. This is not surprising since the ERG has a smaller signal-to-noise ratio than the VEP.

We have used the pattern ERG to evaluate the development of spatial resolution of human infants at a retinal level and to compare it to the development of acuity evaluated from the pattern VEP (Fiorentini et al 1984).

The stimuli were sinusoidal gratings of high contrast reversed in phase at 6Hz (12 rev/sec). The ERG was recorded with a silver wire electrode applied externally on the lower eyelid. To minimize interference with VEP's the reference electrode was set on the lower eyelid of the non-recording eye, that was patched. Details of the experimental procedure are given elsewhere (Fiorentini et al 1984).

162

Data were obtained from 9 infants, 7 weeks to 6 months old. In each infant ERG and VEP were recorded simultaneously. Records were taken at a few spatial frequencies (usually 3 to 4) covering a range of at least one octave. ERG and VEP acuities were evaluated by (linear) interpolation with reference to noise level. The latter was obtained from ERG and VEP recorded while the grating was replaced by a homogeneous, steadily illuminated field.

The data show that ERG acuity increases from about 2-3 c/deg at 7-8 weeks of age to 10-12 c/deg at 5-6 months (Fig 2). The increase in ERG acuity with age parallels the improvement in VEP acuity, indicating that the morphological and/or functional maturation at sites beyond the retina proceed in parallel with the development of retinal acuity.

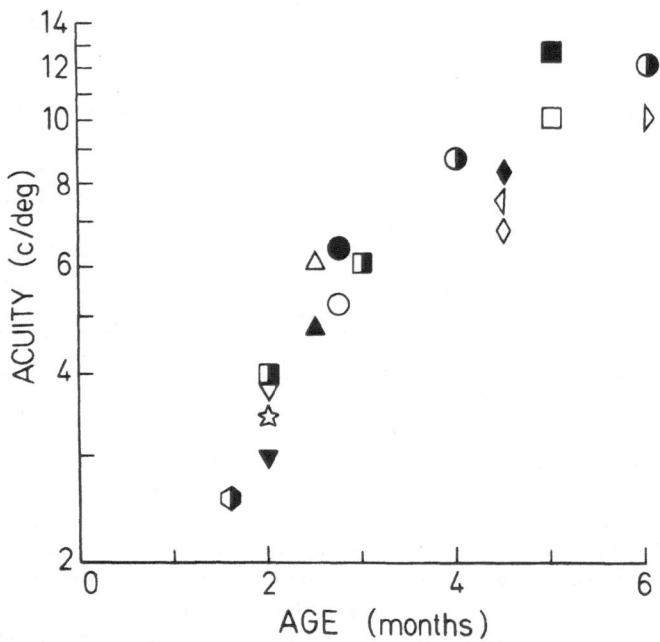

Fig 2 - ERG (open symbols) and VEP (solid symbols) acuities estimated in nine infants and plotted as a function of age. Different symbols indicate different subjects. Two infants were tested longitudinally (squares and circles) (From Fiorentini et al, 1984).

REFERENCES

Fiorentini A, Pirchio M, Sandini G. Development of retinal acuity in infants evaluated with pattern electroretinogram. Human Neurobiol 1984; 3: 93-95.

Fiorentini A, Maffei L, Pirchio M, Spinelli D, Porciatti V. The ERG in response to alternating gratings in patients with diseases of the peripheral visual pathway. Invest Ophthal Vis Sci 1981; 21: 490-93.

Hess RF, Baker CL jr. Human pattern-evoked electroretinogram. J Neurophysiol 1984; 51: 931-951.

Hollånder H, Bisti S, Maffei L, Hebel R. Electroretinographic responses and retrograde changes of retinal morphology after intracranial optic nerve section. A quantitative analysis in the cat. Exp Brain Res 1984; 55: 483-493.

Maffei L, Fiorentini A. Electroretinographic responses to alternating gratings before and after section of the optic nerve. Science 1981; 211: 953-955.

Maffei L, Fiorentini A. Electroretinographic responses to alternating gratings in the cat. Exp Brain Res 1982; 48: 327-334.

Maffei L, Fiorentini A, Bisti S, Hollånder H. Pattern ERG in the monkey after section of the optic nerve. Exp Brain Res (in press).

Porciatti V, von Berger GP. Pattern electroretinogram and visual evoked potential in optic nerve disease: early diagnosis and prognosis. Doc Ophthal Proc Series 1984; 40: 117-126.

DISCUSSION

Spekreijse: In the monkey experiments, since we showed that the pattern response tended to disappear, how well did you control fixation and accommodation?

Fiorentini: The animals were anaesthetised and paralysed. The eye was atropinised and refracted.

Spekreijse: The same treatment also for the other eye?

Fiorentini: Yes. We had contact lenses, 8mm pupils and, if necessary, we had additional lenses for refraction and what we usually did was to choose the lens that gave the best pattern ERGs.

Spekreijse: For the other eye?

Fiorentini: Yes.

Spekreisje: And that lens was applied to the second eye?

Fiorentini: No, not necessarily. Although in most cases we couldn't find any difference in the refraction between the two eyes. There was no apparent change.

Van Norren: Essential to your experiments is the state of the retina beyond the ganglion cell layer. Did you check that? You showed us some pictures of the ganglion cell layers; did you also check for deeper layers? An electrophysiological assessment is possible if you study the oscillatory potentials, they are not generated by the ganglion cells but somewhere deeper but still it is the proximal retina. We did current source density studies and found that the oscillatory potentials have a currrent source in the most superficial part of the retina. Did you check this?

Fiorentini: No, we did not. I think this is a good suggestion and something that could be done quite easily. To answer your first question, we haven't done that on the monkeys yet, but it was done on cats by my colleagues. What they did was to examine the sections of the retina, perpendicular to the retinal surface, and they found that there is no histological change in the deeper layers. Only after a long time, I think 3 or 4 months after optic nerve section, there was a very small shrinkage of the retina something amounting to 10-15% of the original width. There was no other apparent histological change in the deeper layers.

Fielder: Have you an explanation as to why you have to wait so long before the pattern ERG degenerates?

Fiorentini: No, I don't. It is known that ganglion cell degeneration takes a very long time in the cat. As you have seen, in the monkey it is much quicker. But one has to be careful, as there are various aspects to degeneration. In the slide I showed, there was a very obvious disappearance of the ganglion cells, but there may be earlier functional changes. Some clinical cases have been reported in which there was a change in the pattern ERG within one week of the symptoms occurring.

Porciatti: I published some data obtained in patients with optic neuritis. In the acute phase of the illness, the steady-state ERG to alternating sinusoidal gratings is usually normal. The first changes in the pattern ERG occur in most cases within one month after the appearance of the symptoms.

Campos: I would like to comment on the previous paper by van Lith. If I understand correctly the aims of this workshop, the paper by van Lith was one of the most appropriate for this type of meeting and I would encourage the organising committee to have data collected from all laboratories so that we can make a general protocol to find the conditions for which it is advisable for the ophthalmologist to require electrodiagnostic procedures because there is a lot of confusion about this, and van Lith showing his data gave us a lot of insight.

Warburg: Are you suggesting a multicentre approach?

Campos: I suggest at least a data collection by other people as van Lith did in his laboratory, and see whether the reasons for doing electrodiagnostic testing are the same and the results and the answers which can be given are the same. Then discrepancies should be worked out.

Warburg: So you would suggest a sort of protocol to be made and restricted to the various laboratories?

Campos: Clinical laboratories, yes.

van Lith: Thank you for these comments. It is always worthwhile to evaluate what you have done. Usually I do such a thing for the children, but I also did it for glaucoma and optic neuritis then you have to change your protocol. And now I intend to do that, but you talk only of electrodiagnosis. I would be interested also to know of behavioural experiments. How often do you have good results with unselected children? So getting to the question: do you have any results?

Warburg: I wonder how many of us have unselected children?

van Lith: They are never unselected. When the children are selected then they are referred.

Warburg: That is the first selection. And again we might want to have a protocol or at least specific numbers of very specific questions distributed to those working within the field. Is that what you suggest?

van Lith: Yes. That was the reason I suggested specifying three directions. Screening message, simple message for normal children just for detection, another just to find out about visual functions and such diagnostic measures. There are three completely different plans and to discuss all three, then you get confusion.

Warburg: Do you think we might hear about the other concerted Common Market action about health and screening for auditory disorders?

Skupinski: This is a proposal which was accepted two weeks ago and I think they will start. You are talking about the evaluation of screening programmes?

Warburg: Could you tell us more about this?

Skupinski: I think they will not deal with technical problems, but with evaluation of programmes. It is an approach from the COMAC-Health Services Research.

Dubowitz: Just one comment as you asked about behavioural testing. All I can say is that the population is unselected in the sense that I get all the premature babies back at 40 weeks post-menstrual age and perform behavioural testing on them. This is far from ideal as there is about a 40% failure rate.

Warburg: That is tossing a coin, isn't it?

Dubowitz: Yes, that is right. If you can go and get them back another time you can get a much better idea, but unselected at one examination there is a 40% failure rate.

van Hof-van Duin: We have selected children and our success rate is between 80 and 100%.

Dubowitz: Sorry, but what I am saying is about the child who just comes in, and either the child is crying or the mother can't stay so a large part of the screening you want to do is done in 5 or 10 minutes, not in half an hour.

van Hof-van Duin: If we want to test visual acuity only, we need an alert awake baby for 5 minutes, in which time the 'acuity card' procedure is finished.

Dubowitz: These are premature infants, at full term 40 weeks, and I would say that they often come a long distance, and in about 40% I have to tell the mother: "now sit outside, feed your baby, and come back again," but just on one testing we often achieve up to 80% success.

Braddick: When you say your second test, that is on the same visit?

Dubowitz: Yes, but still they sit there for some time.

Mohn: I would like to comment that I think that Dubowitz's population is preselected in a certain sense as they are 40 weeks old. With older children the success rate goes up enormously and we see a great number of neurologically abnormal children between 6 months and 6 years. Then our success rate is about 80% at least.

Dubowitz: Yes, but you are experienced.

Mohn: Sure, but it just shows that the success rate depends on age and other factors.

MEASUREMENT OF VISUAL ACUITY IN INFANTS AND YOUNG CHILDREN BY VISUAL EVOKED
POTENTIALS

Patricia Apkarian, Wim van Veenendaal, Henk Spekreijse

The Netherlands Ophthalmic Research Institute, Amsterdam

INTRODUCTION

Although the electrophysiological assessment of visual function is
routinely performed in both ophthalmology and neurology departments, the
use of electrophysiological measures, particularly the visual evoked potential (VEP), in pediatric ophthalmology or neurology is less common. The
major impediment towards widespread use and full acceptance of the visual
evoked potential as a viable diagnostic aid in neonatal and pediatric
populations stems from the fact that the normal growth function of visual
performance, particularly visual acuity, is yet to be determined. Substantial progress in this direction has been made both by psychophysical procedures, i.e. variants of the preferential looking technique (PLT) (Teller
1979; Fulton et al 1979; Gwiazda et al 1980; Mayer and Dobson 1982; Dobson
1983; van Hof-van Duin et al 1983) as well as by visual evoked potential
measures (Marg et al 1976; Sokol 1978; de Vries-Khoe and Spekreijse 1982;
Moskowitz and Sokol 1983; Norcia and Tyler 1985). However, the lack of
concordance of "normal-for-date" acuity values not only between these two
disciplines but within them as well, severely limits the diagnostic utility
of the acuity estimates thus far reported. The problem of establishing
normative growth values is not restricted to preferential looking techniques nor to visual evoked potential measures but is a long standing
problem inherent to the more conventional behavioral methods of assessing
visual function at least in younger children (Rychener 1958; Woodruff 1972;
Sheridan 1974; Simons 1983).
Topics of discussion across laboratories and within the clinic, range
from differences in acuity estimates derived from various optotypes (Brant
and Nowotny 1976; Friendly 1978) and the complications associated with
grating-Snellen acuity equivalents (Howell et al 1983; Rentschler et al.
1980), or for that matter check size and spatial frequency equivalents
(Kelly 1976; Dobson and Teller 1978), the effects of temporal (Dobson et al
1978a; Moskowitz and Sokol 1980) or spatial (Atkinson et al, 1983; Dobson
et al 1978b; Moskowitz and Sokol 1983) aspects of the stimulus, the effects
of diverse behaviorial (Held et al,1979; Banks and Salapatek 1976;
Atkinson et al 1981) or electrophysiological methodology (Sokol 1978;
Spekreijse 1978; Marg 1976; Pirchio et al 1978) to non-corresponding data
analysis procedures and assumptions (see Sokol and Moskowitz 1985). Several
studies to highlight or disentangle the reported discrepancies have been
attempted (Dobson and Teller 1978; Simons 1983; Sokol and Moskowitz, 1985;
Odom and Green 1985).
Although absolute age-related acuity estimates remain equivocal, the
existing growth functions of visual performance obtained under widely
differing conditions, none-the-less show remarkably similar growth trends
and as a result are beginning to yield important correlations between
visual acuity and underlying anatomical and physiological maturation (for

reviews Fulton et al 1981; Hoyt et al 1982). Recent publications from
Spekreijse (de Vries-Khoe and Spekreijse 1982; Spekreijse 1983) and a
purview of the literature (Fantz et al 1962; Allen 1979; Spekreijse, 1978;
Sokol 1978; Gwiazda et al 1978; Fulton et al 1979; Bauer et al, 1984;
Porciatti 1984) indicates that the growth curve of visual acuity as a
function of age contains three distinct phases of development: 1) an initial phase from birth to 2 months during which improvement in pattern
resolution is unremarkable, 2) a second phase or "fast" phase from about 2
to 8 months during which there is a rapid increase in acuity and 3) a third
or "slow" phase from about 10 months to at least five years or even puberty
during which adult acuity values are finally reached. By examining the
shape invariancy of visual evoked potential amplitude as a function of
check size in a large sample of infants from 2 to 6 months of age,
Spekreijse (de Vries-Khoe and Spekreijse 1982) was able to provide electrophysiological evidence to correlate the fast phase of visual acuity improvement with the morphological maturation of the retina, particularly the
foveal region. Furthermore, by examining the maturation of the contrast
component of the pattern appearance response, evidence was provided to
support the notion that the slower phase of visual acuity development
reflects, in addition to full foveal maturation, more central neural processes. (For a more detailed description of retinal and visual system
development, see Weale 1982; Mann 1949; Magoon and Robb 1981; Abramov et al
1982; Hendrickson and Yuodelis 1984).

Despite the relatively "immature" stage of the field of visual assessment in infants and younger children and the wide variability in acuity
norms within a given age range, the existing growth functions, though not
exact and far from complete, can serve as useful guides when testing visual
function in an individual subject or patient. For regardless of the "state
of art", the clinician is increasingly requested to deal with questions
concerning the visual capacity of the non-verbal patient. Does this baby
see? How well? Is the estimated acuity normal-for-date? Are the left eye
and right eye acuities equal? Though consensus has not been reached as to
the optimum method for attaining answers to these questions, in light of
animal studies and clinical experience, their importance for early detection and treatment of visual pathology is undisputed.
This report attempts to address these questions with a practical
approach to electrophysiological testing. Emphasis is placed on methods of
evoked potential recording in infants and children; the advantages and
disadvantages of one method over another are discussed. This is accom-
plished with the aid of three case studies and three age matched normal
controls. Since state changes in pediatric populations are the bane of
visual evoked potentials, two methods of recording which help to circumvent
the problems of non-stationarity are also discussed.

METHODS

The data presented in this report were derived from three different
stimulus and recording methods, the responses from each of which are designated for convenience 1) standard VEPs, 2) sequential VEPs and 3) sweep
VEPs.

Stimulus

Standard VEPs: For data in figures 2-7, checkerboard patterns of 80%
contrast were generated on a Philips 17" (LDH 2123) video monitor. The mode

of stimulus presentation (unless otherwise stated) was pattern appearance
(40 msec)/ disappearance (460 msec) or pattern reversal (260 msec) at a
constant mean luminance level of 90 cd/m^2. Pattern sizes ranged from about
3' to 194'. Field size was 13°, 10° and 7.5^o at viewing distances of
100, 150 and 200 cm respectively.
    Sequential VEPs: For data of figure 9, checkerboard patterns of nearly
100% contrast were generated on a Sony (CVM-1810E) video monitor. Duration
of pattern appearance was 300 msec, pattern disappearance, 500 msec. Mean
luminance was kept constant at 64 cd/m^2; field size was 20°, viewing distance 100 cm. Check sizes up to six per recording epoch, ranging from 7' to
329', were changed once per 800 msec.
    Sweep VEPs: The stimulus for the sweep VEP (Figure 8) consisted of
vertical sine-wave gratings of 50% contrast generated on a CRT display
(HP1332A;P31). The gratings were switched in counterphase from 12 reversals
per second (rps) to 32 rps. Pattern size decreased logarithmically from 0.5
to 10 c/deg within 12 sec. Mean luminance was kept constant at 48 cd/m^2,
field size equaled 13° and viewing distance, 57 cm.

Recording

    Standard VEPs: Visual evoked potentials were recorded with tinned
copper cup electrodes attached to the scalp with collodion and positioned
one cm above the inion across the occiput with 3 cm spacing in a horizontal
row. Midline positions four and seven cm above the inion were also used.
The minimum number of active electrode sites recorded in a given subject
was three (left, middle and right occiput); the maximum was seven. Reference for all electrodes was linked ears; the common ground was located near
the vertex. Bandwidth of the EEG amplifiers (Nihon Kohden) was set at 0.5-
70 Hz. The high cut-off frequency was set by an anti-aliasing Butterworth
filter (B&S; cut-off frequency 70 Hz) which introduced a phase shift increasing response latency by ca. 7 msec. If the reader wishes to estimate
peak latency from the responses depicted, this correction should be made.
The filtered signals were sampled at a rate of 200 Hz and averaged with an
Apple II microcomputer equipped with an IBS-68000 microprocessor card. All
signals were displayed in real time and stored on disk for further analysis. The number of counts or averages was generally 40 to 200 depending on
the signal to noise ratio.

    Sequential VEPs: The recording procedures for sequential VEPs were
comparable to those described for standard VEPs except that the EEG was
amplified by Medelec/van Gogh amplifiers. Filtered signals were sampled at
100 Hz, first sorted according to stimulating check size and then averaged
by an HP 2100 computer.

    Sweep VEPs: The difference potential of the sweep VEP was recorded
from two gold cupped electrodes attached to the scalp with recording cream
and positioned 3 cm and 6 cm above the inion; the ear served as ground. The
EEG was amplified (Grass), band-pass filtered (Krohn-Hite: cut-off frequency 0.1 log unit above and below the pattern reversal rate) and phase-locked
filtered at the temporal frequency of the stimulus. VEP amplitude as a
function of swept spatial frequency was displayed on-line on an X-Y plotter
and stored for future analysis.

Procedure

Adults and older children were tested while seated comfortably in an electrically shielded room; infants and younger children difficult to test, e.g. with psycho-motor retardation, were seated on the lap of their parent or attending assistant. Recording was interrupted by automatic artifact rejection as well as by an observer who monitored the infant's fixation. Averaging was temporarily halted when a corneal reflex of the stimulus could not be elicited. To help maintain fixation at the stimulus field, the checkerboard presentation as well as averaging procedure was also intermittently interrupted by a cartoon or other popular childrens' video program (see figure 1). This method of interrupting the VEP stimulus and recording intermittently with a cartoon movie presentation has the advantage over the method of cartoon movie-stimulus superposition (Spekreijse 1978) in that the latter introduces an overall reduction of contrast and increases the scatter of normal values; standardization of the film parameters with cartoon superposition is also necessary. In our modified version of movie presentation, when pure checkerboard stimulation replaced the cartoon and recording resumed, the movie sound track, input to an amplifier attached to the back of the stimulus monitor, continued to play. This procedure drew attention to the stimulus by auditory cueing. Attempts to maintain attention were also implemented by "peek-a-boo" games, and dancing, dangling, sound producing toys.

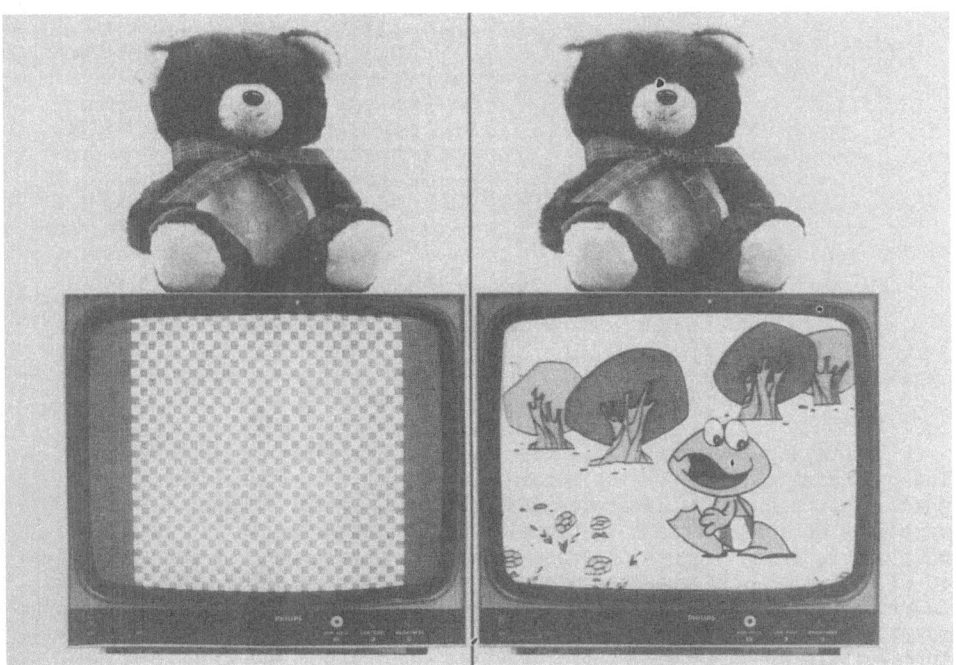

Figure 1. Pattern stimulation, generated on a video monitor, is intermittently interrupted by a children's cartoon movie (generated on the same monitor) to draw attention to the stimulus field. When fixation is appropriate, the checkerboard pattern stimulus and recording are resumed; the movie sound track continues to play.

172

Similar procedures were employed for the sequentially presented checkerboard patterns. For the data of figure 9, however, appropriate fixation
of this subject was maintained by instruction alone.

For the sweep data of figure 8, fixation at the CRT screen was maintained with a dangling toy placed at the distance of the screen.

For all VEP methods, binocular, left eye and right eye responses were
recorded, when possible for each stimulus condition. Monocular recordings
were obtained with total occlusion of the fellow eye. Testing was performed
under ambient low-level illumination.

Subjects

Six normal controls and three patients form the total subject pool for
the data presented in this report. Patient material was obtained from
routine referrals to the electrophysiological unit of the Netherlands
Ophthalmic Research Institute. Patients were referred for electrophysiological assessment of visual function when subjective report was not possible, either because the patient was pre-verbal (fig 7) or psycho-motor
retarded (figs 3 and 5). Patient histories are presented in the result
section.

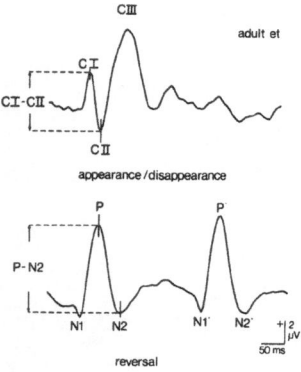

Figure 2.
Upper traces: Pattern appearance
(40 msec) / disappearance (460 msec)
response in adult ET. Note the
presence of three distinct components designated CI, CII and CIII.
Pattern response amplitude is measured beween CI and CII.
Lower traces: Pattern reversal (260
msec per reversal) response in same
adult subject. Pattern response amplitude is measured between P and
N2. Note the presence of two reversal responses every 520 msec.

Data analysis

Before displaying the data for analysis, the EPs were smoothed by a
low pass digital filter which removed mains' hum but did not introduce
phase distortions. The latencies and amplitudes of the real-time averaged
responses were estimated with the aid of a software "cursor" program. For
more mature (figs 3 and 4) pattern appearance waveforms, the peak latencies
of CI, CII and CIII were determined along with the relative response amplitudes between CI and CII. This measurement is characterized in the adult
pattern appearance response depicted in figure 2 (upper trace). For immature pattern appearance response profiles (see figs 5 and 7) latency was
determined, when feasible, by the first major positive peak; amplitude was
taken as the difference between the first major positive peak and "second"
negative peak (P-N). Similar latency and amplitude measures (P-N2) were
taken for the transient reversal response as characterized in the adult
pattern reversal depicted in figure 2 (lower trace). Pattern appearance
responses depicted in figure 6, illustrate a transition between the presence of a single positive peak and the more adult-like triphasic waveform.

The single positive peak in this case, particularly for smaller pattern sizes can be correlated with the CIII component, note the longer latencies; measurement of this peak for acuity estimate is erroneous.

RESULTS AND DISCUSSION

Case study I

The data of figure 3 were obtained from patient Medet, male, born 25 April 1975, who was referred for visual evoked potential assessment of visual function, particularly for an electrophysiological estimate of visual acuity and possible evidence of optic nerve hypoplasia. At the date of test, February 4, 1985, Medet was almost 10 years old. An objective, i.e. VEP, means of procuring an acuity estimate was required since in addition to the final diagnosis of psycho-motor retardation (unknown etiology), a serious language barrier was also present. From general examination Medet was shown to have delayed development. He did not talk before the age of 6 years. At the age of two, a metabolic disturbance (increased β-amino butyric acid) was noted but at the time of VEP examination, metabolic conditions were determined as normal. CT-scan revealed slightly dilated ventricles. Ophthalmological examination revealed alternating divergent strabismus, hypermetropia of +1D and a subjective binocular acuity estimate of about 0.25 (20/80) as determined by a child's recognition test chart (though cooperation was minimal). Anterior segments and optic media were normal while fundus examination revealed small size optic nerve heads (OS, with persisting hyaloid). Nystagmus was also present.

Transient pattern appearance/ disappearance stimulation affords four electrophysiological response parameters for testing functional integrity along the visual pathway: 1) component specificity, 2) amplitude, 3) latency and 4) cortical topography. It is now well established that the triphasic waveform of the mature pattern onset response consists of three major components designated CI (positive), CII (negative) and CIII (positive) (Spekreijse et al 1973; Jeffreys and Axford 1972). The cortical surface distributions of these three components differ as well as the physiological processes which they reflect. CII is the component of interest for visual acuity estimates for relative to CI and CIII, CII is more strongly dependent upon contrast and the structural details of the pattern. In accord, changes in pattern quality such as the introduction of blur, are most sensitively measured by the CII component while CI, the presumptive local luminance response, requires considerably stronger dioptric defocus to produce comparable response attenuation (Spekreijse et al 1973; Jeffreys and Axford 1972). As will be shown in figures 5 through 7, the gradual appearance of the CII component also reflects the maturation of visual resolution capacity (Spekreijse 1978).

The presence of the triphasic waveform in Medet's data is clear (figure 3, left) and when the appearance response is examined as a function of pattern size, response differentiation and the CII component are present to a pattern element size of about 7'. As seen for age matched normal control, Remco with ODS acuities of 1 (20/20), 1 (20/20), VEP resolution acuity for the experimental conditions of this test yield response differentiation to at least 3.5' (the resolution of our video monitor at 228 cm). A conventional method of analysing visual evoked responses to differing pattern sizes is to plot the amplitude of a given response peak as a function of pattern size. For our purposes, with the mature waveform, we plot the difference in amplitude between CI and CII (see fig 2). This

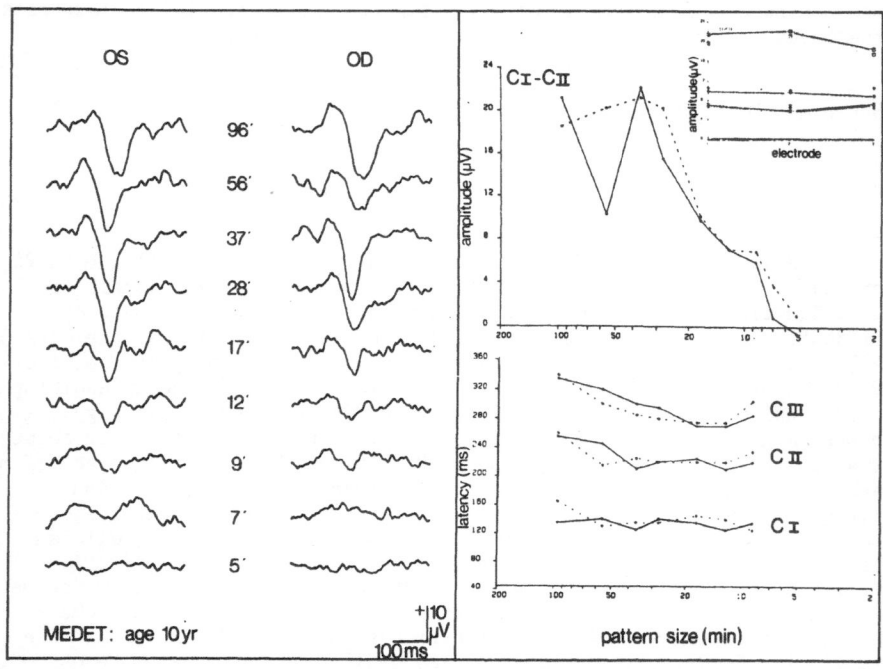

Figure 3.
Left: Left eye (OS) and right eye (OD) pattern appearance responses to
varying check sizes. The distance was 200 cm, field size 7.5°. The minimum
checksize for which a measurable response could be elicited was 7'.
Upper right: Pattern response amplitude plotted as a function of check
size. In this and all remaining figures, right eye responses are depicted
with a solid line, left eye responses with a dashed line. Note that OD and
OS yield comparable responses.
Upper right (insert): Pattern EP amplitude as a function of electrode
position from left (#1) to right (#3) occiput. Responses depicted were
derived from stimulation of check sizes 37' (upper curves), 17' (middle
curves) and 9' (lower curves). These data show hemispheric symmetry.
Lower right: Pattern EP latency as a function of pattern size for components CIII (upper curves), CII (middle) and CI (lower). OD and OS latency
values are comparable but delayed.

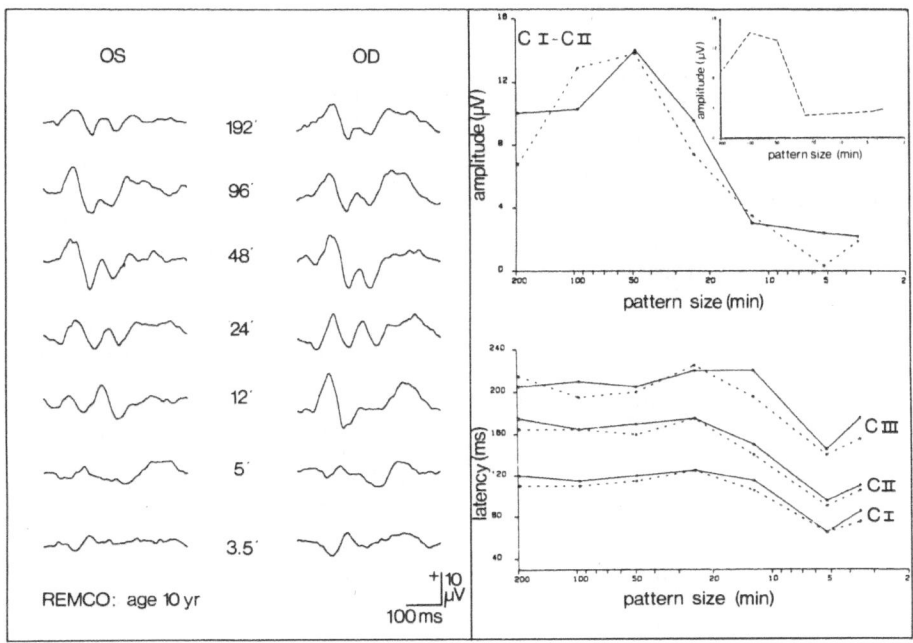

Figure 4.
Left: Note that the minimum checksize for which a measurable response could be elicited was at least 3.5'. For details see figure 3.
Upper right: Response amplitude versus check size plot illustrates the difficulty of zero response extrapolation. Note that response amplitude can remain constant with smaller pattern sizes.
Upper right (insert): Response amplitude versus check size plot derived for the left eye from a left occipital electrode. Note the constancy of response amplitude for pattern sizes smaller than 24'.
Lower right: For details see figure 3. OD and OS latency values are comparable and within normal limits.

procedure eliminates base-line response ambiguity. One of the advantages of presentating data in this form (fig 3, upper right), is that right eye and left eye equality are easily discerned. Note that for Medet, OD (solid line) and OS (dashed line) yield comparable responses with OS responses slightly better than OD. The response plot depicted here was derived from a midline positioned electrode. Comparable functions were obtained across left occipital (electrode number 1) and right occipital (electrode number 3) electrodes. A plot of right eye and left eye response amplitudes as a function of electrode position for three different pattern sizes are presented (fig 3, upper right insert). For Medet, consistent hemispheric symmetry is present and consequent amplitude versus pattern size plots across all electrodes are thus obtained.

If one were to perform a peak amplitude to zero amplitude response extrapolation on the data presented in the amplitude versus check size plot of figure 3, the extrapolated value would be in close approximation to the qualitative estimate obtained by waveform inspection. This correspondence, however, might be considered the exception rather than the general rule, as previously reported (Spekreijse 1980) and again demonstrated here by the amplitude versus check size functions of figure 4. Data from figure 4 (main function) were derived from a right occipital electrode. In this example, a proper estimate of acuity cannot be obtained by extrapolation of the curve to zero response amplitude. Furthermore, this particular subject showed a significant left hemispheric response dominance. Hemispheric asymmetry is not an indicant of a pathological condition, when right eye and left eye responses, following full field stimulation, yield comparable cortical topography. The presence of hemispheric asymmetry simply may reflect individual variability and thus the position of the midline electrode may be at variance with the subject's occipital midline (see Apkarian et al 1983). The plot of evoked potential amplitude and checksize for a left occipital electrode (fig 4, upper right insert) shows that the response amplitude remains constant for progressively smaller check sizes. These data clearly demonstrate that the frequently used extrapolation method described here can lead to serious under or over estimates of VEP spatial resolution. An additional caveat described by Spekreijse et al (1973) concerns the occurrence of polarity reversals as a function of pattern size in the response profiles of some subjects. Their presence also effects the shape of the VEP amplitude versus check size function and vitiates acuity estimates based on extrapolated values.

The remaining electrophysiological parameter to be described for case I is latency. Right eye and left eye latency values for components CI, CII and CIII are presented in figure 3 (lower right) and figure 4 (lower right) for patient, Medet and age-matched normal control, respectively. Medet's data show marked delay across all response components. This result is consistent with the condition of optic nerve hypoplasia in which delayed VEP latencies have been reported in patients with moderate or severe hypoplasia (Sprague and Wilson 1981).

The final VEP conclusions from this case, as reported to the referring clinician were:
1) hemispheric response symmetry;
2) evoked potential acuity estimate of at least 1/3 ODS;
3) abnormally long flash (also included in the test program) and pattern response latency ODS.

Case study II

The data of figure 5 were obtained from patient Raymond, male, born July
30, 1980, who was referred for visual evoked assessment of visual function,
particularly for electrophysiological evidence of pattern perception.
At the date of test, February 4, 1985, Raymond was almost 5 years old.
Because of severe psychomotor retardation (unknown etiology), visual capacity, could not be determined with conventional behavioral methods. As
Raymond was unable to maintain an upright sitting position, VEPs were
recorded while he was seated on the lap of his mother who held him in
gentle restraint. From general examination, Raymond was shown to suffer
from kidney abnormalities and epilepsy. Ophthalmological examination revealed convergent strabismus (OS) and irregular nystagmus. A slightly
pigmented foveal region was noted along with a blond fundus. For the
pattern appearance response of Raymond (figure 5, left), the presence of a
triphasic CI, CII, CIII waveform complex is difficult to discern, though a
single positive peak around 90 msec is clearly present. Normative data from
our laboratory (de Vries-Khoe and Spekreijse 1982; Spekreijse 1983) indicate a nearly 100 % incidence of the contrast component, CII, by the age of
5 years. Raymond's profiles, therefore, appear to show a delayed maturation. None-the-less, if we attend to the responses as a function of pattern
size, we note that the minimum check size for which a measurable response
could be obtained was 12'. The age-matched normal control (fig 6) yielded
a measurable response to at least 3.5', an almost three-fold higher EP
acuity compared to Raymond. If, for the data of figure 5, the relative
amplitude of the earlier major positive peak (peak to peak amplitude, P-N)
is plotted as a function of checksize, (upper right) as with the data of
figure 4, attempted zero response extrapolation for an acuity estimate
would be ambiguous. Further the average responses depicted in this figure
(left most traces) were derived from the dominant or right hemispheric
electrode (number 3). The strong hemispheric asymmetry is illustrated in
the amplitude versus electrode plot (fig 5, lower right). To underscore the
problem of VEP acuity based on a single recording site, the simultaneously
recorded responses from electrodes positioned over the left (number 1) and
middle (number 2) occiput are also depicted for stimulation with the 48'
check size (lower right insert). Note the concomitant response attenuation
in two out of three electrode sites.
    The final VEP conclusions from this case, as reported to the referring
clinician, were:
1) right hemispheric dominance OU, OD and OS;
2) clear presence of flash (also included in the test paradigm) and
    pattern responses OU, OD, OS (binocular data not shown);
3) evoked potential acuity estimate of at least 1/4 ODS.
Recommend retest in 8-12 months to further evaluate waveform maturation and
latency.

    Before turning our attention to the following case study, two addi-
tional points should be noted. A comparison of the responses of figure 6
for the age matched normal control over different check sizes illustrates
an important feature of the transient evoked response, i.e., a large variation in waveshape from small to large check sizes (Spekreijse 1966;
Spekreijse et al 1973). Under these conditions, attempts to plot the amplitude of CI-CII as a function of pattern size (see also methods section) are
not feasible. In violation of this caveat and previous discussion, we,
none-the-less, plot the amplitude of the major response peak (P-N) as a
function of checksize (upper right) for illustrative purposes only. What

178

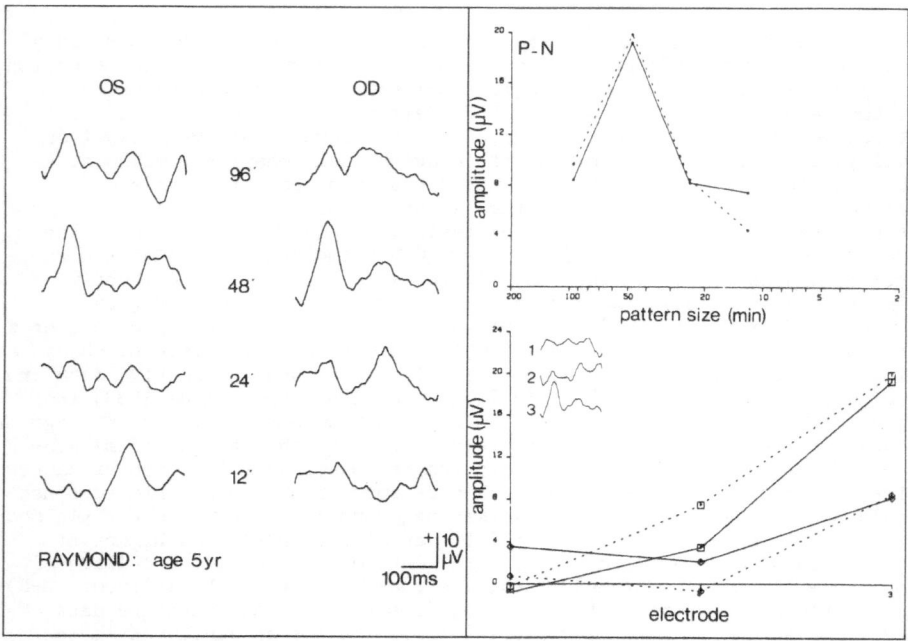

Figure 5.
Left: Pattern appearance responses for varying check sizes. The recording distance was 114 cm, field size 13°. Note that the pattern response consists primarily of a single positive peak.
Upper right: Amplitude of the positive peak (P-N) occurring within ca 150 msec is plotted as a function of check size.
Lower right: Pattern EP amplitude as a function of electrode position from left (#1) to right (#3) across the occiput. Responses depicted were derived from stimulation of check sizes 48' (upper curves) and 24' (lower curves). Near zero and negative values reflect noise.
Lower right (insert): Averaged response to 48' check size for electrodes positioned at left (#1), middle (#2) or right (#3) occiput. Note the right hemispheric response dominance with attendant response attenuation at other sites

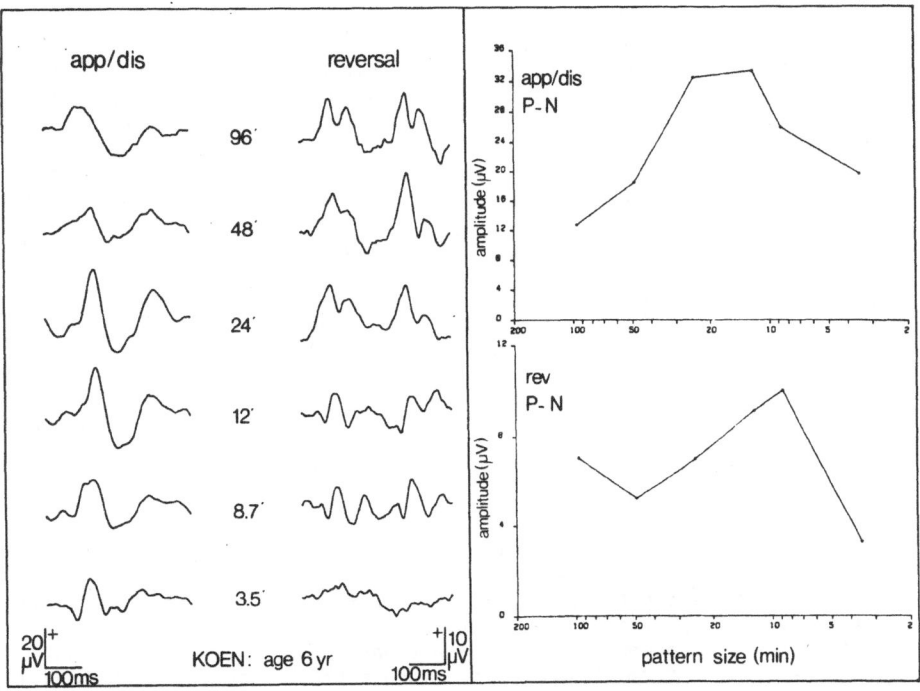

Figure 6.
Left: Right eye pattern appearance (left most traces) and pattern reversal (right most traces) responses for varying pattern sizes. The recording distance was 200 cm, field size 7.5°. Note the dramatic change in waveshape across the range of pattern sizes.
Right: Attempt to plot response amplitudes as a function of pattern size for the averaged responses depicted at the left. Concomitant changes in waveshape and component ambiguity negate the validity of these functions.

becomes immediately apparent is that the underlying waveshape changes render this method of analysing and formatting the data ambiguous at best. And finally, to demonstrate that these problems are not specific to the pattern appearance response, we present an example of similar difficulties encountered with the pattern reversal response. The pattern reversal responses of figure 6 (right most traces) were obtained during the same experimental session as the appearance responses (left most traces). Responses shown are from OD stimulation. The test protocol included careful counterbalancing between those two conditions and thus the lower reversal amplitudes compared to pattern appearance are actual, at least for this subject.

Firstly, note that waveform changes from smaller to larger check sizes result in an apparent maximum response to a pattern size only about one octave from that of the minimum and at the same time substantial response attenuation for larger pattern sizes, a misleading finding compared to visual inspection of the averaged responses.

Secondly, although responses to pattern reversal stimulation are commonly recorded across clinics (this is, at least in part, a result of commercial availability), it is of interest to note that several studies have demonstrated the superiority of pattern appearance recording over pattern reversal, particularly in patient populations in which nystagmus is a frequently occurring symptom, e.g. albinism and multiple sclerosis (Apkarian et al 1983; Riemslag et al 1981).

And lastly, a recent study by Spekreijse et al (1985), highlights the difference between pattern reversal and pattern appearance in terms of the underlying visual processes which they activate, i.e. detectors of motion versus detectors of form and position. Since pattern appearance stimulation enhances the probability of activating primarily contrast mechanisms, it is a preferred mode of assessing visual resolution capacity. That comparisons between behavioral acuity estimates and evoked potential acuity based on appearance responses are more closely related supports this suggestion (Spekreijse 1983).

Case study III

The data of figure 7 were obtained from patient, John, male, born July 7, 1984 and his twin brother, Paul who served as "normal" age matched control and was diagnosed as "normal" ex-premature at the time of test. Gestation period for the twins was 33 weeks; Paul's birth weight was 1870 grams; John's 2500 grams. John was referred for electrophysiological assessment of visual function, particularly for electrophysiological evidence of light perception. An objective, i.e. VEP means of determining visual capacity was requested as no eye contact could be elicited. General examination revealed that John showed delayed maturation. Staff reports state that at times it appeared that John was looking but he did not show tracking behavior nor could his attention be elicited with a strong light source. Ophthalmological examination revealed clear media and no fundus abnormalities. The papillae were somewhat white but normal in size.

For the twin study, six cortical sites were measured with 5 electrodes positioned in a row across the occiput, 2.5 cm apart and 1 cm above the inion; a 6th electrode was positioned 4 cm above the inion. The averaged responses depicted in figure 7 were derived from the midline electrodes. Response distributions for both brothers were generally symmetric with baby John showing a very slight left hemispheric preference. As the clinical question concerned presence of light perception, luminance flash responses (not shown) from 1 to 10 Hz were also measured. Luminance flash responses for John were definitely present but were highly variable and generally lower amplitude than responses from the brother. The temporal frequency series showed following in John from 1 to 6 Hz and in Paul, the "normal" sibling, from 1 to at least 10 Hz.

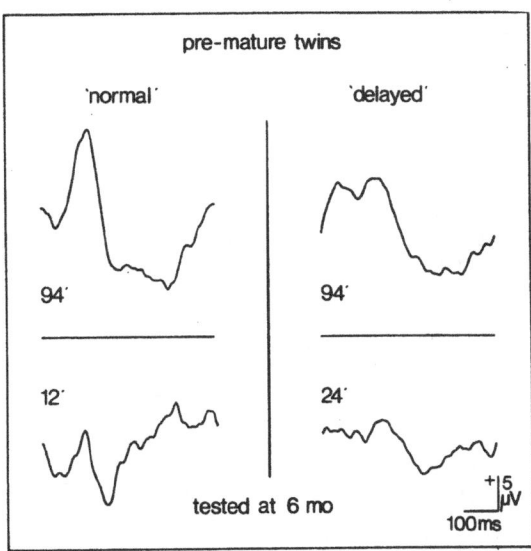

Figure 7. Binocular pattern appearance responses for a "normal ex-premature" twin and his brother who presents with delayed maturation. The minimum check size for which a response could be elicited was 12' and 24', respectively. The recording distance was 150 cm, field size 10°.

Plotted in figure 7 are binocular pattern appearance responses to the largest pattern size tested (94') and the smallest pattern size which yielded a measurable response. The immature waveform complex of these responses, as with the data of figures 5 and 6, do not permit derivation of a meaningful amplitude versus check size plot. In addition, state changes in these infants did not allow reliable left eye response/ right eye response comparisons. The binocular responses, however, show that for John (right most traces), measurable responses were definitely present to about a 24' check size. Evoked responses from the brother, Paul, could be elicited with check sizes at least two times smaller, i.e. 12' checks. The VEP resolution limit in our experimental conditions is at least 3'. John's minimum measurable check size response is 24', about 6 times worse than the possible resolution limit; his acuity is estimated to be at least .12 (20/160). Normative values from our laboratory indicate that Paul's VEP acuity can be estimated at roughly .25 (20/80).

The remaining VEP parameter yet to be discussed is latency. Latency for the single positive peak for Paul's responses, following pattern stimulation, is about 120 msec though, in general, latency values were difficult to determine because of wave shape changes. Comparable measures for John show latency values around 160 to 170 msec. The latter fall outside our normal range. Latencies for luminance flash for John were also delayed.

The final VEP conclusions from this case (for John), as reported to the referring clinician were:
1) hemispheric symmetry;
2) clear presence of flash and pattern response;
3) visual evoked acuity estimate of at least 1/8 (OU);
4) reduced temporal frequency following;
5) significantly delayed latencies for flash and pattern responses.

Sweep VEP

As briefly mentioned in the twin study, state changes are a source of considerable concern when attempting to measure the visual evoked potential. For example, state changes from alert to drowsy may affect accommodation. Though the immature waveform does not consist of the fully developed contrast component (CII) which is most sensitive to blur relative to the CI or CIII components, the immature response none-the-less reflects more than a pure luminance component. Thus fluctuations in accommodation will degrade the response, given that is, that the pattern size falls within the infant's or younger child's resolving capacity (Sokol et al, 1983). In addition, state changes affect the frequency content of the EEG (Prechtl 1968), as well as the VEP. Dramatic phase cancelling and a non-recordable response or response artifact can result.

Attempts to perform VEP acuity estimates within state-stationary recording epochs have led to the introduction of VEP sweep techniques (Regan 1973; 1977; Tyler et al, 1979; Seiple et al 1984). Basically VEP sweep methods involve sweeping through a range of values of a stimulus parameter e.g. pattern size (spatial frequency) or contrast while simultaneously obtaining a running average of EP amplitude. This method takes advantage of the fact that if the stimulus repetition rate is high relative to the time constants of the visual system (greater than about 5 Hz in the adult), the response profile is a waveform considerably simpler than that obtained by transient evoked potential methods. With variants of band-pass filtering techniques a plot of VEP amplitude as a function of pattern size or contrast can be obtained within 10-20 seconds. An example of sweep VEP data obtained from a 12 week old baby under conditions described in the methods section is presented in figure 8. VEP amplitude as a function of bar width was recorded for four different temporal frequencies. At a stimulus repetition rate of 20 rps, a shift in acuity estimates from 12 rps is indicated; by 32 rps the shift is undisputable. The dependence of estimated acuity on temporal frequency suggests that growth functions obtained with spatial frequency VEP sweep techniques are specific to the particular method of measurement and thus, at best, can only provide relative measures of maturation of spatial vision.

Furthermore, it is generally agreed that zero response amplitude extrapolations of VEP amplitude versus contrast show closer correspondence to psychophysically determined contrast threshold than extrapolated values of VEP amplitude versus pattern size (Campbell and Maffei 1970; Spekreijse,1980; Cannon 1983). However, the more traditional procedure for obtaining VEP contrast thresholds requires considerable time prohibiting clinical applicability. Swept contrast thresholds for a given spatio-temporal condition, obtained in less than 20 seconds (Seiple et al 1984) enhances the clinical feasibility of this valuable measure. The speed in obtaining swept VEP functions, in general, makes them rather tempting for clinical application particularly for monitoring the effects of treatment and determining left eye/ right eye equality. None-the-less, the inherent problems outlined in the previous sections for more conventional recording methods apply to sweep VEPs as well and their use must be approached with caution. More detailed discussions regarding the "pros and cons" of VEP sweep techniques have been presented elsewhere (Regan 1980; Tyler et al 1981).

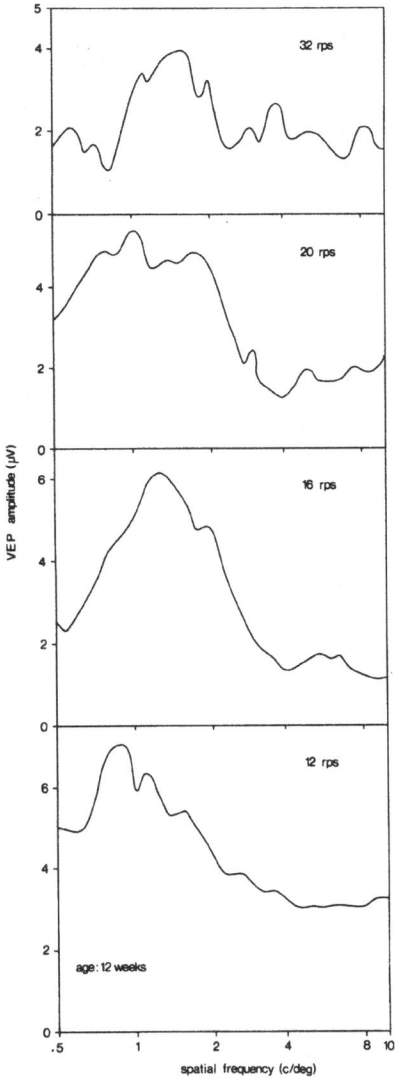

Figure 8.
VEP sweep responses as a function of spatial frequency for four different temporal frequencies. Note that as temporal frequency increases, extrapolated acuity estimates decrease. The dependence of estimated acuity on temporal frequency dictates caution when applying the sweep VEP for monitoring visual system development.

Sequential VEPs

Sequential presentation of varying stimulus parameters is an alternative method of circumventing the detrimental effects of state changes on the VEP (Spekreijse 1980), The data of figure 9, recorded from a five year old child, represent an example of this procedure. The upper traces depict the responses recorded from two separate sequential presentations. During the first series, five different pattern sizes from 7' to 107' were pre-

184

sented in a fixed sequence with each pattern presented for a single sweep (pattern appearance, 300 msec)/ (pattern disappearance, 500 msec). Respective responses per pattern size were sorted and averaged by the computer. The second series proceeded as the first except that only four pattern sizes were presented, ranging from 53' to 329'. The lower traces (solid lines) were recorded with fixed pattern sizes of 13' and 53', respectively. When the sequentially derived responses for comparable pattern sizes are plotted on an expanded time scale and superimposed, the overlap shows that both methods yield similar results. With the sequential method, stable responses to 7 different pattern sizes were obtained in less than 10 minutes. In addition to reducing recording time, this method has the advantage over VEP sweep methods in that waveform and latency information are retained. Both parameters are essential in the investigations of maturational processes of spatial vision.

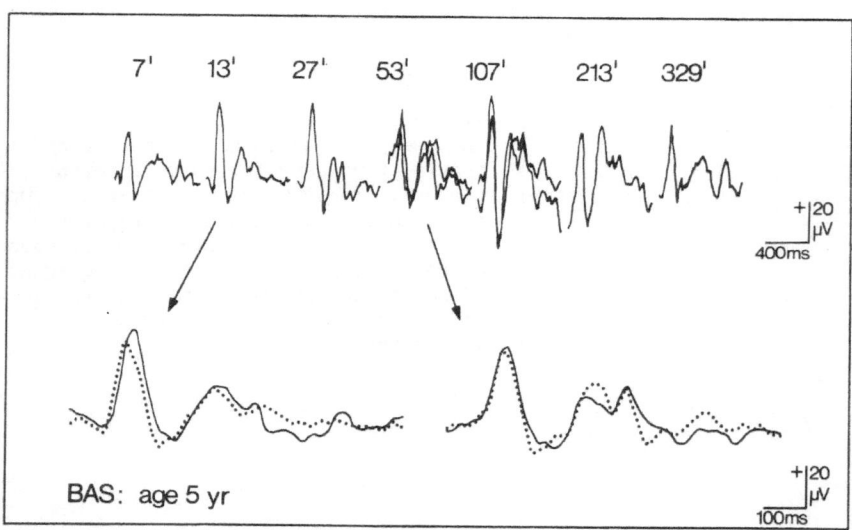

Figure 9. Sequential VEPs for varying pattern sizes (upper traces). Double traces represent the overlap from two separate series. See text for more detail. Responses from pattern sizes (13' and 53') have been redrawn on an expanded time scale (lower traces, dashed line) and superimposed on responses derived from fixed checksize stimulation. Both stimulus conditions yield similar EPs.

CONCLUSION AND SUMMARY

The case studies presented in this report demonstrate that despite the preliminary status of the existing growth functions, clinically relevant information regarding visual capacity, particularly visual acuity is available with visual evoked potential measures in infants and younger children. The electrophysiological parameters of interest are 1) component specificity, 2) amplitude, 3) latency and 4) cortical topography. In combination they provide a powerful clinical tool for assessing visual capacity as well as a steppingstone towards a better understanding of maturation of physiological structures, retinal to cortical, which define the infant's ability to encode spatial distributions of contours. Since the visual evoked potential reflects the developmental process, changes in amplitude or latency as a function of age must be considered only in the context of the underlying components which they measure. Measurement, for example, of a major positive peak which changes shape and complexity not only with age but also as a function of cortical magnification, cortical representation and stimulus parameters, can lead to misleading assumptions and erroneous estimates of the degree and time course of visual acuity maturation. Attempts to plot the presumptive single positive peak as a function of pattern size for acuity extrapolation to zero amplitude response must also be treated with caution. Further, faster rates of pattern stimulation which allow description of the response in terms of one or two harmonics, obscure the underlying evoked potential complexity in addition to introducing additional variables, i.e. motion versus contrast detection in the determination of acuity estimates. Nevertheless, the usefulness of many of these measures, albeit relative in nature, should not be underestimated. An example of their immediate practical applicability has been amply demonstrated in evoked potential amplitude versus patternsize (spatial frequency) funtions in amblyopia (Sokol and Bloom 1973; Apkarian et al, 1981). And lastly, adaptation of VEP measures for the clinic with approaches such as the sweep VEP and sequential VEP promise continuing improvements in infant visual assessment and the eventual establishment of more accurate and reliable visual growth functions.

REFERENCES

Abramov I, Gordon J, Hendrickson A, Hainline L, Dobson V, LaBossiere E. The retina of the newborn human infant. Science 1982;217:265-267.

Allen J, Visual Acuity Development in Human Infants up to 6 Months of Age. Unpublished doctoral dissertation, University of Washington 1979.

Apkarian P, Levi D, Tyler CW. Binocular facilitation in the visual-evoked potential of strabismic amblyopes. Am J Optom & Physiol Optics 1981;58:820-830.

Apkarian P, Reits D, Spekreijse H, van Dorp D. A decisive electrophysiological test for human albinism. Electroenceph clin Neurophysiol 1983;55:513-531.

Atkinson J, French J, Braddick O. Contrast sensitivity function of preschool children. Br J Ophthalmol 1981;65:525-529.

Atkinson J, Pimm-Smith E, Evans C, Braddick OJ. The effects of screen size and eccentricity on acuity estimates in infants using preferential looking. Vision Res 1983;23:1479-1483.

Banks MS, Salapatek P. Contrast sensitivity function of the infant visual system. Vision Res 1976;16:867-869.

Bauer J, Birch EE, Gwiazda J, Shimojo S, Held R. A plateau in the development of grating acuity in human infants during the first year of life. Invest Ophthalmol & Vis Sci Suppl 1984;25:219

Brant JC, Nowotny M. Testing of visual acuity in young children: an evaluation of some commonly used methods. Develop Med Child Neurol 1976;18:568-576.

Campbell FW, Maffei L. Electrophysiological evidence for the existence of orientation and size detectors in the human visual system. J Physiol 1970;207:635-652.

Cannon Jr MW. Contrast sensitivity: psychophysical and evoked potential methods compared. Vision Res 1983;23:87-95.

Dobson V. Clinical applications of preferential looking measures of visual acuity. Behav Brain Res 1983;10:25-38.

Dobson V, Teller DY. Visual acuity in human infants: a review and comparison of behavioral and electrophysiological studies. Vision Res 1978;18:1469-1483.

Dobson V, Teller DY, Belgum J. Visual acuity in human infants assessed with stationary stripes and phase-alternated checkerboards. Vision Res 1978a;18:1233-1238.

Dobson V, Teller DY, Lee CP, Wade B. A behavioral method for efficient screening of visual acuity in young infants, 1.Preliminary laboratory development. Invest Ophthalmol & Vis Sci 1978b;17:1142-1150.

Fantz RL, Ordy JM, Udelf MS. Maturation of pattern vision in infants during the first six months. J Comp Physiol Psychol 1962;55:907-917.

Friendly DS. Preschool visual acuity screening tests. Trans Am Acad Ophthalmol Soc 1978;76:383-480.

Fulton AB, Hansen RM, Manning AB. Measuring visual acuity in infants. Survey of Ophthalmol 1981;25:325-332.

Fulton AB, Manning KA, Dobson V. Infant vision testing by a behavioral method. Ophthalmology 1979;86:431-439.

Gwiazda J, Brill S, Mohindra I, Held R. Infant visual acuity and its meridonal variation. Vision Res 1978;18:1557-1564.

Gwiazda J, Brill S, Mohindra I, Held R. Preferential looking acuity in infants from two to fifty-eight weeks of age. Am J Optom & Physiol Optics 1980;57:428-432.

Held R, Gwiazda J, Brill S, Mohindra I, Wolfe J. Infant visual acuity is underestimated because near threshold gratings are not preferentially fixated. Vision Res 1979;19:1377-1379.

Hendrickson AE, Yuodelis C. The morphological development of the human fovea. Ophthalmology 1984;91:603-612.

van Hof-van Duin J, Mohn G, Fetter WPF, Mettau JW, Baerts W. Preferential looking acuity in preterm infants. Behav Brain Res 1983;10:47-50.

Howell ER, Mitchell DE, Keith CG. Contrast thresholds for sine gratings of children with amblyopia. Invest Ophthalmol & Vis Sci 1983;24:782-787.

Hoyt CS, Nickel BL, Billson, FA. Ophthalmological examination of the infant. Developmental aspects. Survey of Ophthalmol 1982;26:177-189.

Jeffreys DA, Axford JG. Source locations of pattern-specific components of human visual evoked potentials. II.Component of extrastriate cortical origin. Exp Brain Res 1972;16:22-40.

Kelly DH. Pattern detection and the two-dimensional fourier transform: flickering checkerboards and chromatic mechanisms. Vision Res 1976;16:277-287.

Magoon EH, Robb RM. Development of myelin in human optic nerve and tract. Arch Ophthalmol 1981;99:655-659.

Mann I. The Development of the Human Eye. London: British Medical Ass 1949.

Marg E, Freeman N, Peltzman P, Goldstein PJ. Visual acuity development in human infants: evoked potential measurements. Invest Ophthalmol & Vis Sci 1976;15:150-153.

Mayer DL, Dobson V. Visual acuity development in infants and young children, as assessed by operant preferential looking. Vision Res 1982;22:1141-1151.

Moskowitz A, Sokol S. Developmental changes in the human visual system as reflected by the latency of the pattern reversal VEP. Electroencephal and clin Neurophysiol 1983;56:1-15.

Moskowitz A, Sokol S. Spatial and temporal interaction of pattern-evoked cortical potentials in human infants. Vision Res 1980;20:699-707.

Norcia AM, Tyler CW. Spatial frequency sweep VEP: visual acuity during the first year of life. Vision Res (submitted) 1985.

Odom JV, Green M. Developmental physiological optics and visual acuity: a brief review. Experientia (in press) 1985.

Pirchio M, Spinelli D, Fiorentini A, Maffei L. Infant contrast sensitivity evaluated by evoked potentials. Brain Res 1978;141:179-184.

Porciatti V. Temporal and spatial properties of the pattern-reversal VEPs in infants below 2 months of age. Human Neurobiol 1984;3:97-102.

Prechtl HFP. Polygraphic studies of the full-term newborn. II.Computer analysis of recorded data. In: MacKeith R, Bax M, eds. Studies in Infancy. Suffolk: Lavenham 1968.

Regan D. Rapid objective refraction using evoked brain potentials. Invest Ophthalmol 1973;12:669-679.

Regan D. Speedy assessment of visual acuity in amblyopia by the evoked potential method. Ophthalmologica 1977;175:159-164.

Regan D. Speedy evoked potential methods for assessing vision in normal and amblyopic eyes: pros and cons. Vision Res 1980;20:265-269.

Rentschler I, Hilz R, Brettel H. Spatial tuning properties in human amblyopia cannot explain the loss of optotype acuity. Behav Brain Res 1980;1:433-443.

Riemslag FCC, Spekreijse H, van Walbeek H. Pattern reversal and appearance-disappearance responses in MS patients. Doc Ophthalmol Proc Series 1981;27:215-221.

Rychener RO. Vision tests in infants and young children. Pediat Clin North America 1958;5:231-238.

Seiple WH, Kupersmith MJ, Nelson JI, Carr RE. The assessment of evoked potential contrast thresholds using real-time retrieval. Invest Ophthalmol & Vis Sci 1984;25:627-631.

Sheridan MD. What is normal distance vision at five to seven years? Develop Med Child Neurol 1974;16:189-195.

Simons K. Visual acuity norms in young children. Survey Ophthalmol 1983;28:84-92.

Sokol S. Measurement of infant visual acuity from pattern reversal evoked potentials. Vision Res 1978;18:33-39.

Sokol S, Bloom B. Visually evoked cortical responses of amblyopes to a spatially alternating stimulus. Invest Ophthalmol & Vis Sci 1973;12:936-939.

Sokol S, Moskowitz A. Comparison of pattern VEPs and preferential looking behavior in three-month-old infants. Invest Ophthalmol & Vis Sci (in press) 1985.

Sokol S, Moskowitz A, Paul A. Evoked potential estimates of visual accomodation in infants. Vision Res 1983;23:851-860.

Spekreijse H. Analysis of EEG Responses in Man, Evoked by Sine Wave Modulated Light. The Hague:Junk. 1966.

Spekreijse H. Comparison of acuity tests and pattern evoked potential criteria: two mechanisms underly acuity maturation in man. Behav Brain Res 1983;10:107-117.

Spekreijse H. Maturation of contrast EPs and development of visual resolution. Arch Ital Biol 1978;116:358-369.

Spekreijse H. Pattern evoked potentials: principles, methodology and phenomenology. In: Barber C, ed. Evoked Potentials. London:MTP Press 1980.

Spekreijse H, Dagnelie G, Maier J, Regan D. Flicker and movement constituents of the pattern reversal response. Vision Res (in press) 1985.

Spekreijse H, van der Tweel LH, Zuidema Th. Contrast evoked responses in man. Vision Res 1973;13:1577-1601.

Sprague JB, Wilson WB. Electrophysiologic findings in bilateral optic nerve hypoplasia. Arch Ophthalmol 1981;99:1028-1029.

Teller DY. The forced-choice preferential looking procedure: a psychophysical technique for use with human infants. Inf Behav Develop 1979;2:135-153.

Tyler CW, Apkarian P, Levi DM, Nakayama K. Rapid assessment of visual function: an electronic sweep technique for the pattern visual evoked potential. Invest Ophthalmol & Vis Sci 1979;18:703-713.

Tyler CW, Nakayama K, Apkarian PA, Levi DM. VEP assessment of visual function. Vision Res 1981;21:607-609.

de Vries-Khoe LH, Spekreijse H. Maturation of luminance and pattern EPs in man. Docum Ophthal Proc Series 1982;31:461-475.

Weale RA. A Biography of the Eye. Development, Growth, Age. London: Lewis. 1982.

Woodruff ME: Observations on the visual acuity of children during the first five years of life. Am J Optom & Physiol Optics 1972;49:205-215.

DISCUSSION

van Lith: You said that the question was whether the child had pattern perception and now you investigate pattern responses. You may, however, have pattern responses but not pattern perception. I remember a child who was said to be really looking when I put on the light. He looked at the window and he even looked at me, but he never recognised me or even his food. When it did not smell he did not recognise it. But when I made a sound, when I said "food" or "dinner" or something like that, then you could see that he reacted, so that there was very probably no connection between his visual cortex and his memory. So what is visual perception when you have no memory. I suppose we have to be very careful about this. This is what I was trying to say. Often we get no results when the child is suspected of having poor vision and that may be beyond that level. So be careful about saying that there is pattern perception.

Apkarian: The clinical question was: is there pattern perception? And the answer was "we have recorded a pattern response." We also attempt to derive a VEP acuity estimate based on the minimum pattern size to which we obtain a measurable response.

Arden: I would like to put the reverse question. It is quite common to be presented with a child with an apparent unilateral loss of visual acuity and under those circumstances if the evoked potentials are binocular and symmetrical then the difficulty exists anterior to the optic cortex and you refer the child or his parents, not to an ophthalmologist or paediatrician, but to a child psychiatrist and that is a very valuable thing to be able to do.

van Hof-van Duin: My question is the other way round. When you find negative responses, how sure can you be that the results are reliable? Especially when there are neurological problems, like ventricular dilatation on one side. If the location of your electrodes is not correct, it is possible to get false negative pattern evoked potentials. How do you interpret negative results?

van Lith: I don't know enough about this group of children with poor pattern responses, but I do know from adults that when you have good responses they may have low visual acuity. When you have good responses then visual acuity is better than 0.5. There is not a fixed relationship between visual acuity and pattern response, it depends on the diagnosis. If you have an adult with multiple sclerosis or optic neuritis you may have completely absent pattern responses, with a normal Snellen acuity, but perhaps abnormal contrast sensitivity and quite the reverse in demylinating diseases and the optic atrophies. In the atrophies you may have reduced vision, no better than 0.25, with rather good pattern responses, but perhaps Arden can say more about this.

Apkarian: If we get a non-measurable response that is a very difficult situation. We can attempt to repeat the same test until consistent data are recorded; we can also select from a battery of tests an alternative test paradigm.

van Hof-van Duin: How many electrodes do you use?

Apkarian: A minimum of 3 active electrodes.

Atkinson: You should not take the result of one electrodiagnostic technique in isolation; you may need other measures in order to interpret a negative result.

COMPARISON OF RAPID PROCEDURES IN FORCED CHOICE PREFERENTIAL LOOKING FOR
ESTIMATING ACUITY IN INFANTS AND YOUNG CHILDREN

J. Atkinson, J. Wattam-Bell, E. Pimm-Smith, C. Evans,
O.J. Braddick

Visual Development Unit, University of Cambridge

Address for correspondence
Dr. J. Atkinson
University of Cambridge
Department of Experimental Psychology
Downing Street
CB2 3EB

It is over ten years since the method of forced-choice preferential
looking, (FPL) was devised and first used for assessing visual capacities
in human infants (Teller et al 1974; Teller 1979; Atkinson et al, 1974;
Banks and Salapatek, 1976; Gwiazda et al 1978). A number of reviews have
highlighted the similarity of results across different laboratory set-ups
(see Dobson and Teller, 1978, Banks and Salapatek, 1981; Held, 1979;
Atkinson, 1984) but there still remains the question as to which
psychophysical procedure offers the best speed and reliability for
estimating visual acuity. Opthalmological clinics, which are planning to
set up and use FPL routinely with infant patients, need some basis for
selecting the precise statistical procedure (ie. sequence and number of
stimuli present) which should be used to obtain useful clinical results.

The purpose of this study was to investigate empirically the
reliability of various procedures and to devise a reliable but rapid
method, that would be practically feasible for clinical assessments. We
do not discuss in this paper a number of important theoretical
considerations of the FPL procedure which have already been considered
(for example Held et al, 1979, Teller et al, 1982; Banks et al, 1982;
Wolfe et al, 1983). However, it is worth pointing out that theoretical
discussions of psychophysical procedures generally assume that the
subject's behaviour remains stable over time. Experience with infants,
however, suggests that there can be changes in motivation and state over
quite short testing sessions. The effect of this is that theoretical
improvements in statistical reliability, achieved by prolonged testing,
may be more than offset by a decline in the infant's responsiveness. For
this reason we believe that the quality of FPL measures with different
lengths and types of procedure can, in the end, only be assessed
empirically.

Material and Methods

The apparatus and general method ressembled those described by Atkinson et al, 1977, 1982, 1983. Infants were seated on a trained holder's knee 60cm from a pair of circular CRT screens. Each screen subtended 19 degrees at the infant's eyes with the inner edge of each screen 10 degrees from the midline. Between trials both screens displayed a uniform field of luminance 20 cd/m and a set of small coloured flashing LEDs midway between the screens attracted the infant's attention to the centre. A concealed observer watched the infant from a central peephole above the screens and initiated a trial (presentation of a grating pattern on one or other screen) when the infant was looking at the central lights. During a trial one of the screens, selected automatically at random by the controlling microcomputer (Joyce Electronics GRSYSI), displayed a high contrast stripe pattern (with a sinusoidal luminance profile), while the other screen remained uniform and of equal mean luninance. The observer is unaware of which side displays the grating and has to make a forced-choice of this based on observation of the infant's fixations and other behaviour. The duration of the observation period is under the observer's control (with a maximum of 10 sec. which is rarely reached). In the present study a series of stripe widths or spatial frequencies (7 steps in all) were used increasing from 0.48 c/deg. by a factor of 1.6 for each step.

Two different 'staircase' procedures were used, the difference between the two being the number of trials in a 'block' at a particular spatial frequency, on the basis of which the frequency for the next block was selected.

The first procedure, as in our earlier work, used blocks of five trials. If the observer made four or five correct judgments out of five then the frequency was increased (stripes made narrower) for the next block; otherwise it was decreased. This procedure will be called the '5-staircase' in this paper. A 5-staircase was taken as complete when at least 20 trials had been run at each of two adjacent frequencies for which the proportion of correct responses bracketed or included the value of 70% correct. We adopt this number because 70% of 20 trials provides a proportion that is significantly different from chance at the 0.05 level - ie. we are assured that the infant is reliably detecting the pattern. Normally between 50 and 90 trials were needed to meet this criteria. Two 5-staircases were run on each child. To estimate acuity under conditions which were as comparable as possible in terms of the infant's state we used a method of "interleaved staircases" (Atkinson et al 1982). 25 trials of one staircase (ie. 5 blocks) were run followed by 25 trials of the second staircase, followed by 25 trials of the first staircase and so on until each staircase was complete. These two repetitions of the 5-staircase are referred to as "5 R1" and "5 R2".

The second procedure used the same set of spatial frequencies as in the 5-staircases but in this case the spatial frequency was changed according to the 'up down' rule commonly used in psychophysical experiments (Weatherill and Levitt, 1965). That is, if the observer's choice was correct on one trial another presentation of the same frequency was made; if the choice was correct again then a more difficult (higher frequency) grating was presented on the following trial. Any single incorrect choice by the observer caused a lower (ie. easier) frequency to be selected on the following trial. This procedure will be called here the 2-staircase since it involves a maximum block length of two trials. For each infant two 2-staircases were run being interleaved with 25 trials of one staircase being followed by 25 trials of the other until both staircases included at least 20 trials at each of two frequencies which bracketed or included the 70% correct point. The two repetitions of the 2-staircase will be refered to as 2R1 and 2R2. With the up-down rule used the probability of going up or down is equal at a stimulus level that produces approximately 70% correct choices. Thus an alternative way to estimate the 70% point is to take the average of the levels at which the staircase changes direction ('reversals').

To decide the starting point for each staircase the infant was presented initially with the lowest spatial frequency and the frequency increased by one step on each trial until an incorrect choice was made. The starting point was then taken as the highest spatial frequency on which a correct choice was made. (ie. one step down from the first incorrect choice) Both '5R1' and '5R2' staircases were started at the same spatial frequency. The same procedure was begun a fresh to choose a starting point for the 2-staircases and both 2R1 and 2R2 used the same starting point. Half of the infants were tested using the 5-staircases first, and half using the 2-staircases first.

Infants

Twelve infants, from the Cambridge area, volunteered by their parents to help in this study, were tested. All infants had normal birth histories and ranged in age between 12 and 20 weeks. Testing on each infant was completed in a period of two weeks with an average of 3 visits for each child. The times of testing were carefully selected so that the child was in an alert and calm state, usually after a feed.

Results

We take the 70% correct point as a measure of FPL acuity. For each infant there are four estimates of this point one from each of the four staircases 5R1, 5R2, 2R1 and 2R2.

Comparison of the two procedures

Fig 1. shows the acuity values for the two procedures (the 5-staircases versus the 2-staircases) for each child. R1 and R2 has been averaged in each case. As can be seen from this graph there is a high correlation between the two procedures (r = .78) with no difference in the estimated values of acuity between the two procedures.

To test the realiability of the two procedures we calculated the "test- retest" correlation between 5R1 and 5R2 and 2R1 and 2R2. The correlation between 5R1 and 5R2 was r = 0.84 and that between 2R1 and 2R2 was r = .77 The closeness of the values suggests that the two staircase procedures lead to equally reliable estimates of acuity.

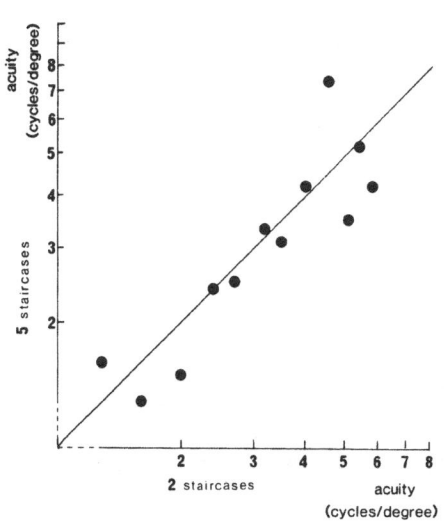

Fig 1. Comparison of acuity values for the two procedures (5-staircases and 2-staircases).

We also compared the number of trials necessary to meet our criteria of completing the staircases for the two procedures and again found no significant differences between the two. This means that both procedures take a similar amount of time which is the time it takes for approximately 50 trials. This is rather longer than an ideal routine clinical test.

Shortened staircase procedures

We therefore decided to examine what information would be available from earlier points in the staircases in terms of the reliability of the acuity estimate and its relation to the estimate obtained from the whole staircase.

For the first shortened session we took the first 20 trials of each staircase (after the initial starting point has been ascertained) and calculated the spatial frequency which would give an interpolated value of 70% correct. The correlation between the acuity estimates from the first 20 trials of 5R1 and 5R2 was $r = 0.88$ and that between the estimate from the first 20 trials of 2R1 and 2R2 was $r = 0.72$. These values are very close to those obtained with the complete staircases: thus we conclude that using twenty trials rather than all the trials is a reasonably reliable way of obtaining a relatively rapid estimate of acuity. Again the results of at test revealed that there is no significant difference between the estimates of acuity based on twenty trials and that based on all the trials, so there is no indication of a systematic bias from use of the early trials. This can be seen in Fig 2 and Fig 3 below where we show the comparison of the acuity values from the first 20 trials and the complete staircases.

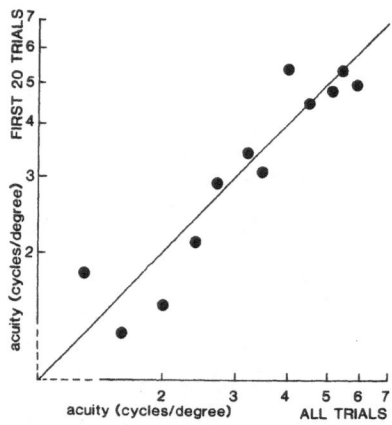

Fig 2. Comparison of the acuity for the first 20 trials and the complete 5-staircases.

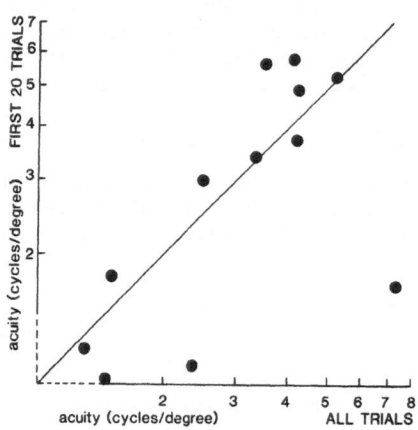

Fig 3. Comparison of the acuity for the first 20 trials and the complete 2-staircases.

A second shortened procedure may be used with the 2-staircases, using the values for reversals in the staircase to estimate acuity. The acuity value was taken as the value at the first reversal, the average of the first two reversals and the average of the first three reversals. The reliability of each of these estimates was once again investigated by calculating the correlation between the values obtained from 2R1 and 2R2. The correlation between the two estimates from the first reversal was .75, from the first two reversals it was r = .88 and from the first three it was r = 0.76. The correlation at the second reversal point is higher than that found for the two complete staircases which suggests that it is giving a good estimate of acuity. On average the second reversal is reached after 8.8 trials which means that only a very short staircase needs to be completed before this estimate can be made.

The shortest procedure of all would merely be to look at the starting points for the staircases to see whether these give a reliable estimate of acuity. However, the correlation between the starting points for the 5 procedure and the 2 procedure, which were obtained independently for each baby, only gave r = 0.31 which is a much lower value, than that obtained when using any of the other abbreviated staircases and differs significantly from them when 2 scores are calculated (Mc Nemor, 1962). On the basis of this result it would not be reliable to estimate an infant's acuity from the starting point alone.

Discussion and conclusions

From the relation between acuity estimates obtained using different procedures with the forced choice preferential looking method, we have found that similar estimates are obtained using either a staircase consisting of 5-trial blocks with the same stimulus or one where the stimulus is changed more frequently according to the up-down rule. When repeated estimates are compared both methods are equally reliable, although both full staircases take a large number of trials (50 to 90) to obtain 20 trials at values bracketing the 70% correct level.

For purposes of clinical assessments, we have tried to find a shortened procedure which gives reliable estimates of acuity. From our results it appears that the best of the shortened procedure is the second procedure where the spatial frequency is changed after every trial or every other trial and the acuity is calculated from the average of the spatial frequencies at the first and second reversal point in the staircase. On average this procedure would take 9 trials after the initial starting point has been obtained. However taking the first reversal point (after estimating the starting point) gives a reasonably reliable estimate of acuity and only takes a very few trials to reach.

For such low numbers of trials the 5-staircase procedure would not be satisfactory since it could only sample very few values of spatial frequency. We would emphasise the importance of the initial procedure to find the starting point rapidly since staircase procedures generally are most efficient when they are close to the threshold value. The starting point procedure is also important in that it provides the infant with the experience of clear and easy initial trials which indicate what is going on; our experience is that infants show less stable behaviour when they

198

have not received some very clearly visible stimuli at the beginning of testing.

We should point out that this study was carried out with infants aged 3-5 months, an age range in which they show quite prolonged attention to FPL stimuli. Older infants, while they may be very alert and show good initial attention, usally show a more rapid decline in attention. For infants of 6 months and older, therefore, the need to use a brief procedure to obtain realistic estimates of visual performance is even more acute than for the younger group. Using the shortened staircases, suggested in this paper should mean that the method can be used clinically to obtain reliable acuity estimates in the future.

Acknowledgements

This work was supported by a grant from the Medical Research Council. We are grateful to the families of our infant subjects for their cooperation.

REFERENCES

Atkinson J. Human visual development over the first 6 months of life. A review and a hypothesis. Human Neurobiol 1984; 3: 61-74.

Atkinson J, Braddick OJ. Acuity, contrast sensitivity, and accommodation in infancy. In Aslin RN. Alberts JR. Petersen MR. (eds) Development of Perception, vol 2: The Visual System. 1981. Academic Press. New York.

Atkinson J, Braddick OJ, Braddick F. Acuity and contrast sensitivity in infant vision. Nature. Lond. 1974; 247: 403-404.

Atkinson J, Braddick OJ, Moar K. Development of contrast sensitivity over the first 3 months of life in the human infant. Vision Res 1977; 17: 1037-1044.

Atkinson J, Braddick OJ, Pimm-Smith E. 'Preferential looking' for monocular and binocular acuity testing of infants. Br J Ophthalmol 1982; 66: 264-268.

Atkinson J, Pimm-Smith E, Evans C, Braddick OJ. The effects of screen size and eccentricity on acuity estimates in infants using preferential looking. Vision Res 1983; 23: 1479-1483.

Banks MS, Salapatek P. Contrast sensitivity function of the infant visual system. Vision Res 1976; 16: 867-869.

Banks MS, Salapatek P. Infant pattern vision: a new approach based on the contrast sensitivity function. J Exp Child Psychol 1981; 31: 1-45.

Banks MS, Stephens BR, Dannemiller JL. A failure to observe negative preference in infant acuity testing. Vision Res 1982; 22: 1025-1032.

Dobson V, Teller DY. Visual acuity in human infants: a review and comparison of behavioral and electrophysiological studies. Vision Res 1978; 18: pp. 1469-1483.

Gwiazda J, Brill S, Mohindra I, Held R. Infant visual acuity and its meridional variation. Vision Res 1978; 18: 1557-1564.

Held R. Development of visual resolution. Canadian J Psychol 1979; 33: 213-221.

Held R, Gwiazda J, Brill S, Monindra I, Wolfe J. Infant visual acuity is underestimated because near threshold gratings are not preferentially fixated. Vision Res 1979; 19: pp. 1377-1380.

McNemar Q. Psychological Statistics. Wiley and Sons Inc 1962.

Teller DY. The forced-choice preferential looking procedure: a psychophysical technique for use with human infants. Infant Behav and Devel 1979; 2: 135-153.

Teller DY, Morse R, Borton R, Regal D. Visual acuity for vertical and diagonal gratings in human infants. Visual Res 1974; 14: 1433-1439.

Teller DY, Mayer DL, Makous WL, Allen JL. Do all preferential looking techniques underestimate infant visual acuity? Vision Res 1982; 22: 1017-1024.

Wetherill GB, Levitt H. Sequential estimation of points on a psychometric function. Brit J Math and Stat Psychol 1965; 18: 1-10.

Wolfe JM, Gwiazda J, Held R. The meaning of non-monotomic functions in the assessment of infant preferential looking acuity. A reply to Banks et al (1982) and Teller et al (1982). Vision Res 1982; 23: 917-920.

VISUAL CROWDING IN YOUNG CHILDREN

J. Atkinson, E. Pimm-Smith, C. Evans, G. Harding, O. Braddick

Visual Development Unit, Department of Experimental Psychology, University of Cambridge

INTRODUCTION

'Visual crowding' or 'lateral masking' is the deleterious effect nearby contours have on the recognition and identification of symbols or letters. Its magnitude has often been estimated by comparing single optotype acuity with acuity for multiple arrays. In adults, the effect was described for peripheral vision some time ago (Ehlers, 1936; Woodworth and Schlosberg, 1954; Bouma, 1970) with a smaller similar effect being described for the fovea (Flom et al., 1963). In a number of studies of amblyopes a large crowding effect has been described (Stuart and Burian, 1962; Oliver and Nawratzki, 1971; Hilton and Stanley, 1972; Tommilla, 1972; Weiss, 1973; Youngson, 1979; Beyerstein and Freeman, 1977). To assess the degree of abnormality in amblyopes it is necessary to know the size of the crowding effect in children with normal vision. Here we report two studies using novel tasks to assess crowding in children with normal vision. The results of this study are to serve as a baseline against which to measure abnormality. Relatively naive adults have also performed the tasks for comparison purposes.

Study 1 - 'C' and 'O' discrimination in 5-6 year olds and adults

The task is a matching task with the symbol to be matched being one of two letters, a 'C' or an 'O'. We originally planned to test two age groups (3½ year olds and 5-6 year olds) to find out whether there was a reduction in crowding over the preschool years. However, after preliminary testing, it was decided that the task was too cognitively taxing for the younger pre-school children. Numerous verbal and visual confusions were demonstrated in pilot studies with 3 year olds, even with the use of very large letters. Confusions using similar discriminations (for example, the illiterate E) had already led to poor and variable acuity estimates in pre-school children (Stuart and Burian, 1962; Tommilla, 1972; Hedin, Nyman, and Derouet, 1980) and so it was decided that only the older age group (5-6 year olds) would be given the 'C' and 'O' discrimination task. An easier, less confusing test was designed and used for testing the younger age group in Study 2.

Subjects

All children were volunteered by their parents for testing in our Visual Development Unit. 14 children were tested between the ages of 5 years 3 months and 6 years 2 months with a mean of 5½ years. 9 of the mothers of the children acted as adult subjects (all adults were between 30 and 40 years, had recently had their eyesight checked and were wearing an adequate correction where necessary). All the children had normal refractions (all could accommodate accurately and had not more than 0.5D astigmatism in either or both eyes) as measured using photorefraction (Braddick, Atkinson, French and Howland, 1979).

Stimuli

The stimuli are shown below.

C O

a

O C C O C O

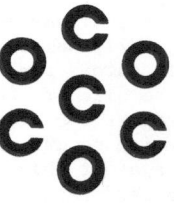

b   c

Figure 1. Stimuli used for acuity testing of 5-6 year olds.
(a) single optotype. (b) linear array (only the central four symbols used for testing). (c) circular array (only the central symbol used for testing).

They consisted of black C's and O's on a white background. Three different arrangements were used, these being:- (a) a single C or O, (b) a line of C's and O's (linear array), (c) a circular arrangement of C's and O's (circular array).

For (b) and (c) a random placement of the 3 C's and 3 O's was used. For (a) an equal number of C's and O's were used. Six different cards of each type were made up so that they could be randomly presented and any artefactual cues (marks on the cards) were minimized. The letters were made out of Letraset sheet no. 247 (Avantgarde Gothic Bold). The gap between the letters for the (b) and (c) arrangements was set at half the letter width, so that in (c) all symbols were equidistant.

These stimuli were than photographically reduced so that the gap size in the letter C was 1 min arc at 3 metres (i.e. equivalent to 6/6 Snellen vision).

Procedure

The children and adults viewed the stimuli in a corridor, well illuminated by fluorescent strip lighting (luminance 30 cd/m^2). They sat on a chair at the appropriate distance from the test card which was held vertically at the eye level of the subject. For each card either a verbal response was given or the child could point to either the 'C' or the 'O' on a demonstration card held in their hand. Extensive practice in the task was given at a close distance before testing proceeded. 11 different distances were used from 1.5 m to 8.4 m, these being in a constant ratio so that each step was equivalent to half the difference between Snellen rows (i.e. the gap size decreased by 19% on each step). Testing started at 2.5 metres. Throughout testing the tester used a fine pale grey knitting needle to point to the letter to be identified. Every attempt was made to keep the knitting needle a constant distance (i.e., half one letter width) below or above the letter to be identified.

At least two sessions (separated by several weeks) were arranged for each child. On the first session the single letter condition (a) and the linear array (b) were used, half the children being first tested with (a) and half with (b). A separate staircase procedure, described below, was run for each condition and interleaved so that the child had 20 presentations with either (a) or (b) and then 20 presentations of the other, followed by 20 of the original stimuli, until both staircases were complete.

In the second session, the single letter stimuli (a) were interleaved with the circular array (c) in a similar manner to the first session.

Staircase procedure

A similar procedure has already been described for two different visual tasks (Atkinson, French and Braddick, 1981; Atkinson, Braddick and Pimm-Smith, 1982). The trials were run in blocks of 4 for each particular distance, each trial being the identification of a letter on the chart, with only the middle 4 letters being used on the linear arrays (the end letters were excluded to maintain constant crowding in this condition). The distance was varied between blocks according to a modified staircase procedure, based on the subjects proportion of correct choices in the preceding block. Much encouragement was given to the children with sweets and sticky stars being given as rewards every 5-10 trials. Frequent breaks were given so that testing was only for approximately 10 minutes at a time.

If the child got 3 or 4 correct in a block the stimuli were moved one distance step further away. If they got 2 correct another block was initiated at the same distance until three blocks at 50% correct had been run; then a distance step nearer was used. If they got only 1 or 0 correct then the stimulus was moved one distance step nearer. The staircase was continued until 20 trials were obtained for at least 2 distances with performance at or above 70% correct at one distance and below at the other (70% = 14 correct out of 20 trials). The distance at which the observer gave 70% correct was interpolated from a graph of per cent correct as a function of distance and was called the <u>threshold distance</u>. The crowding effect was then calculated as the ratio of threshold distance on multiple targets (either (b) or (c)) to that for a

204

single target (a). The equivalent acuity for the threshold distance was
also calculated.

Results

Figure 2 shows a comparison of the single optotype acuity for each
child with that on (b) and (c).

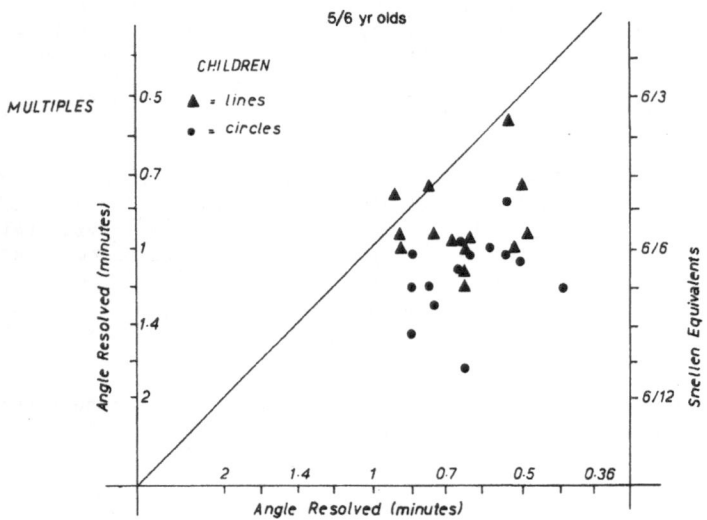

Figure 2. Comparison of single optotype acuities with acuities for the
multiple ("crowded") symbols, for individual 5-6 year old children.
Triangles: multiple symbols in linear array. Circles: multiple symbols
in circular array. The diagonal line indicates equality.

If acuities were equal on these tasks then the points should all fall on
the 45° line. A clear "crowding" effect is demonstrated for many of the
children with the acuities being lower in (b) and (c) than in (a). Some
children show a much larger effect than others.

Figure 3 shows the same comparison for adults. Again a crowding
effect is shown for many adults, although the points are closer to the 45°
line than in Figure 1, showing in general a smaller effect for adults than
for children. A t-test confirmed that the acuity estimates for both
multiple arrays were significantly lower than for single letters (p <
0.05) for the children; the difference for adults only reached
significance for the circular array (c) compared to the single letters
(a). With the linear array (b) the mean crowding ratio for children was
1.46 whereas for adults it was 1.04. With the circular array (c) the mean
ratio was 1.78 for children and 1.33 for adults.

A further statistical comparison revealed that the crowding effect
was larger for the circular array than for the linear in children and

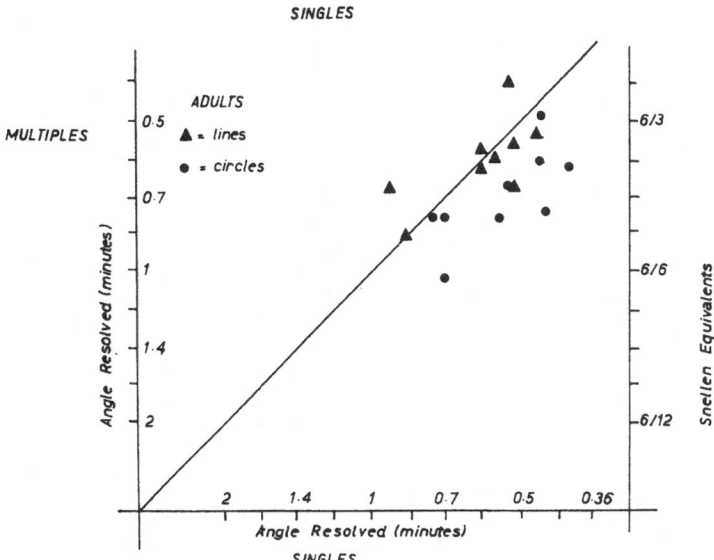

<u>Figure 3</u>. As Figure 2, for adult subjects.

adults (p < 0.05). It is interesting to note that although the circular array produced a larger crowding effect than the linear array, this result was not in agreement with subjective reports of either the adults or children. Both commented that the circular array was much "easier" because they did not have to maintain fixation and position, as in the linear array. For the children more frequent breaks were necessary when using the linear array to keep motivation high.

Reliability

The data was analysed to check within-subject reliability across the two tests by looking at the single optotype acuities on the first session and the second. The correlation coefficient for the children was 0.87 (p < 0.05) showing that there was no significant change in performance on the repeat test. For the first session using the single letter, the threshold distance was 4.61 m and in the second session it was 4.73 m. This is equivalent to an average acuity of 6/4.5 in Snellen terms.

Single optotype acuity

A comparison of the single optotype acuity for children and adults showed that there was no significant difference between the two. The children's single optotype acuity was as good as the adults, at around 6/4.5.

Discussion

Many other studies, using a variety of stimuli, of the single optotype form, show acuity in 6 yr olds to be at 6/6 or better (Weiss, 1973; Oppel, 1974; Woodruff, 1972; Smorvik and Bosnes, 1976); line acuities are in general around 6/7.5 (Slataper, 1950). From the present results the average single optotype acuity was 6/4.5, for a linear array it was 6/6 and for the circular array it was 6/7.5.

The results also show significantly greater crowding effects for the children compared to the adults, with some children showing much greater effects than others. At present we have no explanation for this dichotomy in the children's group. No significant correlation with acuity was found, i.e. those with higher acuity did not show a greater or lesser crowding effect. Nor was the extent of crowding correlated with age, some of the younger in the group showed smaller crowding effects than the older children. It is possible that the extent of crowding relates to other visual skills such as reading, but at present we have no independent measures of these skills on these children.

It appeared that by 6 years some children have a visual system which is close to the adults', whereas the majority still show some immaturity. This immaturity does not seem to relate well to an idea of simple 'sharpening' up of acuity to explain the reduced effect in adults.

It is possible that some cognitive differences account for those children showing big effects and those showing small, but if this is so it was not indicated by the motivational state of the children, or the comments made by adults and children alike that the linear array was more 'difficult' than the circular array. It has recently been suggested that the fine eye movement control of children is poorer than adults (Kowler and Martins, 1982). This explanation of the extent of crowding seems unlikely because in our present study better eye movement control was probably required for identifying letters in the linear array than in the circular array, but the crowding effect was larger in both adults and children in the circular array rather than the linear array. The effort required for accurate control of eye movements to judge position in the linear array may be the reason for the subjective 'difficulty' of this task, but does not explain the magnitude of the crowding. It seems that in the circular array the additional letters above and below the central one, produce additional crowding.

Because of the failure of reliable results on 3½ year olds on the 'C' and 'O' task, and the difficulty of linear arrays even for 5 and 6 year olds, we designed a second set of stimuli using a greater variety of letters, although the letter to be identified was always an O.

Study 2 - Identification of 'O' in a crowding task for 3½ year olds and adults

Subjects

All 15 children were volunteered by their parents to take part in tests in our Visual Development Unit. The children's age range was 3 years 1 month to 4 years 1 month with the average age being 3 years 3 months. 8 mothers of the children were tested as adult controls, as in

the previous study. One child did not complete testing because of
scheduling problems and one did not cooperate. The results of the other
13 children are reported here.

Stimuli

A typical stimulus card is shown in Figure 4.

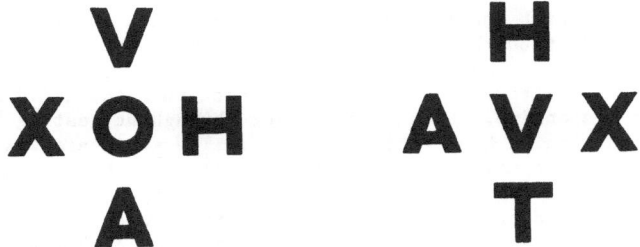

Figure 4. Examples of multiple stimulus arrays used in the testing of 3½
year old children. The child was required to distinguish whether the
central symbol was '0' or another letter. Single optotypes were similar
but included only the central symbol.

The letter '0' was arranged in the centre of a display with the letters X,
A, T, V, H, randomly arranged around the central letter. Half the
displays had an '0' in the centre and half had another letter in the
centre. The same Letraset type face as in the previous study was used.
The stimulus arrays were photographed at different magnification so that a
series of 6 sizes (comparable to the half rows of a Snellen chart) could
be viewed, all at 3 metres, the largest being equivalent to 6/24.

The cards were mounted on the inner surfaces of transparent acrylic
cubes (7.6 cm high by 8.9 cm wide) which were photographic display cubes.
Each cube was packed with polyurethane foam, with a small piece cut out of
the base of the foam so that a reward could be concealed under the cube.
Sweets, crisps, adhesive gold stars or teddy bears were used as rewards.

Procedure

The procedure was the same as that used in a previous study on preschool children (Atkinson, French and Braddick, 1981). Two of the cubes were placed on chairs at a distance of 3 metres from the child with the face displaying the letters facing the child. A material barrier was placed from between the cubes to the child so that the child looked first at the cube down one side of the barrier and then to the other side. Only one of the two cubes on each presentation had the letter 'O' on it (either on its own, or in the centre of a multiple array) and the task for the child was to go to either the cube on the left or right of the barrier which displayed the 'O' and get the reward from under the cube. After very little practice, all the children except one got the idea of the test and were happy to run up and down the 3 metres many times. To remind the child about the shape of the 'O' a card displaying an 'O' was held by the child for comparison.

Two staircase procedures were used, one for the single letters and one for the multiple arrays. The staircases were interleaved, half the children starting with the single letters and half with the multiple. The staircase started with the largest letters (equivalent of 6/24) and if the choice was correct then the next smaller letter was used, and so on until an incorrect choice was made. At this point a "dummy" run was inserted where the largest letter was used again to check that the child was still motivated and responsive. From time to time throughout testing "dummy" trials were inserted to keep motivation high. The staircase was run in blocks of 5 trials starting at one letter size larger than the first incorrect choice. At the end of 5 trials, if 4 or 5 choices were correct the letter size was decreased. If 3 or less trials were correct the letter size was increased. A staircase terminated when twenty trials had been run at two letter sizes when one size of letter yielded at least 14 out of 20 trials correct and the next smaller letter size yielded less than 14 out of 20 trials correct. The 70% correct was used as the estimate of acuity and interpolated from the staircase results.

When the mothers were tested they were simply asked to tell the tester which cube displayed a letter 'O', with a similar staircase procedure being used, and an acuity being estimated similarly.

Results

3½ year olds

All 13 children had higher equivalent acuity on the single optotypes than the multiple, showing a crowding effect. These results are plotted in Figure 5 and show that all the points are above the 45° line. The average single optotype acuity was 46.6 c/deg (equivalent to 6/4) on this task, while the average on the multiple arrays was 22.7 c/deg. equivalent to (6/8). This crowding effect was significant on a t-test (p < 0.05). If these two results are compared the crowding ratio, in terms of distance threshold is, 2.0.

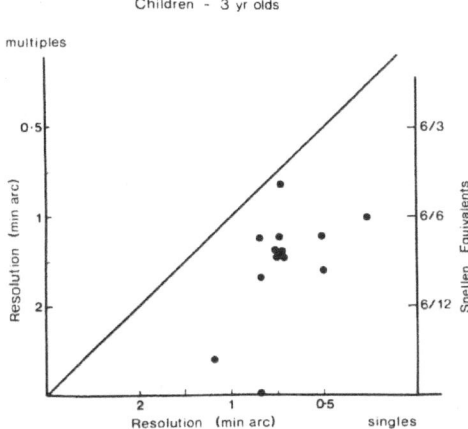

Figure 5. Comparison of single optotype acuities with acuities for multiple "crowded" symbols, for individual 3½ year old children. The diagonal line indicates equality.

Adults

Most of the adults detected correctly the smallest single 'O' available (equivalent to 6/3) and so an exact measure of their threshold cannot be made. On the multiple array the average adult acuity was 50 c/deg (equivalent to 6/4). The comparison of the two conditions is shown on Figure 6. A crowding effect, represented as displacement away from the 45° line, is shown for most of the adults.

Discussion

A large crowding effect has been demonstrated in 3½ year olds. The stimulus producing crowding is similar in the second study to the first but not identical. In the first the choice is between a 'C' and 'O', whereas in the second study the task is discrimination between an 'O' and one of the other letters. As the other letters are all made up of straight lines, they would appear to be more dissimilar to an 'O' than the 'C' of the first study. This would mean that the choice task in the second task should be easier than in the first, although the differences in the ease of the task could be offset by surrounding angular letters crowding an angular central letter more than an 'O'.

In general the crowding effect is larger in the 3½ year olds than in the 5-6 year olds with a number of the older children showing no crowding effect, which is unlikely to be due to the differences between the two tasks. It seems as though the crowding effect gradually reduces in the

210

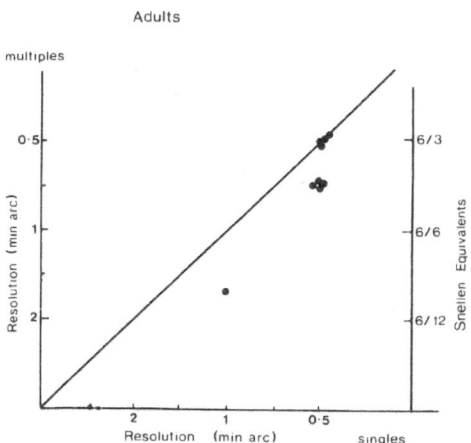

<u>Figure 6.</u> As Figure 5, for adult subjects tested with the stimuli used
for 3½ year olds.

preschool years as part of normal vision development, but until both age
groups have been tested on exactly the same task the relative crowding
across ages cannot be measured. Such a study is underway in our Unit at
present.

The results of this study show that children with normal vision have
a single optotype acuity which is at least equivalent to 6/6 vision at 3½
years, and for some of these preschool children is better than 6/6. This
result is in line with the data from previous studies (Nordlow and
Joachimsson, 1962; Sheridan, 1963; Woodruff, 1972; Weiss, 1973; Brant and
Nowotny, 1976; Smørvøk and Bosnes, 1976; Atkinson, French and Braddick,
1981). On stimuli where crowding is induced, the average equivalent
acuity for 3½ year olds is 6/8, whereas for adults it is still at least
6/6 or better. For older children the crowded stimuli gave acuity values
equivalent to 6/4.5 for the linear array and 6/7.5 for the circular array,
which was significantly worse than the adults on the same test.

If a test which is useful for detecting amblyopia is to be devised,
it must take into account the magnitude of crowding in children with
normal vision and this would seem to be a function of the child's age.
Some of the 5-6 year olds showed significant amounts of crowding in our
present tests, failing to show at least 6/6 vision (which would be
regarded as normal on a Snellen chart). However, as at present there is
considerable variation in spacing of the letters and row of letters among
the charts used in hospital eye clinics and in community health clinics,
it may only be possible to state that a child's vision (under 7 years of
age) is likely to be in the normal range if it is at least 6/6. If it is
6/7.5 or worse then it could be that the particular chart that is employed

is maximising crowding and that the child is still visually immature along this dimension. If however the chart used in school checks has such widely spaced letters and rows that it is effectively similar to the single optotype chart, then vision of 6/7.5 would be abnormally poor for the child's age.

The results from the above study point to the necessity of standardising in terms of crowding, all charts that are used for school entrance children in school eye checks and for devising new preschool tests to include crowding effects. These tests must be adapted to the cognitive ability of the preschool child and will have to be validated on a large group of preschool children before being put into general use. We are at present deriving and devising norms for such a test which could perhaps be used in future preschool vision screening programmes rather than the single optotype test, which is presently used.

Acknowledgements

This research was supported by the Medical Research Council of Great Britain. We would like to thank Jackie Day and John Wattam-Bell for assistance with some of the testing and analyses.

REFERENCES

Atkinson J, French J, Braddick O. Contrast sensitivity function of preschool children. Brit J Ophthal 1981;65:525-529.

Atkinson J, Braddick O, Pimm-Smith E. 'Preferential looking' for monocular and binocular acuity testing of infants. Brit J Ophthal 1982; 66:264-268.

Beyerstein BL, Freeman R. Lateral spatial interaction in humans with abnormal visual experience. Vision Res 1977;17:1029.

Bouma M. Interaction effects in parafoveal letter recognition. Nature 1970;226:177-178.

Braddick OJ, Atkinson J, French J, Howland HC. A photorefractive study of infant accommodation. Vision Res 1979;19:1319-1330.

Brant J, Nowotny M. Testing of visual acuity in young children: An evaluation of some commonly used methods. Develop Med Child Neurol 1976;18:568.

Ehlers H. The movement of the eyes during reading. Ophthalmologica 1936;14:56.

Flom MC, Heath G, Takahaski E. Contour interaction and visual resolution: contralateral effect. Science 1963;142:979-980.

Hedin A, Nyman KG, Derouet B. A modified letter matching chart for testing young children's visual acuity. Journal of Paediatric Ophthalmology and Strabismus 1980;17:114-118.

Hilton AF, Stanley JC. Pitfalls in testing children's vision by the Sheridan Gardiner single optotype method. Brit J Ophthalmol 1972;56: 135-139.

Kowler E, Martins AJ. Eye movements of preschool children. Science 1982;215:997-999.

Nordlow W, Joachimson. A screening test for visual acuity in four year old children. Scand J Psychol 1962;17:122-

Oliver M, Nawratzki I. Screening of pre-school children for ocular anomalies. Brit J Ophthal 1971;55:462-466.

Oppel O. On the development of visual acuity in children of the preschool age. Klin Mbl Augenheilk 1964;145:358.

Slataper FJ. Age norms of refraction and vision. Arch Ophthalmol 1950; 43:568-576.

Smørvik D, Bosnes, O. Assessment of visual acuity in preschool children. Scand J Psychol 1976;17:122.

Stuart JA, Burian HM. A study of separation difficulty: its relationship to visual acuity in normal and amblyopic eyes. Amer J Ophthalmol 1962; 53:471.

Tommilla V. A new chart for testing line acuity in amblyopia. Acta Ophthalmologica 1972;50:565-569.

Weiss JB. Mesure de l'acuite visuelle du jeune enfant. Vision Res 1973; 13:1139-1149.

Woodworth RS, Schlosberg H. Experimental Psychology. New York: Holt. 1954.

Youngson RM. Anomaly in visual acuity testing in children. Brit J Ophthalmol 1979;59:168-170.

THE DEVELOPMENT OF PREFERENTIAL-LOOKING VISUAL ACUITY IN HUMAN INFANTS. A CORRELATION WITH ANIMAL MODELS.

Ruxandra Sireteanu[1], Klaus-Peter Boergen[2]
and Regina Kellerer[2]

[1]Max-Planck-Institut für Hirnforschung,
D-6000 Frankfurt 71, FRG
[2]Augenklinik München, D-8000 München 2,
FRG

INTRODUCTION

It is well established that visual acuity develops
dramatically during early infancy. Less understood, however,
are the mechanisms which underlie this development of acuity.
In human infants, it was speculated that acuity development is
determined by the postnatal emergence and maturation of the
fovea (Mann, 1964; Abramov et al., 1982; Hendrickson and
Yuodelis, 1984). On the other hand, the development of acuity
could be due to postnatal changes in the optical and
geometrical properties of the eye or to the maturational
processes which take place at different levels of the neural
visual pathway (for a recent review see Garey, 1984).

The experiments reported in this paper attempt to give an
answer to these questions. To define the role of the fovea, in
a first group of experiments we determined the development of
acuity in the peripheral visual field of human infants. We
then compared this development to the development of acuity in
the central visual field, using a modification of the
preferential-looking technique (Sireteanu et al., 1984; for a
complete description of this technique, see Teller, 1979). In
a second experiment, the preferential-looking method was used
to determine the development of visual acuity in very young
kittens (Sireteanu, 1985). A comparison of these results with
the developmental events known to take place at different
levels of the visual pathway suggests that the development of
acuity is determined at the retinal level, but is not entirely
due to the maturation of the fovea.

RESULTS

Experiment I. The development of visual acuity in human
infants.

a.) "Best" visual acuity. In this experiment, we used the preferential looking technique to determine the development of visual acuity in the central part of the visual field. The infants were seated on their mother's lap, facing a screen on which a pair of stimuli was projected. The stimuli were a square-wave grating and a uniform grey surface of equal mean luminance. The infants were encouraged to compare the two stimuli. A naive observer was forced to guess the side of presentation of the grating, basing her observation on every available cue from the infants. The proportion of correct responses was then cumulated for all tested infants at each spatial frequency. The visual acuity of the age group was then determined by interpolation. Acuity was defined as the spatial frequency which yielded 70% correct responses from the observer. Sixty-eight infants participated in this experiment.

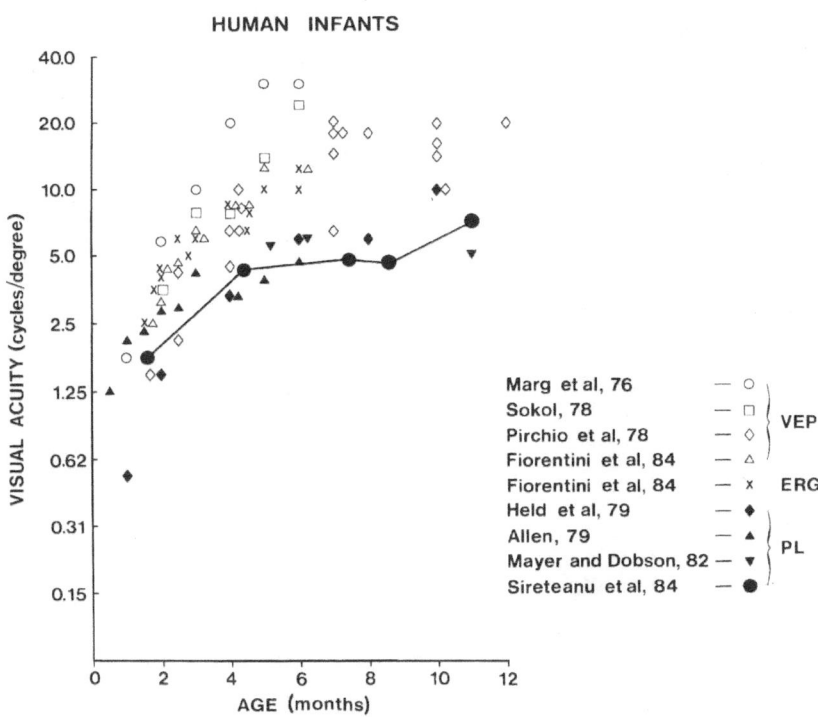

Fig. 1 Development of visual acuity in human infants. Closed symbols: acuity determined with the preferential looking technique. Open symbols: acuity determined by extrapolation of the visually evoked potential. X-symbols: acuity determined with the pattern-evoked electroretinogram.

216

The results are shown by filled circles in Fig. 1. "Best" acuity develops clearly during the first half of the first year of life, and more slowly afterwards. These results agree closely with other longitudinal data reported in the literature (shown by filled symbols in Fig. 1). It is remarkable that acuity determined with the preferential-looking method is consistently lower (by 1-2 octaves) than acuity determined by extrapolation of the visually evoked potential (shown by open symbols in Fig. 1) or with the pattern-evoked electroretinogram (indicated by crosses in Fig. 1).

b). Peripheral visual acuity. The experimental conditions were identical to those of the previous experiment, except that the attention of the infant was attracted to the midline before the beginning of each trial. The task of the observer was to record the direction of the infant's first saccade from the midline to the peripheral stimulus. The results were then processed in exactly the same way as in the previous experiment. Seventy-four infants participated in this experiment.

HUMAN INFANTS

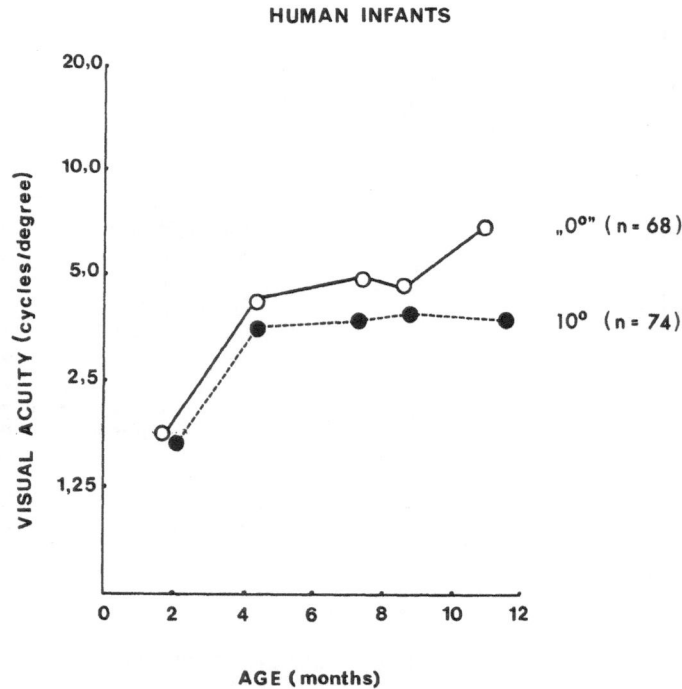

Fig. 2   A comparison of the development of "best" acuity (open symbols) and peripheral acuity (closed symbols) in human infants.

The results are summarized in Fig. 2. It is evident that, at all ages tested, peripheral acuity (shown by filled symbols) is lower than the visual acuity obtained under free-viewing conditions (open symbols). Moreover, peripheral acuity clearly develops between 2 and 4 months of age, after which it reaches a plateau, while the visual acuity of the central visual field continues to show a slower development.

This finding of a clear development of visual function in the peripheral visual field suggests that the development of acuity in human infants cannot be due entirely to the maturation of the fovea.

Experiment II. The development of visual acuity in infant kittens.

In this experiment, the preferential looking technique was used to evaluate the development of visual acuity in very young kittens. The kittens were hold by an experimenter on a table, while a second naive observer presented the stimuli in front of the kitten. This observer was also forced to guess the side of presentation of the grating, by using every available cue from the kitten ("best" visual acuity). Twenty-six kittens participated in this experiment.

The results are shown by large filled circles in Fig. 3. It can be seen that, like in human infants, the preferential looking method tends to produce lower acuities than those obtained with the visually evoked potential (shown by open symbols in Fig. 3). On the other hand, visual acuity obtained with the visually evoked potential shows a good agreement with the mean acuity of single cells from the area centralis in the retina and the lateral geniculate nucleus (shown by X-symbols and crosses in Fig. 3).

This good agreement between retinal and cortical acuity is seen in both kittens and human infants (compare Figs. 1 and 3) and suggests that, in both species, visual acuity is already determined at the level of the retinal ganglion cells.

CONCLUSIONS

The results presented in this paper show that the method of forced-choice preferential looking can be successfully applied to evaluate the visual acuity of young infants and kittens. In both species, the visual acuity estimated by a criterion of 70% correct is lower than the visual acuity estimated by the extrapolation of the visually evoked potential. However, if a more lenient criterion is employed, the discrepancy between these two methods disappears. In young kittens, preferential looking acuity estimated with a 58% correct criterion (small closed circles in Fig. 3) comes very close to the acuity of the best-resolving single cortical cells (shown by star symbols in Fig. 3), thus suggesting that even young kittens are able to use the acuity of their best cortical cells in a behavioural task.

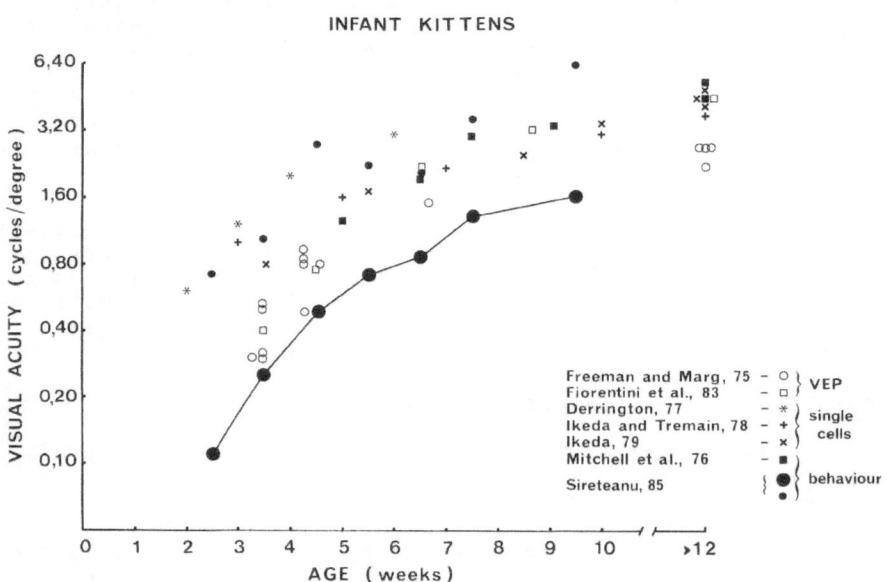

Fig. 3   Development of visual acuity in young kittens. Closed symbols: acuity determined behaviourally. Open symbols: acuity determined by extrapolation of the visually evoked potential. X-symbols: mean acuity of retinal ganglion cells from the area centralis. Crosses: mean acuity of cells in the lateral geniculate nucleus (input from the area centralis). Star synmbols: spatial resolution of the best-resolving single cell in the striate visual cortex.

Our results on human infants suggest that the development of acuity cannot be due entirely to the postnatal maturation of the fovea. This conclusion is supported by the finding of a similar development in the cat, an afoveate species. On the other hand, the good agreement between the development of retinal and cortical acuity suggests that, in both humans and kittens, the development of acuity has to be determined at or before the level of the retinal ganglion cells. In the adult

cat, acuity is inversely related to the size of the dendritic
fields of the ß-cells described by Boycott and Wässle (1974).
Surprisingly, however, in the young kitten, the dendritic
fields of identified ß-cells are not larger, but smaller than
in the adult (Russoff and Dubin, 1977; Mastronarde et al.,
1984). Therefore, the low acuity of retinal ganglion cells in
young kittens may be due to an abnormally extensive excitatory
input onto single ganglion cells or to the lack of inhibitory
synapses onto these cells. The postnatal maturation of these
mechanisms might provide the neural basis of the development
of acuity reported in this paper.

REFERENCES

Abramov I, Gordon J, Hendrickson A, Hainline L, Dobson V,
LaBoissiere E. The retina of the newborn infant. Science
1982;217:265-7.

Allen J. Visual acuity development in human infants up to 6
months of age. Unpublished doctoral disseration. University of
Washington. 1978.

Boycott BB, Wässle H. The morphological types of ganglion
cells on the domestic cat's retina. J Physiol
1974;240:397-419.

Derrington AM. Development of selectivity in kitten striate
cortex. J Physiol 1977;276:46-7P.

Fiorentini A, Pirchio M, Spinelli D. Development of retinal
and cortical responses to pattern reversal in infants: a
selective review. Behav Brain Res 1983;10:99-106.

Fiorentini A, Pirchio M, Sandini G. Development of retinal
acuity in infants evaluated with pattern electroretinogram.
Human Neurobiol 1984;3:93-5.

Freeman DN, Marg E. Visual acuity development coincides with
the sensitive period in kittens. Nature 1975;254:614-5.

Garey LJ. Structural development of the visual system of man.
Human Neurobiol 1984;3:75-80.

Hendrickson AE, Yuodelis C. The morphological development of
the human fovea. Ophthalmology 1984;91:603-12.

Held R. Development of visual resolution. Canad J Psychol/Rev
canad Psychol 1979;33(4):219-21.

Ikeda H. Physiological basis of visual acuity and its
development in kittens. Child care health Develop
1979;5:375-83.

Ikeda H., Tremain KE. The development of spatial resolving
power of lateral geniculate neurones in kittens. Exp Brain Res
1978;31:193-206.

220

Mann I. The development of human eye. British Medical Association, London. 1964.

Marg E, Freeman DN, Peltzmann P, Goldstein PJ. Visual acuity development in human infants: Evoked potential measurements. Invest Ophthalmol Vis Sci 1976;15:150-3

Mastronarde DN, Thibeault MA, Dubin MW. Non-uniform postnatal growth of the cat retina. J Comp Neurol 1984;228:598-608.

Mayer DL, Dobson V. Visual acuity development in infants and young children, as assessed by operant preferential looking. Vis Res 1982;22:1141-51.

Mitchell DE, Giffin F, Wilkinson F, Anderson P, Smith ML. Visual resolution in young kittens. Vis Res 1976;16:363-6.

Pirchio M, Spinelli D, Fiorentini A, Maffei L. Infant contrast sensitivity evaluated by evoked potentials. Brain Res 1978;141:179-84.

Russoff AC, Dubin MW. Kitten ganglion cells: dendritic field size at 3 weeks of age and correlation with receptive field size. Invest Ophthalmol Vis Sci 1978;17:819-21.

Sireteanu R. The development of visual acuity in very young kittens. A study with forced-choice preferential looking. Vis Res 1985; in press.

Sireteanu R, Kellerer G, Boergen K-P. The development of peripheral visual acuity in human infants. A preliminary study. Human Neurbiol 1984;3:81-5.

Sokol S. Measurement of infant visual acuity from pattern reversal evoked potentials. Vis Res 1978;18:33-9.

Teller DY. The forced-choice preferential looking procedure: a psychological technique for use with human infants. Infant Behaviour and Development 1979;2:135-53.

PREFERENTIAL LOOKING ACUITY IN NORMAL AND NEUROLOGICALLY ABNORMAL INFANTS AND PEDIATRIC PATIENTS

Gesine Mohn and Jackie van Hof-van Duin

Department of Physiology I, Erasmus Universiteit Rotterdam
P.O.Box 1738, 3000 DR Rotterdam, The Netherlands

INTRODUCTION

Even the simplest acuity charts used in pediatric ophthalmological practice, whether based on outline drawings of common objects, E-hooks or Landolt-C's, require a fair amount of comprehension and verbal capacity from the patient for a successful acuity assessment, and are thus restricted to normal children from at least 3-4 years of age.

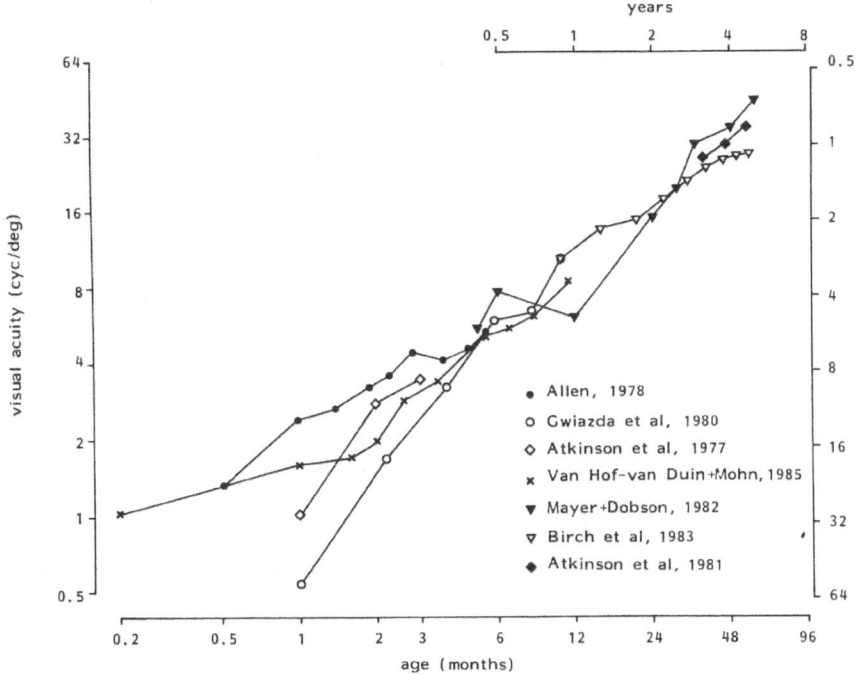

Fig.1: The development of grating acuity in normal fullterm infants and children as measured with the forced-choice preferential looking technique (FPL) and its operant variation (OPL) in various laboratories.

The advent of the preferential looking technique, based on the apparently inborn preference of infants for a pattern over a uniform stimulus, for the first time allowed the behavioural assessment of acuity in preverbal infants practically from the moment of birth (Teller et al 1974). Studies of the development of preferential looking acuity for grating targets in normal fullterm infants and children have yielded remarkably consistent results despite the variations in apparatus and methods used in different laboratories, and indicate an approximately ten-fold increase of acuity during the first year of life (see Fig.1). On the basis of these normative data, it has become possible to detect and assess impairments of visual development at this hitherto inaccessible age. Several studies (Jacobson et al 1981,1983; Mohindra and Van Hof-van Duin 1983; Dobson 1983; Mayer et al 1985; Boergen 1985; Lennerstrand 1985) have reported acuity measurements in infants with ophthalmological disorders such as congenital strabismus, cataracts, or retinal degeneration. A second clinical population with a high incidence of visual defects consists of infants born prematurely. Preterm infants not only more often have ophthalmological disorders like retinopathy of prematurity, myopia and strabismus, but also frequently suffer a variety of perinatal complications , such as asphyxia or hypoxia, the respiratory distress syndrome requiring mechanical ventilation, convulsions and intracranial hemorr hages which may lead to abnormal neurological development and also visual impairment(for a review, see Van Hof-van Duin and Mohn 1984).

Finally, since the preferential looking technique requires only minimal cooperation and no verbal capacity, it has proved useful for assessing acuity also in older children with neurological disorders, who due to developmental retardation often cannot be assessed by standard ophthalmological tests (Mohn and Van Hof-van Duin 1983; Mayer et al 1983; Lennerstrand et al 1983).

Below we describe our results of preferential looking acuity measurements during the first year of life in preterm infants with normal and abnormal neurological development, as well as further findings in infants and children with a variety of congenital and acquired neurological disorders.

SUBJECTS AND METHODS

Acuity was assessed in 121 preterm infants born 3-14 weeks prematurely. Age at testing ranged from 5 to 57 weeks postnatal age, or minus 4 to 65 weeks of age from the expected term (corrected age). The infants were divided into three groups according to the severity of perinatal complications and absence or presence of neurological defects as follows:

1. A group of 35 infants with normal neurological development and with minimal perinatal complications as defined by the following criteria: normal birthweight for gestational age; an Apgar score of > 6 at 5 minutes; no other indications for perinatal or postnatal hypoxia; mechanical ventilation and/or phototherapy for no longer than one week; no surgery for patent ductus arteriosus or necrotizing enterocolitis; no retinopathy of prematurity; no convulsions ; no or only very minor intracranial hemorrhage as assessed by ultrasound scans.
2. A group of 67 infants with one or more of the above perinatal risk factors, who were developing normally until the age of testing.
3. A group of 19 infants with one or more of the above risk factors and evidence of abnormal neurological development. This consisted either of rather mild deficits like hypertonia or mild developmental delay, or more serious symptoms like (beginning) spastic quadriplegia or

surgically relieved hydrocephalus.

All these infants were tested at the Sophia Children's University Hospital, Rotterdam, either before leaving hospital after birth, or, in the great majority of cases, during outpatient visits for developmental check-ups.

Assessment of acuity was further attempted in 94 infants and children with a wide variety of congenital and acquired neurological disorders and varying degrees of psychomotor retardation, often with accompanying ophthalmological disorders like strabismus, spontaneous nystagmus or structural ocular abnormalities (see also Van Hof-van Duin and Mohn, this volume). Since the present report is primarily concerned with the general usefulness of the preferential looking technique in these patients rather than results obtained in patients with specific neurological disorders, no further specification of the disorders will be presented. Age at testing ranged from 2 months to 23 years, with 82 of the 94 patients younger than 6 years of age. The patients were referred to us for extensive assessment of visual functions, and were examined at the Department of Physiology, Rotterdam.

Acuity for high contrast square wave gratings was assessed using the two-alternative forced choice preferential looking technique (Teller et al 1974). The apparatus and the "staircase" method used for presenting gratings of different stripewidths have been described previously (Teller et al 1974; Ma yer et al 1982; Mohn and Van Hof-van Duin 1983). Older infants and patients were often tested with the operant preferential looking technique, in which the infant is rewarded for a correct response of the observer by the appearance of an animated toy from behind an otherwise darkened glass screen. When acuity assessment could not be completed in neurological patients, due to insufficient cooperation, it was nevertheless often possible to estimate a "minimal acuity" on the basis of the finest grating which was judged correctly in 80% or more of at least 6 trials, which may or may not have corresponded to the actual acuity threshold.

RESULTS

The development of visual acuity in the low-risk preterm infants with minimal perinatal complications and normal neurological development is compared to that of normal fullterm infants in Fig 2.

The age of the preterm infants is plotted either according to age from birth (postnatal age) or age from the expected term date (corrected age). When postnatal age was used, the preterm infants lagged behind the fullterm infants up to an age of approximately 8 months, while acuity in two groups is very similar at all ages when using corrected age. The preterm infants in fact had consistently slightly higher mean acuities than fullterm infants of the same corrected age, but the difference was statistically not significant.

Results obtained in the high-risk preterm infants with one or more perinatal risk factors and either normal or abnormal neurological development are presented in Fig.3.

224

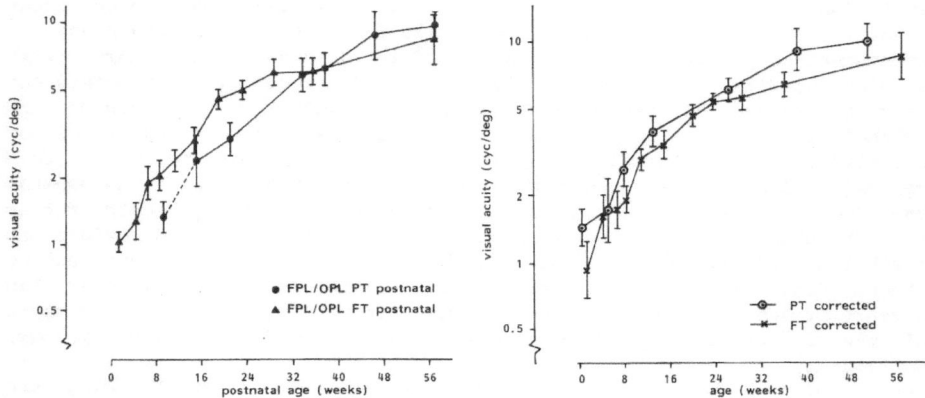

Fig.2: The development of preferential looking acuity in normal fullterm (FT) and low risk preterm (PT) infants. Age of the preterm infants is given either from birth postnatal age (postnatal age: left side) or from the expected date of term (corrected age: right side). Good agreement is seen between fullterm and preterm infants of the same corrected age.

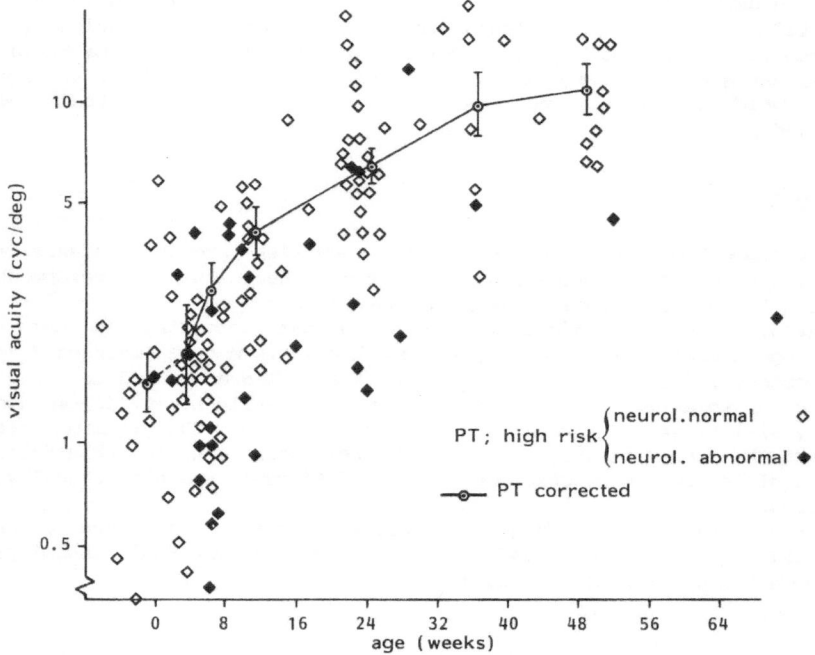

Fig.3: Acuity development in high risk preterm infants with normal and abnormal neurological development, compared to the mean acuity of low risk preterm infants.

Many of the infants with normal neurological development had lower than normal acuities during the first 3-4 months post-term, suggesting that the perinatal complications had temporarily slowed down their visual development to some extent. By 6 months corrected age, however, their acuities generally clustered symmetrically around the mean acuity of the low-risk infants. Of the neurologically abnormal infants, those with mild neurological symptoms mostly had acuities close to those of the low-risk infants, while in infants with serious disorders, acuity was only half or less of the mean low-risk acuity. Nevertheless, within the group of neurologically abnormal infants, older infants usually had higher acuities than younger infants, suggesting that visual development, similar to their neurological development, was slowed down, but not arrested.

The results of acuity assessments in 36 neurological patients referred to us between the ages of 2 months and 2 years are shown in Fig.4.

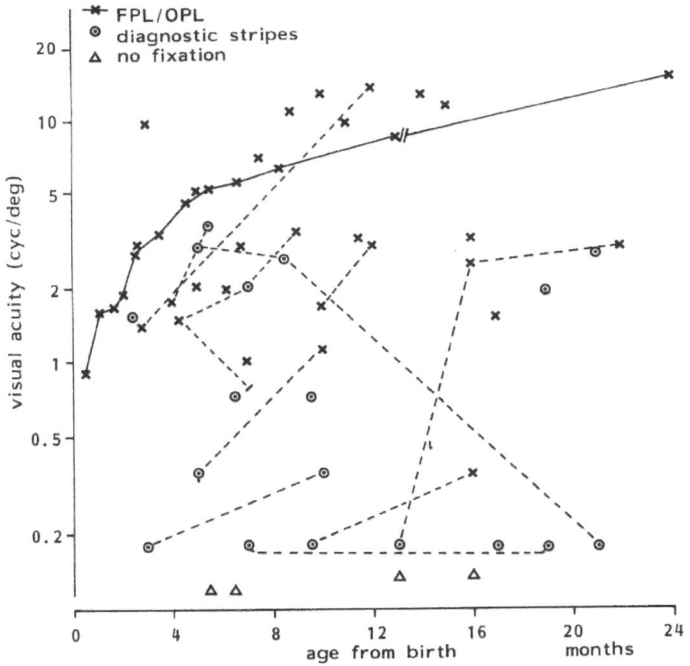

Fig.4: Preferential looking acuity estimates obtained in pediatric neurological patients under the age of 2 years. The line indicates mean acuity of normal fullterm infants (Mayer and Dobson, 1982; our results). Diagnostic stripes: "minimal acuity" estimate only.

As with the preterm infants, a number of infants of this group had normal
acuity for age at the initial examination. In most of the patients,
however, acuity was between 1-2 octaves (i.e. by a factor of 2-4) lower
than the age norm. Six infants initially only fixated the grating with the
widest stripe width, while 3 showed no fixation at all, and appeared to be
blind. Repeated examination in most cases revealed an increase in acuity
parallel to improvements in neurological development, but with the
exception of one infant, acuity remained abnormally poor. One severely
retarded infant with poor acuity at 5 and 8 months of age was no longer
testable at 21 months, and at this time only reacted to the widest stripes.
Qualitatively similar results were obtained in older neurological patients.
Acuity generally varied with the severity of the neurological disorder and
psycho-motor retardation, with normal or near-normal acuity only in
patients with mild disorders. Acuity was, of course, also affected by
ophthalmological defects like strabismus, cataract, etc.

TABLE I

Neuropeadiatric patients (FPL/OPL)

	n
Acuity < widest stripe (0.2 c/deg)	6
Not testable	13
"Minimal acuity": >.....c/deg	5
Reliable acuity estimate	70
Total	94

Table I: Success rate of acuity assessment with the preferential looking
technique during initial examinations in 94 pediatric neurological
patients, aged 2 months to 23 years.

Table I gives an overview of the quality of acuity assessment at the first
examination in all of the 94 patients seen. Six patients appeared to be
blind and did not react even to the widest stripewidth presented. For 70
of the remaining 88 patients (80%), a statistically reliable acuity
assessment was obtained, while a minimal acuity could be estimated in a
further 5 patients. In only 13 patients (15%), acuity assessment was
impossible either due to insufficient cooperation, or because the fixation
pattern could not be judged. Only 14 patients could also be tested with a
letter matching task.

DISCUSSION

The results of the low-risk preterm infants show that the development of
behavioural acuity is closely related to conceptional or post-term
(corrected) age rather than age from birth. This is in agreement with
previous studies of preferential looking acuity in preterm infants which

used less quantitative methods (Fantz and Fagan 1975; Dobson et al 1980), and confirms our earlier results (Van Hof-van Duin and Mohn 1984). Although the preterm infants here appeared to be slightly superior to the fullterm infants of the same age from term, it is clear that for clinical purposes, preterm infants should be expected to have the same acuity as fullterm infants of the same corrected, rather than postnatal age. Very similar development in normal fullterm and preterm infants of the same corrected age is also seen for a number of other visual functions, such as monocular optokinetic nystagmus (OKN), the visual threatening reflex, and visual field size (Van Hof-van Duin and Mohn, this volume).

Perinatal complications, even in the absence of neurological symptoms, often seemed to slow down acuity development until the corrected age of 3-4 months. Relatively poor acuity in this age range may thus not be a reliable indicator of later development in such infants. By 6 months, however, acuity was generally within the normal range except in infants with neurological abnormalities. In the latter group, visual acuity was related to the severity of the neurological disorder, with poorest acuity in clearly abnormal infants. Poor acuity has previously been described in preterm infants with early neurological abnormalities, tested before or at term (Morante et al 1982; Dubowitz, this volume). The present results extend these observations to the first year after term. The high-risk infants of the present study also often show delays in the development of monocular OKN, visual threat and visual field size, particularly when neurological development was abnormal (Van Hof-van Duin and Mohn, this volume).

A relation of acuity to the severity of the neurological disorder and accompanying psychomotor retardation, with additional effects of ophthalmological defects, was also seen in the pediatric neurological patients. The results, as well as the 80% success rate of acuity assessment, are similar to those described in earlier studies of preferential looking acuity in young neurological patients (Lennerstrand et al 1983; Mayer et al 1983; Mohn and Van Hof-van Duin et al 1983).

In conclusion, the development of visual acuity as well as other visual functions in normal preterm infants with minimal perinatal complications is very similar to that of fullterm infants when age is corrected for prematurity. High-risk preterm infants often show a delay in acuity development even when neurological development is normal. The preferential looking technique not only allows the early detection of visual impairments in infants too young to be examined by other tests, but is also a very useful tool for assessing acuity in older neurological patients, whose behavioural visual capacity so often cannot be assessed by the standard tests, and might be a prognostic tool in predicting later neurological impairments.

ACKNOWLEDGEMENTS

We are grateful to the staff of the Department of Neonatology, Sophia Children's University Hospital, Rotterdam, for their cooperation. We thank A.Evenhuis-van Leunen, H.Frenkel and F.Groenendaal for their help in testing the infants, and A.Gispen-van Dobbenburgh for administrative assistance.

REFERENCES

Allen JL. The development of visual acuity in human infants during the early postnatal weeks. PhD Dissertation , Univ.Washington, Seattle. 1979.

Atkinson J, Braddick O, Moar K. Development of contrast sensitivity over the first 3 months of life in the human infant. Vision Res 1977b;17:1037–44.

Atkinson J, French J, Braddick O. Contrast sensitivity function of preschool children. Br J Ophthalmol 1981;65:525–29.

Birch EE, Gwiazda J, Bauer JAJr, Naegele J, Held R. Visual acuity and its meridional variations in children aged 7 to 60 months. Vision Res 1983;23:1019–24.

Boergen KP. Preferential looking for detection of early amblyopia and monitoring early therapy. 1985; this volume.

Dobson V. Clinical applications of preferential looking measures of visual acuity. Behav Brain Res 1983;10:25–38.

Dobson V, Mayer DL, Lee CP. Visual acuity screening of preterm infants. Invest Ophthalmol Vis Sci 1980;19:1498–1505.

Dubowitz LMS. Visual function in premature babies. 1985; this volume.

Fantz RL, Fagan JF. Visual attention to size and number of pattern details by term and preterm infants during the first six months. Child Develop 1975;46:3–18.

Gwiazda J, Brill S, Mohindra I, Held R. Preferential looking acuity in infantsfrom two to fifty-eight weeks of age. Am J Optomet Physiol Opt 1980;57:428–32.

Jacobson SG, Mohindra I, Held R. Br J Ophthalmol 1981;10:727–35.

Jacobson SG, Mohindra I, Held R. Age of onset of amblyopia in infants with esotropia. Doc Ophthalmol Proc Ser 1981;30:210–16.

Jacobson SG, Mohindra I, Held R. Monocular visual form deprivation in human infants. Doc Ophthalmol 1983;55:199–211.

Lennerstrand G, Axelsson A, Andersson G. Visual testing with 'preferential looking' in mentally retarded children. Behav Brain Res 1983;10:199–203.

Lennerstrand G. Visual development in children with congenital cataract operated early. 1985; this volume.

Mayer DL, Fulton AB, Sossen PL. Preferential looking acuity of pediatric patients with developmental disabilities. Behav Brain Res 1983;10:189–99.

Mayer DL, Fulton AB, Hansen RM. Visual acuity of infants and children with retinal degenerations. Ophthal Ped Gen 1985; in press.

Mayer DL, Dobson V. Visual acuity development in infants and young children as assessed by operant preferential looking. Vision Res 1982;22:1141-52.

Mayer DL, Fulton AB, Hansen RM. Preferential looking acuity obtained with a staircase procedure in pediatric patients. Invest Ophthalmol Vis Sci 1982;23:538-43.

Mohn G, Van Hof-van Duin J. Behavioural and electrophysiological measures of visual functions in children with neurological disorders. Behav Brain Res 1983;10:177-89.

Mohindra I, Jacobson SG, Held R. Binocular visual form deprivation in human infants. Doc Ophthalmol 1983;55:237-49.

Morante A, Dubowitz LMS, Levene M, Dubowitz V. The development of visual function in normal and neurologically abnormal preterm and fullterm infants. Devel Med Child Neurol 1982;24:771-84.

Teller DY, Morse R, Barton R, Regal D. Visual acuity for vertical and diagonal gratings in human infants. Vision Res 1974;14:1433-39.

Van Hof-van Duin J, Mohn G, Fetter WPF, Mettau JW and Baerts W. Preferential looking acuity in preterm infants. Behav Brain Res 1983;10:47-51.

Van Hof-van Duin J, Mohn G. Vision in the preterm infant. In: Prechtl HFR, ed. Continuity of neural functions from prenatal to postnatal life. Spastics Int Med Publications, Oxford, Blackwell Sci Publ 1984; Clinics in developmental medicine 94:93-114.

Van Hof-van Duin J, Mohn G. Visual field measurements, optokinetic nystagmus and the visual threatening response: normal and abnormal development. 1985, this volume.

PREFERENTIAL LOOKING FOR THE DETECTION OF EARLY AMBLYOPIA AND
MONITORING EARLY THERAPY

Klaus-P.Boergen*, Gina Kellerer*, Christina
Bauernfeind-Kaliwas**, Ruxandra Sireteanu***

*   Augenklinik der Universität München
**   Institut für Med.Psychologie, München
*** Max-Planck-Institut für Hirnforschung,
     Frankfurt

INTRODUCTION

Amblyopia due to congenital or early acquired unilateral
ocular changes such as monolateral squint, cataract, ptosis etc.
is a widespread clinical problem. It is well known from clinical
experience that early detection and treatment of amblyopia improves the final functional outcome of this entity. Clinically
it is not difficult to detect amblyopia in cases characterized
by large angle squint or gross unilateral ocular pathology, because it is indisputable that such eye changes influence visual
development in the involved eye. But there are also cases where
small angle squint or slight ocular changes like pupillary ectopia
angle kappa, or nystagmus makes it difficult or impossible to
decide clinically whether amblyopia is present or not (presumed
amblyopia).

The detection of amblyopia in these ambigious cases may be
facilitated by the employment of preferential looking. Additio-
nally, therapeutic regimes employed in the treatment of amblyopia
may be monitored by utilizing this techniques. Until recently,
knowledge about amblyopia therapy during infancy has been very
limited. Traditional therapy has always stressed occlusion of
the good eye, although little is known regarding the optimal
occlusion frequency. This optimum is important in the developing

visual acuity in the amblyopic eye without sacrificing acuity
in the good eye through occlusion - induced deprivation as
shown by MOHINDRA et al. (1983). Purely clinical observations
regarding the appearance of free alternation in monolateral
squint patients are not sufficient for monitoring amblyopia
therapy during the pre-verbal period since alternation may
be due to a visual reduction in the good eye with only slight
visual increase in the amblyopic eye. Quantification of the
therapeutic effect and comparison to the age norm is therefore
mandatory. For this purpose, preferential looking promises to be
useful tool for the clinician. It was the diagnostic (detection
of early amblyopia) and therapeutic (monitoring of early therapy)
aspect of the amblyopia problem that encouraged us to start clinical studies in infants with apparent or presumed amblyopia. In a
previous paper (BOERGEN et al., 1983), results of study performed
with the classical forced-choice-PL method (TELLER, 1979) were
published with stimulus presentation according to a constant
stimulus procedure. As this turned out to be too time consuming,
we switched to a stair-case method (ATKINSON et al., 1982; MAYER
et al., 1982). Some preliminary results will be presented in the
following paper.

MATERIAL AND METHODS

Subjects:

The infants tested (Tab.1)
were routine out-patients
of the University Eye Clinic
in Munich,referred from
ophthalmologists, pediatri-
cians or other clinics. Each
infant had a thorough orthoptic
examination and PL-testing performed by the same orthoptis
(G.K.). Ocular pathology was
diagnosed and ruled out by an
experienced ophthalmologist
(K.P.B.). Retinoscopy under
cycloplegica was done in every

Total number of cases :	75
1. normal infants :	44
2. squinting infants :	22
- divergent	2
- convergent	20
* alternating	7
* monolateral	13
3. others :	9
- pupillary anomalies	5
- angle K	1
- nystagmus	3

Tab.1: see text.

infant. Only when PL-testing could be done in both eyes during
the same session was the infant included in the study.

Apparatus and testing procedure:

The PL-technique employed in the study was a modification of the
forced-choice-PL-apparatus described by GWIAZDA et al. (1978).
Details are given elsewhere (SIRETEANU et al., 1984). Like all
PL-techniques, it is based on the asumption that an infant exposed
to both a patterned (e.g. a square wave grating) and a blank stimulus of equal mean luminance will preferentially fixate upon the
patterned one provided it is able to discriminate between the two.
In our set-up, the stimuli were projected from behind onto semi-
transparent screens. Using automatic projectors allowed the observer to operate the projection, observe the infant through a
peep-hole, and record the data concurrently. All our experiments
on clinical cases were performed in this manner. Only for our
'based-line' experiments on normal infants did two persons, an
experimentor and a separate observer, perform the tests. All our
clinical cases were tested during office hours. Therefore only a
limited time of 30 minutes maximum was available for each infant.

Data-Analysis:

Our normal infants were divided into age groups (Fig.1). In our
clinical cases, only differences in grating acuity between the
two eyes were of interest according to the outlined context. Therefore, age was neglected in the presentation of the results. The
data was analyzed according to a modified procedure described by
MAYER et al. (1982).

RESULTS

Normal infants:

44 normal infants were
tested monocularly. The
other eye was occluded by
a disposable patch. As expected, the results showed
that the development of
grating acuity is equal in
both eyes and is in good

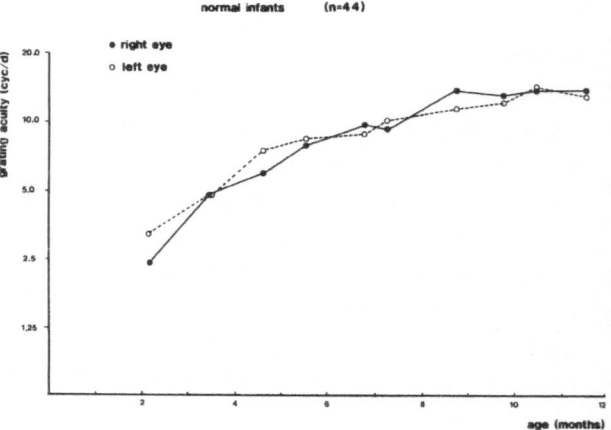

accordance with the binocular results of BOERGEN et al. 1983 and SIRETEANU et al., 1984, as well as those reported in the literature (DOBSON and TELLER (1978).

Fig.1:
Results of monocular PL-testing in normal infants.

Alternating squint:
7 primarily alternating infants revealed surprisingly slight differences in grating acuity between two eyes (Fig.2). Despite these re-sults, no therapy was applied to these infants as the danger of subsequent amblyopia seemed to be mini-mal. Nevertheless, one of them (*1) showed a signifi-cant drop of acuity in the left eye when tested again (*2). This corresponded to a left esotropia. Occlusion therapy had to be started and the infant is still under controll.

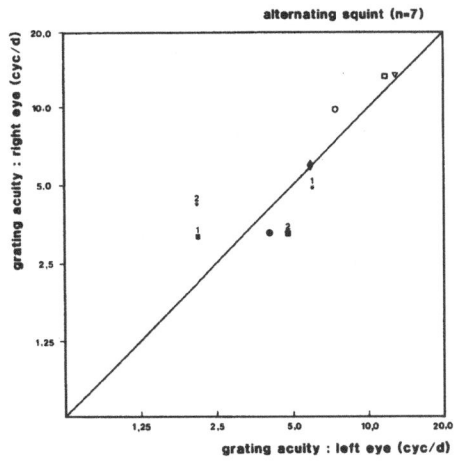

Fig.2: Alternating squint: nearly equal grating acuity in both eyes; in one case (*) within two months a left esotropia appeared ($^2_*$), in another (■) there was a shift of dominance from the right (♦) to the left eye ($^2_■$).

Monolateral squint (untreated):
Divergent squint
Congenital divergent squint is a very rare condition. Until recently, we were able to test two such cases sucessfully. Where-as the fixating eye showed a grating acuity within the age norm, the divergent eye showed a 'temporal preference', i.e. it con-stantly looked to the temporal side during testing.

Convergent squint
In only one out of 6 infants with monolateral untreated convergent squint could both eyes be tested regularly, which showed a slight difference in acuity between the two eyes (Fig.3). Only the fixa-

234

ting eye could be tested in
the other five. On occlusion,
the squinting eye showed a
constant 'nasal preference'
as has already been des-
cribed in our previous paper
(BOERGEN et al., 1983). Two
of these infants were controlled under occlusion
therapy. One showed an improvement exclusively in the
acuity of the fixating
(□1, □2), the second also
in the squinting eye
(O2,O3).

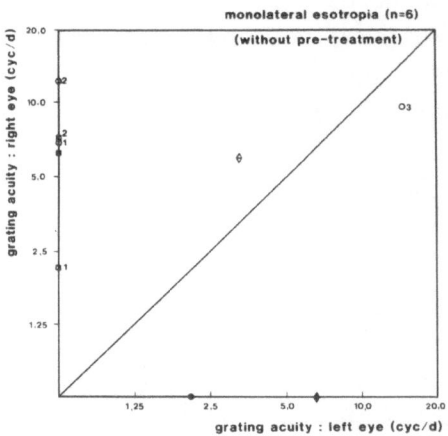

Fig.3: Monolateral untreated esotropia
only one infant could be tested (♦)
in both eyes, in the others the squinting eye showed 'nasal preference'.
Occlusion of 6 weeks (1 h/day) in one
case (♦) did improve grating acuity in
the left eye (^2_O = after 4 weeks, ^3_O =
after 6 weeks). The other cases are
still under therapy.

Monolateral squint
(pre-treated):

Out of seven patients who
were tested under treatment
and in whom no PL was performed before therapy, three
had equal grating acuity
even though no alternation
had appeared (Fig.4). In
four other infants who
clinically presented in the
same way (strict monolateral
squint), acuity in the fixating eye developed according
to the age norm. However, the
squinting eye sill revealed
a lower grating acuity necessi-
tating the continuiation of
occlusion therapy.

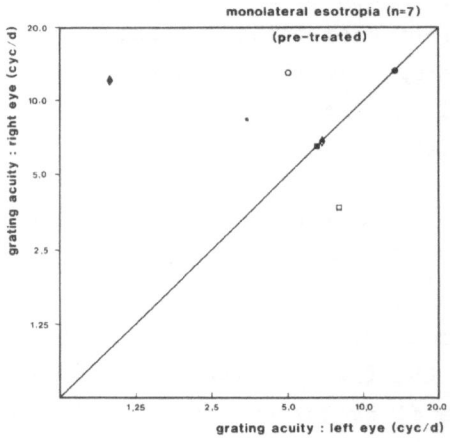

Fig.4: Monolateral esotropia under
occlusion therapy: in three cases
(■,♦ ,●) equal grating acuity has
been achieved after occlusion of
three months (1 h/day). No alternation
is present in these cases. The other
four are still under therapy.

Presumed amblyopia:
pupillary anomalies:

Grating acuity in three cases with pupillary displacement or anisocoria (Fig.5) was nearly equal in both eyes, allowing therapy to be excluded. Two other infants showing a marked difference in acuity had to be occluded. Both had a congenital corectopia and it was impossible to detect amblyopia in these cases by routine clinical diagnosis.

Angle kappa:

A positive angle kappa may mimic convergent squint. In one such case we were able to demonstrate equal visual acuity in both eyes and rule out amblyopia (Fig.6).

Nystagmus:

Nystagmus cases may prove difficult in ruling out additional squint and unilateral amblyopia. In three cases we found reduced but equal acuity in both eyes. In one case, monocular was worse than binocular acuity due to a latent component of nystagmus becoming manifest on occlusion.

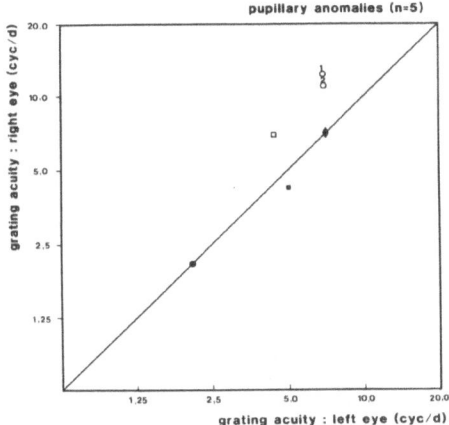

Fig.5: Presumed amblyopia (pupillary anomalies): in three cases (● = iris coloboma of the left eye; ■, ◆ = anisocoria) grating acuity is nearly equal; in one case with ectopia of the left eye was reduced; in another with the same diagnosis, a reduction of acuity was found on two successive examinations ($^4_0$, $^2_0$).

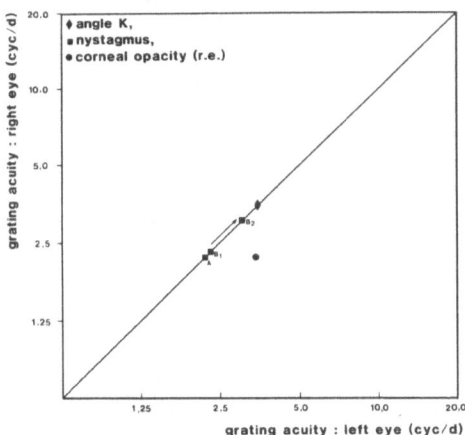

Fig.6: Other cases with presumed amblyopia: in one case with a positive angle kappa (◆) mimicing left esotropia no amblyopia could be detected; in another with a right corneal opacity, grating acuity was reduced in the involved eye (●). In two nystagmus cases (A and B), grating acuity was reduced in both eyes compared to the age norm (6 and 10 months) but equal in both eyes. B_2 indicates the result of binocular testing.

DISCUSSION

In the present study, preferential looking with stimulus presentation according to a stair-case method was applied to normal, squinting and presumably amblyopic infants under clinical conditions.

The stair-case procedure proved to be more suitable for clinical tests than the classical constant stimulus method, since it requires less time. Our special interest was early detection of amblyopia, especially in cases with presumed amblyopia due to slight anatomic eye changes, where traditional clinical diagnostic tools like corneal reflexion were insufficien for amblyopia diagnosis. A further problem was the question on whether PL is a useful instrument for monitoring early amblyopia therapy.

Monocular testing of normal infants revealed that patching of one eye does not influence looking preference. This has been demonstrated previously for the constant stimulus method (BOERGEN et al., 1983), and the stair-case procedure (ATIKINSON et al., 1982).

For alternating squint patients we found nearly equal gratin acuity in both eyes as expected. But equal acuity is not always accompanied by alternation. Two infants in the monolateral eso-tropia group (Fig.4) still had a marked dominance of one eye although grating acuity was equalized. These cases especially show that PL-testing can help in monitoring occlusion therapy. As already demonstrated in a previous paper (BOERGEN et al.,1983) untreated monolateral esotropic infants showed a high incidence of so-called 'nasal preference'. This finding has been substan-tiated by the results of this study (five out of six infants). Surprisingly, two divergent cases showed the opposite: a 'tempo-ral preference'. One possible explanation for the nasal preferenc might be a dominance of the nasal retina in congenital esotropic patients (HARCOURT, 1984). The reverse may be true for congenital exotropias. As to the optimal occlusion frequency, a final eva-luation cannot be given at the moment. In the treated group, the good eye developed according to the age norm under occlusion of 1 to 3 hours per day. But under this occlusion regime, visual acuity in the amblyopic eye only gradually improved over one to

two months. We shall therefore increase the occlusion time
with caution, as some studies (MOHINDRA et al., 1983) indicate
a high sensitivity of the good eye for the depriving effect of
occlusion.

For cases of presumed amblyopia, PL-testing is especially
useful. Grating acuity was equal in seven out of nine cases,
which allowed therapy to be excluded. Had we relied only on
clinical signs, a prophylaxtic treatment would have been started.

SUMMARY

A modified forced-choice preferential looking procedure with
stimulus presentation according to a stair-case method was applied
to normal (44), squinting (22), and infants with presumed amblyopia
(9) in order to determine the feasibility of PL as a clinical
tool in the detection of early amblyopia and monitoring of early
therapy. The normal infants were tested monocularly and visual
acuity in both eyes were equal. The same was true for alternating
squint patients as expected. In five out of six cases with untreated monolateral esotropia, the squinting eye could not be
tested but showed a constant nasal preference. Two divergent
squint patients had a temporal preference in the squinting eye.
In seven cases of esotropia, occlusion of 1 to 3 hours per day
had been applied before PL-testing. Three had equal visual acuity,
though a constant monolateral squint was still present. The other
four showed marked differences in acuity of both eyes, indicating
that amblyopia therapy has to be continued. In nine infants,
amblyopia was presumed according to unilateral pupillary anomalies,
angle kappa or nystagmus. In only two of them were acuity differences present, whereas the others showed equal acuity, making
occlusion therapy unnessessary.

PL-testing can help the clinician in therapeutic evaluation,
amblyopia detection, and therapy monitoring.

REFERENCES

ATKINSON J, BRADDICK O, PIMM-SMITH E. 'Preferential looking' for
monocular and binocular acuity testing of infants. Br J Ophthalmol 1982;66:264-268.

BOERGEN KP, BAUERNFEIND-KALIWAS C, SIRETEANU R. Preferential looking in normal and squinting infants. Transact 5th Int Orth Congr Lyon: Lips, 1983:47-52.

DOBSON V, TELLER DY. Visual acuity in human infants: A review and comparison of behavioural and electrophysical studies. Vis Res 1978;18:1469-1483.

GWIAZDA J, BRILL S, MOHINDRA J, HELD R. Infant visual acuity and its meridional variation. Vis Res 1978;18:1557-1564.

HARCOURT B. Some aspects of early onset esotropia. Australian J Ophthalmol 1984;12:233-238.

MAYER DL, FULTON AB, HANSEN RM. Preferential looking acuity obtained with a stair-case procedure in pediatric patients. Invest Ophthalmol 1982;23:538-543.

MOHINDRA I, JACOBSON SG, ZWAAN J, HELD R. Psychophysiological assessment of visual acuity in infants with visual disorders. Behav Brain Res 1983;10:51-58.

SIRETEANU R, KELLERER G, BOERGEN KP. The development of peripheral visual acuity in human infants. A preliminary study. Human Neurobiol 1984;3:81-85.

TELLER DY. The forced-choice preferential looking procedure: A psychophysical technique for use in human infants. Infant Beh Dev 1979;2:135-153.

DISCUSSION

Warburg: That was encouraging, wasn't it?

Campos: Were the children tested one eye at a time or both eyes together?

Atkinson: These were binocular results, but we do both. Monocular testing takes you longer, you spend less time on the test and more time in between trials, and the failure rate is higher.

Campos: I realise that crowding is present at this age. There should be a difference in crowding between the two eyes, and in amblyopia the crowding phenomenon should be significantly more important in affected eyes.

Atkinson: Yes, that is so. We tested a group of normal children monocularly for the crowding and the crowding is the same in the two eyes in 3 to 5 year old children.

Campos: Sireteanu made an important point on the development of the peripheral retina. This is another factor in favour of early operation in congenital monolateral cataract which generally gives a poor visual prognosis. Probably there could be at least a benefit as far as peripheral function is concerned.

Fielder: I would like to comment on Sireteanu's paper. I think she said that the fovea was fully developed at 4 to 5 months. Was that correct?

Sireteanu: I think so, for new histological data has shown that the fovea is not developed at birth. I think the end point of development is not so definite, but it is not before 4 months.

Fielder: There are two recent studies, one indicating that the fovea is still quite immature at a year, the other that it is not fully developed until about 45 months.

Sireteanu: I meant 45 months.

Atkinson: What was that an exact measurement of? If you say the fovea was mature by that stage, there are differences of criteria between those two studies that look very important.

Fielder: I do appreciate that you cannot necessarily correlate histology with function, but it is an indication and something that can at least be taken into account.

Atkinson: Yes, but I think that in those two histological studies there are differences in criteria as to what they looked at to come to their conclusions as to whether the fovea was complete or not. In one case you were talking about presence by the appearance of the beginning of a foveal pit and in the other you were talking about the total movement of the ganglion cells.

Fielder: No, the latter study looked at all those aspects.

Atkinson: Yes but depending very critically on exactly which aspect you take you would get a range from somewhere around six months to a year and a half.

Fielder: But central migration still takes place up to 45 months.

Atkinson: Yes, but I am saying that it is different saying that there is a beginning of migration at 4 to 5 months.

Fielder: All I am saying is that it was not necessarily mature at six months.

Kommerell: If we check for crowding we want this as a predictor of the ability to read later in life, and therefore I would suggest validating this in adult amblyopes who have difficulties in reading. Applied to your test it should be interesting to know whether people who have difficulties in reading a line also have diffculty in detecting the symbol.

Atkinson: That is going on at the moment, but we haven't got enough cases for this to be clear cut. In our normal 5 to 6 year olds there were two groups. There was the one group that showed a bigger crowding effect, and another who looked rather like the adults with a very small crowding effect. Now whether we could make some prediction about the reading ability of those children based on the crowding effect is an interesting question, but we don't know the answer.

Haase: Atkinson, there is a small difference in the result of the amount of crowding. Maybe this is due to the different interspacing between the symbols, and have you tried different spacings?

Atkinson: We tried that in empirical studies in adults and in some normals, but we haven't done it on a big enough group. We used a constant spacing which is half the letter width.

Braddick: Constant in a different sense. Yours is constant in minutes, ours is constant in proportion to the lettersize.

Haase: It is a little bit like Snellen.

Atkinson: After we had done this study we looked at Snellen cards to find out exactly what the spacing was, and I now have 8 different Snellen charts. So before anybody says that Snellen has a standard, they ought to look at the particular charts that they are using because they are all different.

Haase: I am glad that you confirm that. Can you differentiate normal children from amblyopes with such a crowding test?

Atkinson: When we are looking at children who are suspected amblyopes coming out of our screening programme, we have also discovered that the refractive correction has to be extremely accurate before you say that the child is amblyopic because about 0.75 D of astigmatism will reduce vision by one line.

van Lith: Concerning the remarks you made about Snellen acuity cards, years ago there was a Dutch ophthalmologist who used different charts and showed how different they were. He proposed a standardised card, but even now it is not used because it is difficult for ophthalmologists to use all these tricky cards.

Harcourt: Could I ask two simple questions? Boergen showed very nicely that preferential looking is a tool that can be used to differentiate visual function in the two eyes. Did he find by correlating that quite complicated method of assessment that it was superior to the extremely simple tests of fixation which most ophthalmologist use as their indicator of the difference of vision between one eye and the other? The other question is to those people who do preferential looking. As we see methods coming along whereby these tests may be useful in an average clinical situation, what is the minimum level of skill and sophistication of the technician who is making the judgements? For instance, should it be possible for anybody who is trained as an orthoptist to be able with certainty to get reliable result using these testing procedures and get them at fairly rapid speed, and how long a training programme would be required?

Dubowitz: A good nurse can do it on a full-term infant.

Fielder: Using the card procedure a non-ophthalmical trained nurse can get results which, in early infancy, correlate well with my own findings.

Mohn: I think it also depends on the mental level of the children. If it is a neurological patient, a retarded child or a child with low vision, these are much more difficult to assess and I think then it takes some experience. But with normal children it is quite easy.

Atkinson: I would agree. If there are any abnormalities of mental or physical development, you need a highly skilled specialised person to get a sensible result.

Dubowitz: The point is you can screen. A good nurse can screen, and your highly specialised person can go and do the rest.

Bagley: May I speak as an orthoptist? If you are looking to the person who is going to do this sort of assessment and if you are considering orthoptists in this role, you have to look at the training of orthoptists, as there is not a standard throughout Europe. Speaking as a British orthoptist we have a standardised training. I would say as one responsible for teaching orthoptists that they are competent. Whether it is a waste of their time or not is something else.

Lennerstrand: I just wanted to make a comment with regard to Boergen's talk on using preferential looking in the management of amblyopia. It is useful to get an idea of how long it takes for amblyopia to recover. What we found, a bit surprisingly, is that if you occlude the good eye full-time and measure vision every day, it would take only a week in a 9-month-old child to get to the same level of grating acuity in both eyes. But there is another thing to this and that is how well grating acuity and letter acuity agree. My experience is that there is certainly an overestimation of acuity with gratings and that when you do the testing with letter matching tests, the acuity is much lower.

Harcourt: This is pattern fixation behaviour.

Lennerstrand: Yes, that was my impression from the treatment. The major question is how well grating acuity works.

Atkinson: I think it is measuring something different. It isn't worse or better or more sensitive. In one case you are measuring acuity and in the other case you are measuring eye movement. They may be two entirely separate things.

Harcourt: I agree entirely. What we were talking about was a method of decision making, what you are actually going to do with the child in terms of what type of occlusion therapy or how long you persist with the therapy and whether one is superior as a determinant of treatment over the other. The fact that they are different does not make any difference as to whether one is better than the other.

Atkinson: I would question how good the fixation data is.

Boergen: I would like to answer Lennerstrand. I agree that it is difficult to assess grating acuity, because what do we measure with grating acuity? We do not use the whole-day occlusion because we have the impression that if we occlude for a whole day and then we open again for a whole day we might reduce the grating acuity in the occluded eye.

Dubowitz: It becomes more and more important to compare the development of pre-term infants directly with full-term infants. Now what Mohr has shown is that in premature babies development is delayed. She then said that there was a difference at about 9 months of age when the prems were apparently better than full-term infants. Can she comment whether this was statistically significant? My guess is that if she has got enough infants it will be statistically significant. The importance of it is that if your premature infant is at the level of the full-term infant, it is, in fact delayed. This is something that one should remember when you test prems.

COMPUTER ASSISTED EVALUATION OF VISUAL FUNCTIONS IN NON VERBAL CHILDREN

Charlier Jacques[1], Nguyen Duc Dung[1], Hugeux Jean-Pierre[1], Paris Vincent[1], Bocquet Xavier[1], Defoort Sabine[2], Hache Jean-Claude[2].

(1) U.279 INSERM, 15 rue Camille Guérin - 59800 Lille, FRANCE
(2) Exploration fonctionnelle de la vision, CHR de Lille, Place de Verdun - 59037 LILLE CEDEX, FRANCE

ABSTRACT

This paper presents a computerized system specifically designed for the evaluation of visual functions in non verbal children.

Tests used for preferential looking, visual attraction, visual pursuit, optokinetic nystagmus as well as flash and pattern visual evoked potentials are generated by a cathode ray tube system.

Eye movements are recorded with a near infrared television system. Eye orientation is determined from the position of the corneal reflex relative to the pupil. This measurement is independant from head movements and is performed every 20 ms.

The recording and processing of visual evoked potentials and electroretinogram include artefact rejection algorithms and a statistical analysis. These features are extremely important in children examination for which the lack of cooperation limits the reliability of averaged data.

INTRODUCTION

Computers find many applications in ophthalmic diagnostic. They have been introduced in automated refractors, computer assisted perimeters, electrophysiological units, etc...
Such developments are due to several interesting features :

1) a reduction of operator's involvement resulting from the use of standard, reproduceable protocols.

2) a decrease in examination duration and consequent reduction of patient's fatigue (and improvement of equipment availability).

3) an increased quality of examination due to the introduction of reliability criteria.

Problems affecting the visual evaluation of non verbal children are quite similar and often even more acute than those involved in these clinical examinations. In this domain, the application of computers can be a valuable tool for clinical investigations.

METHODOLOGY

Many methods have been proposed for visual testing of non verbal children. Each of them involves a specific combination of stimulus and response (Table 1). Each of them can also be used for testing different modes of visual functions, i.e. for evaluating responses to light, pattern and binocular stimulations. For instance, visual poursuit can be elicited from a moving spot of light, a moving pattern such as a checkerboard or even from a shifting dynamic random dot stereogram (SIMONS and MOSS, 1981).

These methods have their specific interests and limitations. They provide correlative and complementary informations and their confrontation should be extremely valuable for the establishment of a diagnosis.

TECHNIQUE	STIMULUS	RESPONSE
preferential looking	Static local presentation	Duration of eye fixation
visual attraction	Static local presentation	Orientation of eye fixation
visual pursuit	Constant motion local presentation	Eye movements
optokinetic nystagmus	Constant motion fullscreen presentation	Eye movements
V.E.P.	transient fullscreen presentation	vertex to occiput biopotential

TABLE 1
Stimulus-response combinations used in
non verbal children visual tests.

CATHODE RAY TUBE (CRT) STIMULATOR

CRT technology offers a large amount of flexibility as far as image structure and animation are concerned. However, it presents several drawbacks. Spatial and temporal resolutions are restrained by the electron beam scanning process. A compromise must be made between resolution and background field dimensions. Light spectrum, luminance and contrast are limited by the opto-electronic conversion process.

The CRT stimulator is built from a 20 inches, P31 white phosphor tube. The electron beam scanning rate is 100 frames per second with 200 non interlaced horizontal lines per frame. Time resolution is therefore 10 ms. The screen sustains a 44 degrees horizontal by 32 degrees vertical angle at a viewing distance of 0.5 meter. With this set-up, the maximum resolution is 10 minutes of visual angle. Higher resolutions require a different set-up. For instance, a 1 minute resolution is obtained with a reduced scanning area of 4 degrees horizontally by 3 degrees vertically at a viewing distance of 2 meters.

246

Image structure and timing are generated by a LSI graphic controller circuit. This solution offers optimal flexibility, reliability and cost compared to magnetic storage techniques.

For the preferential looking and visual attraction procedures, the stimulus is displayed either on the right side or on the left side of the screen. It is made of a checkerboard pattern of programmable size and contrast whose average luminance matches the background luminance (Figure 1).

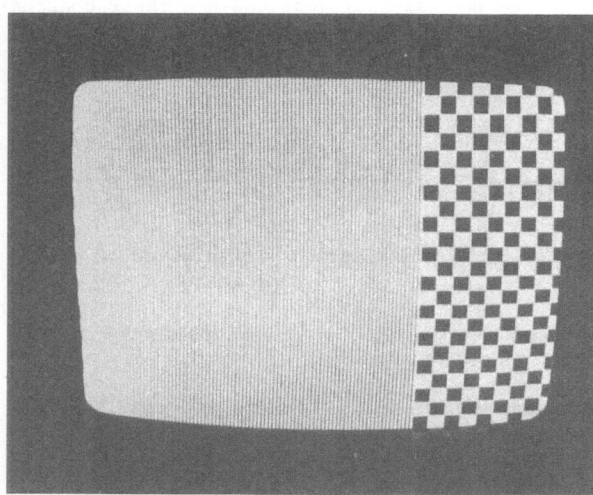

Figure 1 :
Stimulus used in preferential looking and visual attraction procedures.

In visual pursuit procedures the stimulus is made of a small square area filled with a vertical grating.(Figure 2).

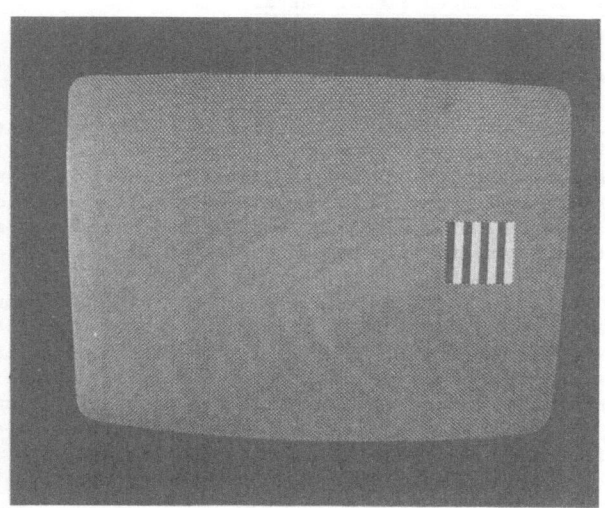

Figure 2 :
Stimulus used in visual pursuit procedures.

The stimulus average luminance matches with the background luminance. It sustains a 6 degrees visual angle and is put in motion along the horizontal axis at constant velocity programmable from 0.5 up to 10 degrees per second.

In optokinetic nystagmus, a vertical grating is generated over the center screen and is put in motion at a constant velocity (Figure 3).

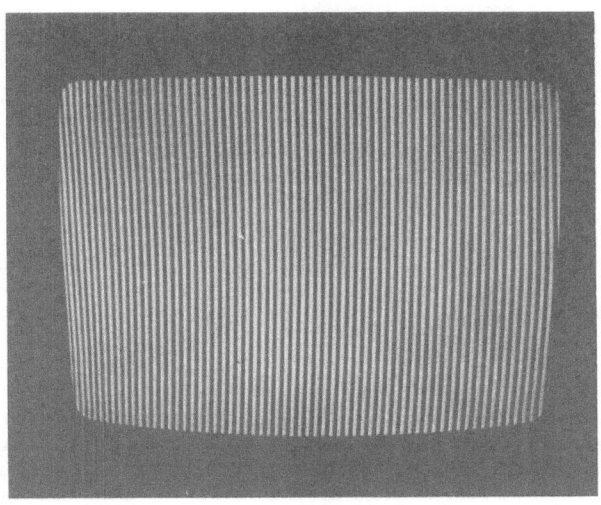

Figure 3 :
Stimulus generated for optokinetic nystagmus procedures.

EYE MOVEMENTS RECORDING AND ANALYSIS

The image of the child's eye is recorded from a television camera located under the CRT screen (Figure 4).

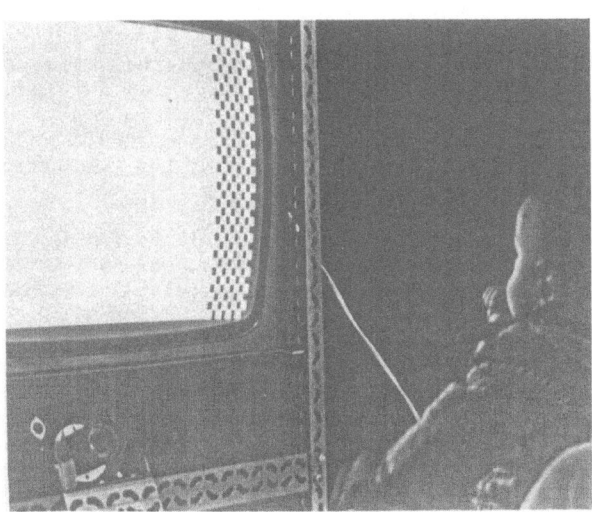

Figure 4 :
Relative location the CRT screen and of the television camera.

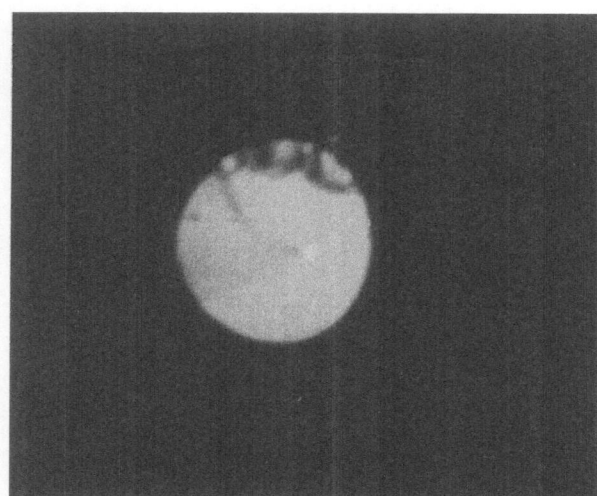

figure 6 :
Image recorded for the
automated analysis of
eye movements.

Relatively low cost is possible thanks to the use of large scale integrated technology. However, a compromise has to be made between the
precision of measurement and the control volume which is the allowable
head motion in all directions. Present control volume is 10 cm^3. This is
not really enough for applications such as work on young children.
Solutions have been proposed for increasing this control volume up to
10.000 cm^3. However these performances are only obtained by using
expensive mechanical positioning systems (YOUNG and SHEENA, 1975).

BIOELECTRIC SIGNAL RECORDING AND ANALYSIS

One area in which computer applications can bring usefull improvement is the processing of bioelectric responses recorded in vision
tests, namely VEP and ERG.

Several approaches have been made in order to improve the examination
reliability when performed under clinical conditions.

Many artefacts which contaminate electrophysiological recordings are
characterized by specific waveforms (HUGEUX et al., 1985). This allows for
the detection and rejection of artefacted signals associated with body
movements, eye movements, eye blinks, etc...

The automated analysis of averaged responses includes detection of
peaks and quantification of their amplitude and latency. The probability
for having an evoked response significantly different from the averaged
"noise" is also computed from the means and standard deviation of the
detected peaks (Figure 7). This feature appears to be very useful for
young children evaluation. It provides a reliable criteria for stopping
the examination as early as possible and for deciding whether an evoked
response exists.

The television camera is equipped with a silicon vidicon tube which presents a peak of sensitivity in the near infra-red spectrum.

Illumination is provided by an array of light emitting diodes producing totally invisible near infra-red light (869 nm).

Analysis of responses is performed by visual examination of recorded data. For this purpose, several additional informations are super-imposed upon the image of the child. A cursor indicates stimulus position and several figures allow for the identification of stimulus spacial resolution and timing (Figure 5).

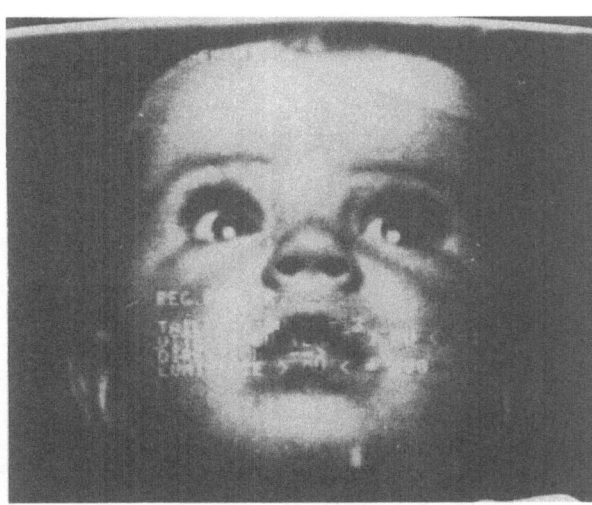

Figure 5 :
Image recorded for the for the analysis of eye movements.

Direct eye movements analysis from recorded pictures requires a large amount of skill and is very dependent upon many subjective factors. Automated analysis would be of great interest for clinical applications. A suitable eye movements sensor would be non invasive, easy to implement, highly reliable and also available at an accessible cost.
Such an oculometer is currently under development, based upon the measurement of the corneal reflex position relative to the pupil. This appears to be one of the most suitable techniques as it provides a measurement of eye orientation which is independent of head position. The optical axis of the camera and of the illumination are made coincident, so that light entering the eye is reflected by the retina and back lightens the pupil.

This arrangement produces a "bright pupil effect", i.e. the pupil appears as a bright disk over a dark background, allowing for a better detection of the eye position (Figure 5).

With adults measurements of eye orientation with a precision better than 1 degree have been obtained.. Specific hardware and processing algorithms have been implemented in order to eliminate adjustements and obtain reliable measurements even with such problems as eye lashes, eye lids, eye blinks or even parasite reflections (CHARLIER et al., 1984).

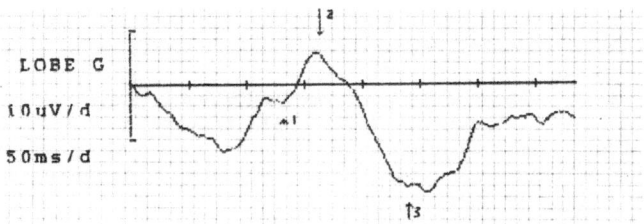

LOBE G

No	ms	uV	%
1	132 5	-3 3	75
2	164 5	5 8	100
3	240 7	-19 1	100

Figure 7 :
Automated   analysis of averaged electrical responses.

CONCLUSION

Clinical evaluation of this new equipment is currently under process at Lille Medical Center. 20 electrophysiological examinations of non verbal children are performed every week. The statistical analysis has been used for more than 3 years and proved to be very useful in providing clinicians with a reliability criteria.

Behavioral tests are still at an early stage of evaluation. Only about 160 children have been tested with a successfull rate of about 50 percent among non preselected children.

REFERENCES

Charlier J, Bariseau JL, Chuffart V, Marsy F, Hache JC. Real time pattern recognition and feature analysis from video signal applied to eye movement and pupillary reflex monitoring. In: applications of optical instrument in medicine. Medical image production, processing, display and archieving. Schneider RH ed., Spie, Bellingham WA, USA.

Defoort S. Méthodes d'étude clinique de la vision binoculaire chez le jeune enfant. Thèse de Doctorat en Médecine, Université de Lille II.

Hugeux JP, Charlier J, Hache JC, Moschetto Y. Validation et traitement assistés par ordinateur des signaux électrophysiologiques recueillis en clinique ophtalmologique chez les très jeunes enfants. Innov. Tech. Biol. Med.,

Nguyen DD, Charlier J, Hache JC, Defoort S, Moschetto Y. Dispositif de présentation de tests vidéo pour l'examen de la vision chez le nourrisson. Innov. Tech. Biol. Med.,

Simons K, Moss A. A dynamic random dot stereogram-based system for strabismus and amblyopia screening of infants and young children. Comp. Biol. Med 1984;11:33-46.

Young LR, Sheena D. Survey of eye movement recording methods. Behaviour Research Method and Instrumentation 1975;7:397-429.

Acknowlegdment :
This work was partly supported by grant P.R.C. N° 125045 from the INSERM.

DISCUSSION

Braddick: I wonder if you could explain a bit more when you say you get good results following them with PL. Is this with comparable stimuli, that is with gratings in both cases?

Charlier: Yes, it is by using gratings in both cases.

Braddick: Can you verify the detectability of your grating pattern under, for instance, conditions of degraded acuity? I think that there is a risk that with a sharp-edged patch you are introducing detectable features even with very blurred vision.

Charlier: I think it should be the opposite way if what you say is correct, because the edges introduce higher frequencies, so I don't think it is correct.

Braddick: Do you have an empirical check of those frequencies present in your test.

Vital-Durand: I have the feeling that colour, the chromatic component of the stimulus, was not the same in your screen when there was a pattern.

Charlier: No, this was due to the processing of my slides.

Fells: What means did you take to control the head fixation and how young a child could you examine?

Charlier: This has been used in children from 2 months up to 12 months of age. We are not at present using any control of head movements but if we are able to implement our eye monitoring technique we have the data on the head position.

Atkinson: When you said that you got results on 50%, was the other 50% because their eye went out of the frame? Was that the problem?

Charlier: No, this data was not obtained without automated processing. We use a wide-angle lens on the camera.

Atkinson: Yes, but that only includes the face.

Charlier: No, the problem is that children do not participate in the examination.

Atkinson: I don't understand.

Charlier: It was a technical and a psychological problem. The children did not want to look at that screen.

Atkinson: What is the visual angle? Can they move their head and eyes throughout?

Charlier: Well maybe you could compute it from the slide.

Atkinson: It looked to me as though you were restricted in head and eye movements in order to get the two eyes into your frame. If the baby moved 2 cm to one side you would lose the eyes.

Charlier: This was not a problem. You adjust the child's position.

VISUAL ACUITY ASSESSMENT WITH 'PREFERENTIAL LOOKING' IN YOUNG CHILDREN
TREATED FOR OPACITIES OF LENS AND VITREOUS; A LONGITUDINAL STUDY

Gunnar Lennerstrand*, Peter Jakobsson** and Annette Axelsson**

*Department of Ophthalmology, Karolinska Institute, Stockholm
and ** Department of Ophthalmology, Linköping University
Hospital, Sweden

INTRODUCTION

Animal experimentation on visual deprivation has demonstrated the
existance of a sensitive period in visual development after which the
neuronal effects of deprivation are irreversable (Hubel & Wiesel 1965,
Blakemore and van Sluyters 1973).   Although the sensitive
period in humans has not been exactly delineated, it is known that in order
to avoid stimulus deprivation amblyopia, dense opacities of the lens and
vitreous occurring in the newborn child has to be removed at an early age.
It is generally agreed that children with bilateral cataracts may gain good
visual acuity if the cataracts are operated before 2-4 months of age (Taylor
et al 1979,Gelbart et al 1982) and the aphacia corrected with contact lenses
immediately post-operatively. In cases with monocular opacities at birth,
treatment (including operation, contact lens fitting and occlusion therapy)
must be started even earlier, and probably not later than at 6 weeks of age
(Bellar et al 1981).

A few studies report visual acuity development in children treated for
congenital opacities using visual evoked potentials (Gelbart et al 1982) or
psychophysical methods, i.e. 'preferential looking' (Jacobson et al 1981).
We have performed a longitudinal study of visual acuity in five children
treated for congenital cataracts. In two of them vitreous opacities were also
present. We assessed visual acuity with the forced choice and operant preferential looking (FPL and OPL) techniques described by Teller (1979) and
Mayer and Dobson (1982). We report briefly the visual results during a follow-
up time of 1-2.5 years and describe different factors that influenced the
visual outcome.

MATERIAL AND METHODS

The five patients studied were all boys. The ophthalmological and pediatric
diagnosis as well as particulars of the treatment in each case are shown in
Table I. In three of the boys the diagnosis was made during the first weeks
of life, in the other two at a later age. In all of them extracapsular
cataract extraction was performed and contact lenses fitted with an over-
refraction of 2-4 diopters. Visual acuity was tested with the preferential
looking (PL) technique of Teller and Dobson (Lennerstrand et al 1983).
Depending on the results of visual acuity testing and/or an orthoptic
evaluation, occlusion therapy was instituted, monitored and adjusted.

TABLE I.   Summary of clinical findings and ophthalmological treatment.

Patient	Diagnosis	Age at							Remarks
		diagnosis	operation		CL fitting		occlusion		
			RE	LE	RE	LE	RE	LE	
E.E.	Hereditary, bilateral cataracts and nystagmus	1 w	3 w 3.5 m	4.5 w	1 m	1 m	–	4.5 m -12.0 m	Op.sec. cat. RE at 3.5 m. Corneal vessels RE. Occlusion LE stopped at 12 m. ET RE.
J.B.	Mb Down. Oesophagus atresia Bilateral cataracts	3 w	4 w	5.5 w	7 w	7 w	–	–	EP -> alt ET Photophobia
C.S.	Bilateral cataracts	9 m	10 m	10.5 m	11 m	11 m	–	–	ET before operation. EP -> alt. ET after.
R.P.	Right eye cataract and persistant arteria hyaloidea	1 w	2 w 1.5 m	–	2 w	–	–	4 m -10 m	Op. sec. cat. RE at 1.5 m XT RE and nystagmus on fixation attempt.
A.G.	Left eye cataract and persistent arteria hyaloidea	2.5 m	–	14 m	–	14.5 m	3.5 m -32 m	–	XT LE -> XP at 4 m ET LE at 32 m.

secondary opacities, heterotropia, nystagmus, photophobia etc. However, poor cooperation on behalf of the child was also a contributing factor, particularly in the 1 - 2 year age range (Dobson 1983).

The results in each of the five patients exemplifies different aspects on treatment in congenital ocular opacities. Early removal of dense opacities is required in order to obtain fairly normal visual development as seen in patient J.B. up to 12 months of age. (Beyond that age other problems made assessment difficult in this boy with Down's syndrome).The visual development after cataract removal in this patient is in accordance with the reports of Jacobson et al (1981) and Atkinson and Braddick (1983). Treatment has to be instituted during the sensitive period which in humans probably extends to 4 - 6 years of age. However, the visual system is more vulnerable to stimulus deprivation at lower ages. The recommendation based on animal experimentation and clinical experience is to start treatment for bilateral congenital cataracts at age 4 months at the latest and for monolateral cataracts even before 6 weeks of age. Patient R.P. with monolateral opacities was not treated optimally until age 4 months when occlusion therapy was instituted in addition to aphacia correction, and the result with regard to visual acuity was poor. In patient C.S. the cataracts did probably not develop until after birth and the abnormality was not evident until some 9 months of age. This is probably beyond the most critical period of visual development, since in this patient vision was normal for his age already 1 month postoperatively.

Children with partially occluding monocular opacities can be treated conservatively, as shown for patient A.G. with persistent arteria hyaloidea in his left eye. Patching of the good eye under control of visual acuity restored normal vision in both eyes until the lens opacities in the left eye increased and had to be removed. Binocular imbalance and esotropia in the postoperative aphacic period reduced vision in the affected eye in comparison with the normal eye in spite of proper contact lens fitting and occlusion therapy. It is well known that the visual dysfuntion in monocular opacities is due not only to form deprivation of the eye involved but also to abnormal binocular interaction i.e. inhibition from the good eye (von Noorden 1978). This was probably also the cause of persistant visual reduction in patient E.E., where a secondary cataract developed in one eye and was removed at the age of 3.5 months. Since this patient already had the binocular vision reduced by congenital nystagmus, occlusion therapy was tried but not persued rigorously in order not to interfere with the visual development of the better eye.

SUMMARY

Visual acuity was tested regularly with preferential looking technique in 5 infant boys with congenital opacities of the lens. Two had monocular cataract and persistent arteria hyaloidea in one eye. The others had binocular cataracts. Three of the boys were operated within 1 month postnatally. The other two had partial opacities and were operated later, one with monocular cataract after a period of occlusion.All were fitted with contact lenses immediately postoperatively.

Visual development during the first 1 - 2 years was almost normal in one boy operated early for bilateral cataracts, as well as in another boy with partial bilateral cataracts and in a third boy with partial monocular cataract, both operated later. A secondary cataract in a boy with bilateral cataracts operated early lead to monocular deprivation amblyopia in spite of occlusion treatment. Irreversible amblyopia occurred in another boy

RESULTS

Patient E.E. (Fig. 1A). As seen in the Table this boy was operated during the first month of life. A secondary cataract developed in the right eye at the age of 3 months. In spite of immediate operation and occlusion therapy, the right eye never recovered the same vision as the left eye. A hereditary nystagmus also reduced vision in both eyes. The nystagmus was blocked in convergence. Contact lens fitting was difficult due to the small eye globes with reduced corneal diameter. At age 32 months binocular visual acuity with a letter matching test was 0.1, i.e. the same as with PL.

Patient J.B. (Fig. 1B). This boy with Down's syndrome was operated upon for oesophagus atresia at 1 week of age and for congenital cataract within 3 weeks of life. His visual acuity developed normally during the first year, but the visual acuity values dropped during the second and third years due to poor cooperation at testing and photophobia of unknown etiology. He also developed an undulating nystagmus. The psychomotor development progressed in spite of the visual problems.

Patient C.S. (Fig. 1C). This boy developed an esotropia at age 9 months and subsequently bilateral cataracts were discovered. After operation and contact lens fitting there was at first a right sided esotropia. With occlusion visual acuity became normal for his age at 14 months and 22 months, with a reduction of visual development in between, probably due to contact lens problems and eye infections.

Patient R.P. (Fig 1D). This case shows that monocular visual deprivation is much harder to treat than binocular problems. In spite of an early removal of left eye opacities by vitrectomy and lens extraction at 2 weeks of age, contact lens fitting at the same age and removal of a secondary membrane at age 1.5 months, visual acuity remained much reduced in the affected right eye. A right exotropia persisted from age 4.5 months. From age 10 months the boy objected strongly to visual examination. Probably the visual deprivation had progressed too far when PL testing was done and left eye occlusion instituted at age 4 months, and the amblyopia had become irreversible.

Patient A.G. (Fig. 1E). Opacities in the left eye were discovered at age 3 months but the visual obstruction was partial and with occlusion treatment the visual acuity improved. An intermittent exotropia was changed into an exophoria. Acuity in the left eye developed slower than in the normal right eye and started to decrease when the lens opacity increased in the left eye. The cataract was extracted at 14 months of age. With contact lens and continued occlusion therapy, vision in the left eye could be retained, although it was reduced in comparison with right eye acuity. At 32 months of age esotropia was seen. The left eye acuity at this age was 0.3 with PL but only 0.1 with a letter matching test. The acuity of the right eye was 0.45 with letter matching.

DISCUSSION

Visual acuity testing with preferential looking proved useful in assessing visual development after treatment for lens and vitreous opacities in very young children. By means of these tests, effects of optical correction and occlusion therapy could be evaluated and the treatment adjusted. This should allow optimal visual results in each eye and reduce the risk for deprivation amblyopia by occlusion or by abnormal binocular interaction, in the phase of treatment after the operation. Reduced visual acuity, unaccounted for by poor contact lens fitting, could usually be related to ocular pathology, i.e.

258

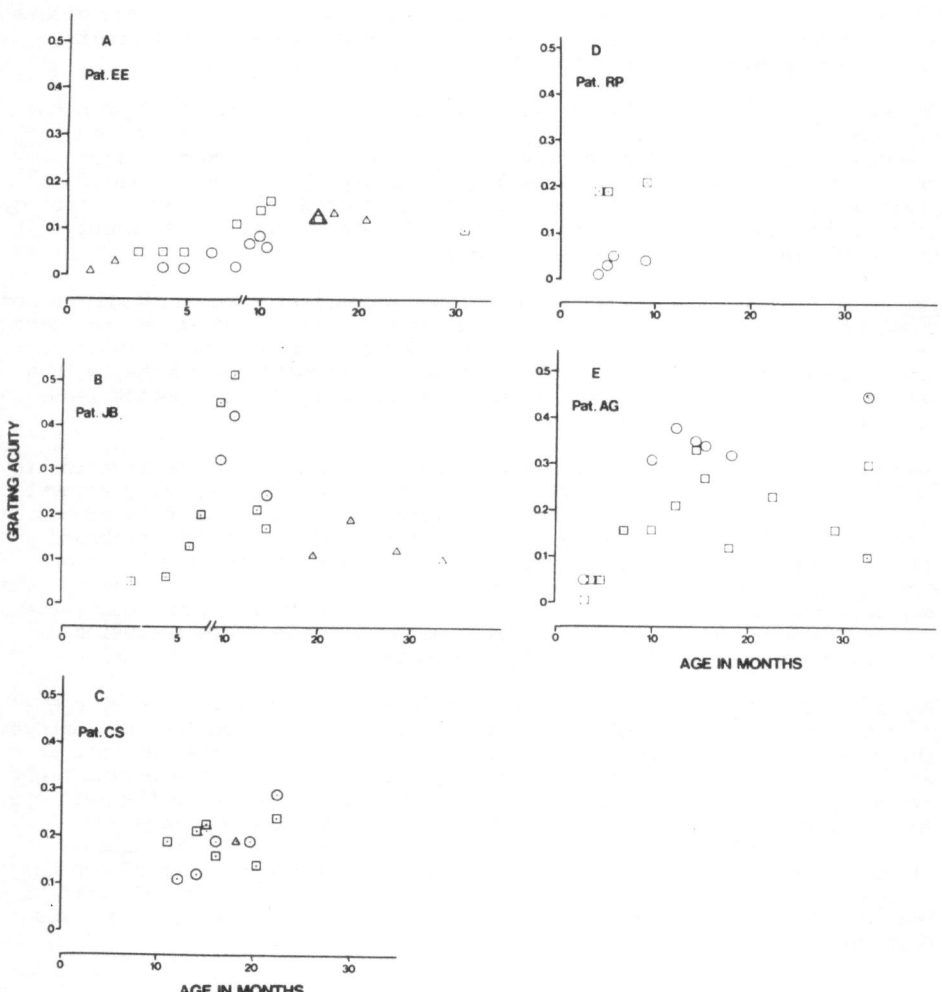

Fig. 1. Visual acuity determined with PL (open symbols) and with a letter
matching test (filled symbols) plotted against age, in each of the patients.
Values obtained binocularly are marked with triangles, in the right eye with
circles and in the left eye with squares.

operated early for monocular cataract in whom occlusion therapy was delayed.

Infants with congenital cataracts must be followed closely and treated from an early age, in order for fairly normal visual development to occur. Visual acuity determination with preferential looking has proved very useful in monitoring effects of treatment and visual progress.

ACKNOWLEDGEMENTS

This study was supported by grants from the Swedish Medical Research Council (no 4751) and the First-of-May-Flower Foundation.

REFERENCES

Atkinson J, Braddick O. Assessment of visual acuity in infancy and early childhood. Acta Ophthalmol (Copenh) 1983; Suppl 157: 18-26.

Beller R, Hoyt CS, Marg E, Odom JV. Good visual function after neonatal surgery for congenital monocular cataracts. Am J Ophthalmol 1981; 91: 559-65.

Blakemore C, van Sluyters RC. Reversal of the physiological effects of monocular deprivation in kittens: Further evidence for a sensitive period. J Physiol 1973; 237: 195-216.

Dobson V. Clinical application of preferential looking measures of visual acuity. Behavioural Brain Res 1983; 10: 25-38.

Gelbart SS, Hoyt CS, Jastrebski G, Marg E. Long-term visual results in bilateral congenital cataracts. Am J Ophthalmol 1982; 93:615.

Hubel DH, Wiesel TN. Binocular interaction in striate cortex of kittens reared with artificial squint. J Neurophysiol 1965; 28: 1041-59.

Jacobson SG, Mohindra I, Held R. Development of visual acuity in infants with congenital cataracts. Br J Ophthalmol 1981; 65: 277-35.

Lennerstrand G, Andersson G, Axelsson A. Clinical assessment of visual functions in infants and young children. Acta Ophthalmol (Copenh) 1983; Suppl 157: 63-7.

Mayer DL, Dobson V. Visual acuity development in infants and young children, as assessed by operant preferential looking. Vision Res 1981; 22: 1141-52.

Taylor D, Vaegan , Morris JA, Rodgers JE, Warland J. Amblyopia in bilateral infantile and juvenile cataract. Relationship of timing of treatment. Trans Ophthalmol Soc UK 1979; 99: 170-5.

Teller DY. The forced-choise preferential looking procedure: A psychophysical technique for use with human infants. Infant Behav Dev 1979; 2:135.

Von Noorden GK. Amblyopia: Basic concepts and current treatment. In: Symposium on Strabismus. Trans New Orleans Acad Ophthalmol St Louis: CV Mosby, 1978: 1-14.

REFRACTIVE CHANGES AND RETARDED VISUAL DEVELOPMENT IN APHAKIC CHILDREN
AFTER OPERATION FOR CONGENITAL CATARACT

Elisabeth Schulz, M.D.

University Eye Clinic Hamburg/FRG

INTRODUCTION

In the year in which Wiesel and Hubel's (1963) first publication on
the effect of visual deprivation in animals appeared Hatfield stated that
11,5 % of blindness in preschoolage was due to congenital cataract. Ten
years later   Frey et al (1973) reported on visual function in monolateral
and early operated congenital cataracts. To our knowledge this was the
first paper to show some patients with relative fair visual acuity in case
of early operation and consequent orthoptic treatment and contactlens
correction.

Since the early 70ies we have tried to encourage early surgery in
congenital cataract, give accurate contact lens correction and consequent
orthoptic follow-up. At that time there were a couple of questions, some
of which still remain unanswered:

1. How long is the sensitive period for total visual deprivation in
humans? Would there be a chance for visual development after three, six or
even nine months of congenital cataracts or should an operation be performed in the first weeks of life?

2. There was general agreement that cataractous eyes in babies are
small and   hyperopic. Nothing has been known about the real amount
of refractive power in the first months of life and nothing about possible
changes in refraction after early operation.

3. There is some insufficiency in the optical correction which
theoretically should immitate a clear and accommodating lens:

- The optical correction (contact lens) can have only one focus.
Which distance would be best?

- Accommodation is not possible (bifocal contact lenses will not be
appropriate in babies).

- Astigmatism might not be corrected using soft contact lenses.

- Irregular and decentered pupils will contribute to blurred image.
How much do all these factors interfere with visual development?

4. In unilateral cataract the phakic eye should be occluded. What
would be the appropriate occlusion time to be effective in amblyopia
treatment but harmless for the phakic eye?

5. How good could the visual acuity results really be?

In general our observations are comparable to those of other authors
(Beller et al, 1981, Gelbart et al, 1982, Rogers et al, 1981, Taylor 1982,
Treumer, 1983). So only additional data concerning refractive development
and experience contributing to visual development shall be mentioned here.

MATERIAL

Children operated in our clinic until the age of 2 years for congenital
cataract in the time from 1976 to 1983 have been evaluated. There were 21
patients with monolateral cataracts and 32 patients (=64 eyes) with
bilateral congenital cataract. For data in refraction any available and
reliable refractive measurement out of[a] 10 years' statistics (von Domarus
et al, 1984) and up to the age of 8 years has been taken. Only few of the
children have been referred to our clinic before the age of 3 months. But
there is a tendency to early referral and thus early operation in the recent
years (table I),

Table I.:

CONGENITAL CATARACTS

(University Eye Clinic Hamburg 1976 - 1983)

Operation up to age (months)	bilateral	monolateral
2	6 eyes	-
4	22 "	5 eyes
6	22 "	2 "
9	3 "	4 "
12	4 "	6 "
18	2 "	3 "
24	5 "	1 "
Total	64 eyes	21 eyes

this being due to educational effect in ophthalmological and paediatric
courses.

RESULTS

1. Refraction

Bilateral cataracts in the first months of life have a (spectacle -)

refractive requirement between +15 and +25 dpt (fig. 1).

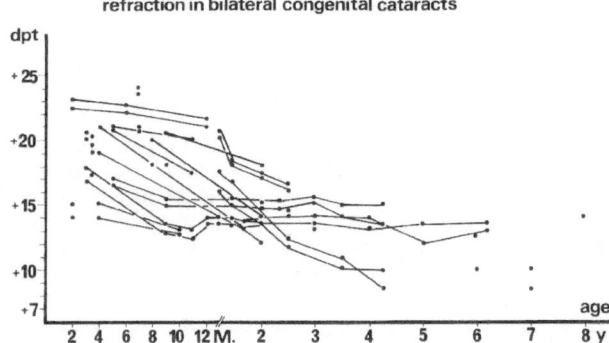

<u>Fig. 1:</u>

Refraction in bilateral congenital cataract - spectacle correction for far
distance. Follow up data of the same eyes are combined by lines. Note
expanded scale in the first year.

In general there is a decrease in plus power in the first year of life.
In some cases the loss of plus-refraction is tremendous - up to 7 dpt
in the first year - and continues in the following years. Especially in
Down-syndrome there is the highest regression.

Monolateral cataracts show the same maximum refractive power (+25 dpts)
in some cases, but in most less hyperopia and even rapid myopic development was present (fig. 2).

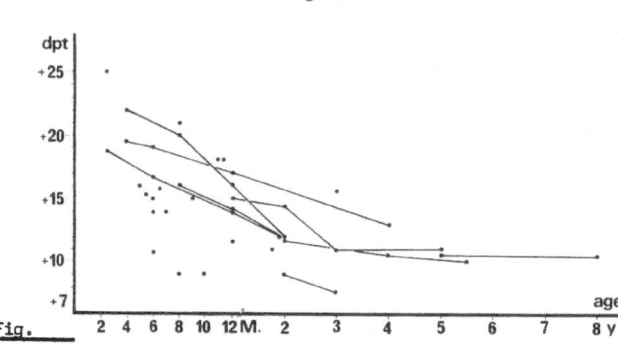

<u>Fig.</u>

Refraction in monolateral congenital cataract (phakic eyes only).
Note expanded scale in the first year.

2. Visual acuity

a) Monolateral congenital cataracts

Visual acuity levels better than 0,1 (or foveal fixation respectively) have
been achieved in 7 out of 21 monolateral cataracts. These patients have
been operated in the first 4 months of life with 1 exception (fig. 3).

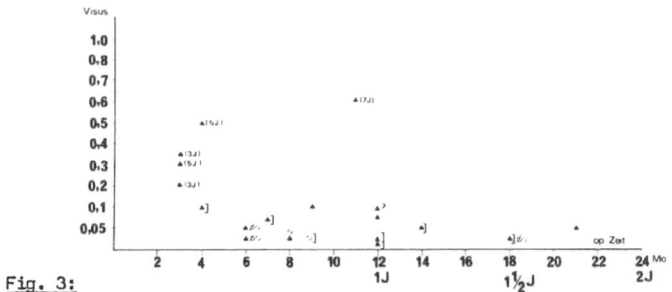

Fig. 3:

Monolateral cataracts: visual acuity versus age at operation. Only
children operated in the first 4 months show visual acuity better
than 0,1. In operations at a later age wearing of contact lens (J)
or occlusion (∅ 0) stopped.

At different ages visual acuity ranges between 0,1 and 0,6 for the aphakic
eye. Visual acuity results depend on the age of testing. The first <u>verbal</u>
visual acuity assessment (usually at the age of 2 to 3 years) is
disappointingly poor. But the striking phenomenon is an increasing visual
acuity with ongoing therapy and age (fig. 4). This "retarded" visual
development involves the phakic eye as well.

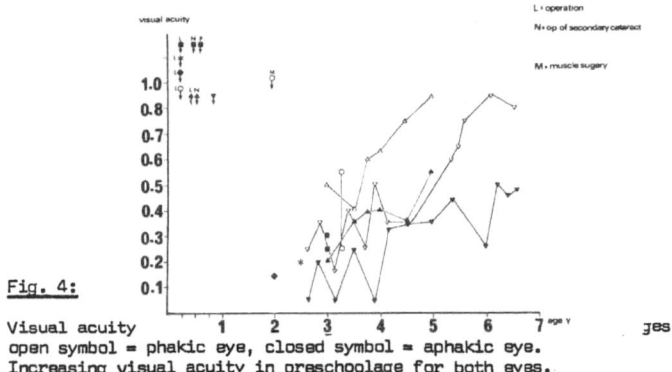

Fig. 4:

Visual acuity
open symbol = phakic eye, closed symbol = aphakic eye.
Increasing visual acuity in preschoolage for both eyes.

b) Bilateral congenital cataracts

Similar results can be given in bilateral congenital cataracts. Reliable
visual acuity results could be achieved in 10 out of 32 patients (others
were either mentally retarded or too young to give exact data), some
patients could not be followed up. The "sensitive period" seems to be
limited to the first 6 months beyond which there is no better visual acuity
than 0,1 (fig. 5). As in monolateral congenital cataracts there is a retarded visual development showing visual acuity below 0,2 at the age of 3 years
but increasing up to early schoolage (fig. 6).

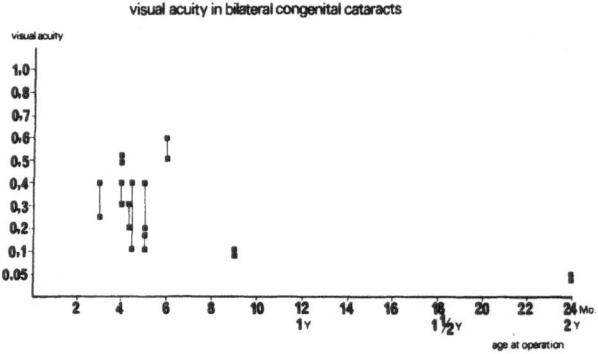

<u>Fig. 5:</u>

Bilateral congenital cataracts: Visual acuity versus age at operation.
Right and left eye of the same patient are combined. Visual acuity better
than 0,1 only in patients operated before the age of 6 months.

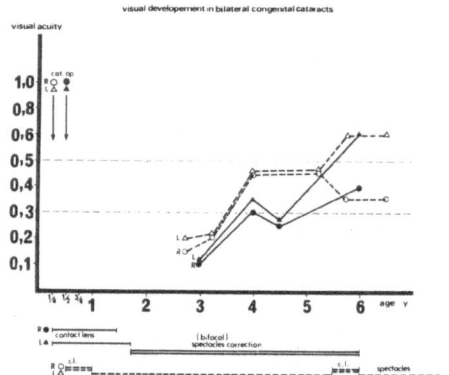

<u>Fig.6</u> :

Visual development in bilateral congenital cataracts (two patients
as an example). Increasing visual acuity up to early schoolage.

c) Sensitivity to therapy

In monolateral cataracts there is a high sensitivity to therapy in both
phakic and aphakic eye.Loss of bifocals e.g. (and atropine in the phakic
eye) will reduce visual acuity in both eyes, stop of occlusion or penali-
sation in the phakic eye will reduce visual acuity in the aphakic eye
(fig. 7).

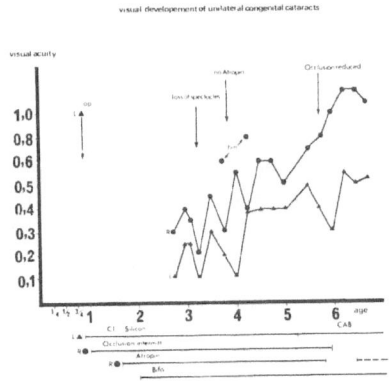

<u>Fig. 7:</u>

Visual development in monolateral cataract and reaction to therapy.
bin = binocular visual acuity. Loss of v.a. after loss of spectacles
in both eyes and after stopping atropin or occlusion in the aphakic eye.

DISCUSSION

Refractive changes from high hyperopia in eyes aphakic after congenital
cataracts to   myopia could be expected but have not been demonstrated up to now. Objections to early surgery, which might stop the growth of
the eye, are thus ruled out. The refractive development in a single case
cannot be predicted. This and the still lacking information about refractive
requirements and development before the age of 2 months limits to our
opinion the value of refractive surgery in congenital cataracts like
intraocular implants (Aron 1983)   and epikeratophakia (Morgan et al 1984).
The sensitive period in humans (or other words: the chance for fair visual
results in dense congenital cataracts) seems to be limited to the age of 4
or 6 months in monolateral or bilateral cataracts respectively. As in most
cases of later detection of an infantile cataract it is doubtful, whether it
is really congenital, and in case of increasing density later surgery might
be successful. This could have been the fact in our patients who's monolateral cataract has been operated at the age of 9 months and who proved
to achieve a visual acuity of 0,6.

The striking phenomenon is the initially poor but during preschoolage increasing visual acuity in both mono- and bilateral congenital
cataracts. The reduced visual results certainly are due to improper

correction and adjacent problems during early childhood. But this moderate form of deprivation seems to keep a visual system with the ability for further development. Retarded visual development in late correction of refractive errors, like high hyperopia and large astigmatism, is known to ophthalmologist and orthoptist and can occur even in schoolage. Conditions in congenital cataract have been worse with lack of accommodation and precedent total light deprivation. In spite of this the ability of the visual system for further development is evident. There is evidence for retarded visual development in preferential-looking-data of congenital cataract (Jacobson et al, 1981) compared to those of normal babies (Dobson and Teller 1978).

The retardation of visual development effects phakic (and part time occluded) eye as well. But the occlusion effect does not result in permanent visual impairment.

The sensitivity to changes in orthoptic treatment is another phenomenon we should be aware of . Amblyopia treatment seems to be necessary, for probably more than a decade, to prevent regression. Thus indicating that the visual system is still pliable.

SUMMARY

- highest refractive changes in 1st year of life
- operation in congenital cataract should be performed up to the age of 4 (6) months latest in monolateral (bilateral) congenital cataract
- visual development is retarded but can improve till early schoolage (no experience later than that)
- visual acuity results of 0,6 to 0,8 can be obtained
- there is no permanent visual impairment (occlusion effect) in the phakic eye.

Literatur:

ARON, J.J., ARON-RESA, D.: Intraocular lens implantation in unilateral congenital cataract. A preliminary report. Am. Intra-ocular Implant. Soc. J. (1983), 306 - 308.

BELLER, R., HOYT, CS, MARG, E., ODOM, J.V.: Good visual function after neonatal surgery for congenital monocular cataracts. Am. J. Ophthalmol., 91 (5), 559-565 (1981).

DOBSON, V., TELLER, D.Y.: Visual acuity in human infants: A review and comparison of behavioral and electrophysiological studies. Vis. Res. 18 (1978) 1469 - 1483.

von DOMARUS, D., SCHULZ, E., PABST-HOFACKER, M.: Lens aspiration in children. Paper presented European Ophthalmology Society-Meeting Helsinki (1984).

FREY, T., FRIENDLY, D., WYATT, D.: Re-evaluation of monocular cataract in children. Amer. J. Ophthalmol. 76 (1973), 381.

JACOBSON, SG., MOHINDRA, I., HELD, R.: Development of visual acuity in infants with congenital cataracts. Br. J. Ophthalmol, 65 (10), 727 - 735 (1981).

MORGAN, K.S., ASBELL, P.A., MAY, J.G., LOUPE, D.N., KAUFMAN, H.E.: Pediatric epikeratophakia. Strabismus II (R. Reinicke edt.) p 937 - 942 (1984). Grune and Stratton.

ROGERS, GL., TISHLER, CL., TSOU, BH., HERTLE, RW., FELLOWS, RR: Visual acuities in
        infants with congenital cataracts operated on prior to 6 months of age.
        Arch. Ophthalmol, 99 (6), 999 - 1003 (1981).

TAYLOR, D.S.I.: Risks and difficulties of the treatment of aphakic in infancy.
        Trans. ophthal. Soc., UK (1982).

TAYLOR, D.S.I.: Treacher Collins Prize Essay (1982): Developments in the treatment of
        cataract. Trans. Ophthalmol. Soc. UK, 102 (Pt 4), 441 - 453 (1982).

TREUMER, H.: Funktionelle Resultate nach Frühoperation der angeborenen Katarakt. Ein
        Beitrag zur Entwicklung des visuellen Systems. (Functional results
        following early surgery of congenital cataract. A contribution to the
        development of the visual system.) Fortschr. Ophthalmol, 80 (3),
        261 - 264 (1983).

WIESEL, T.N., HUBEL, D.H.: The effects of visual deprivation on morphology and physiology
        of cells in the cat's lateral geniculate body. J. Neurophysiol. 26 (1963)
        978.

WIESEL, T.N., HUBEL, D.H.: Single-cell responces in the striate cortex of kittens
        deprived of vision in one eye. J. Neurophysiol. 26 (1963), 1003.

DISCUSSION

De Laey: I was impressed by Lennerstrand's ability to test visual acuity, especially in the postoperative period when inflammatory diseases may occur. How far is the method he used to determine visual acuity by preferential looking applicable to normal children and to children with visual disturbances? I was very impressed by Schulz's marvellous results, even in late cases, which I never observed except in those cases where the cataract was not very marked in early life, and in cases where the operation could be delayed to the age of 4, 5 or 6 years. I wonder whether the cases which she presented, with visual acuities up to 6/10, 8/10 and even 10/10, were not cases where the cataract operation could be delayed?

Lennerstrand: The question was whether preferential looking could measure visual acuity. There are studies of comparing visual acuity with preferential looking, grating acuity and ordinary letter testing. I think that these have to be continued and expanded in this field of ocular pathology and amblyopia. My feeling is that there is not complete agreement, particularly not in amblyopia due to abnormal binocular interaction. I think that although preferential looking values might not be accurate, it still gives you an idea of the general level of vision, and also diffferences between the vision in each eye, which is important for treatment.

Schulz: To answer your question, there is at this time no quantititave assessment of measuring the density of the deprivation factor in certain congenital cataracts. At the time of operation these cataracts operated on were so dense that it would be a severe obstacle to foveal vision. It was not the decision of only one surgeon.

De Laey: Yes, I quite agree, but you have cases at the age of 4 or 5 years?

Schulz: If there is late detection, you never can say exactly what the position would have been at birth.

Campos: In my experience patients with monocular congenital cataract often have other associated abnormalities, particularly micophthalmos. This creates a further problem if visual restoration is possible. I am surprised by Schulz's results because they were associated with a persistent hyaloid artery, and also the occlusion was started late. In my experience, although studies exist in the literature claiming improvement in visual acuity in monolateral congenital cataract, there is only one such study which gives magnificent results from an American author. Nobody was able to see his patients and to confirm his results. A lot of us deal with bilateral cataracts. Usually we don't operate on both eyes at the same session; we first do one eye and after about 2 days the second eye. In the intervening time we patch patients binocularly in order to avoid a possible imbalance between the two eyes. Strabismus frequently develops in these patients so I don't know what happens, particularly as secondary cataract is prevented by posterior capsulotomy.

Warburg: We were asked if somebody had tried the correlation between
optotypes and preferential looking. In my clinic we examined 35 children
with Down's syndrome and most of them could be tested with optotypes.
There was good correlation between the PL acuity and picture optotypes. In
those who were impossible to test with picture charts, it was clear that
the preferential looking technique was superior. In cases of nystagmus,
picture charts gave low acuity in monocular cases of nystagmus while this
was not so in preferential looking.

Fielder: For clinicians who are interested in preferential looking this
must be an important clinical use, because without using preferential
looking how can one assess the density of a cataract, to determine which
lens requires removal.

De Laey: I wish to ask whether in Warburg's cases with nystagmus visual
acuity for near was quite good, because these children can block their
nystagmus. Could this be related to the fact that preferential looking was
much better than conventional Snellen acuity?

Warburg: I will go back home and examine this.

Campos: What I do to assess the density of a cataract is to look at the
fundus with an ophthalmoscope. If I see the macula I can delay surgery.
If I don't see the macula I assume the child is unable to see through the
cataract.

van Lith: I think preferential looking is a very good method from what I
have heard today for control of these children who have cataracts. Before
surgery, how can you know when you have low vision due to the cataract or
to amblyopia. I don't think you can decide only by preferential looking.
So the simple message is: "how dense is the cataract?" I always use
ophthalmoscopy and see through an undilated pupil how well I can see the
macula. But how can you do this on little children, because you don't know
if the reduced vision is caused by the cataract or by amblyopia.

Lennerstrand: In monocular opacities you can use occlusion and test the
visual acuity after a while. If vision improves it was probably amblyopia
and not the cataract.

Taylor: I am intrigued because we found the same in a few of our patients,
not the same sort of proportion as yours, and our reaction was to wonder
whether we have got it wrong. But I don't think that is the case, I think
there is something that happens late in these children. I want to see
somebody publish a technique that doesn't work (ie most people's experience
with monocular congenital cataract). My experience is the same as most of
yours, that monocular truly congenital cataract has a terrible visual
prognosis despite the ones that we have had early, before 2 months. We
have only had 3 that have fulfilled the criteria to be operated on and
optically corrected before 2 months, and wore a contact lens and did some
patching and they had brilliant fixation. As small children they did
everything. They could pick up their hundreds and thousands (their little

sweets), they had steady eyes, no squint and we knew from their visual
behaviour that they were going to have good acuity. They did, and two had
1/60 and one had 3/60 vision. I would like to see one patient from
anywhere with a truly congenital cataract with good acuity. It is
economically, socially, and personally an insignificant disease and so far
we don't influence it by treatment and it is only under very special
circumstances that I think we should be treating it.

Schulz: It is difficult to treat bilateral aphakic children and monitor
them carefully, and that is why we need preverbal vision testing to decide
which are going to be amblyopic and which not. We get selected patients
with monocular congenital cataracts because these are the patients who were
refused operation and the mother demanded that something should be done.
They will do so regardless of what you tell them, and they are highly
motivated. I am quite sure that when we encourage early operation in every
patient we get poor results. What I don't know in monocular cataract is
whether the vision will last. How long do we go on with our therapy, and
do aphakic eyes go down in visual acuity some years later if you stop doing
anything?

Taylor: I am not saying that one shouldn't operate. You have to in some
circumstances. It is the parent's decision after you have given them all
the information as you see it. They still say you must do something and
you can't say: "go somewhere else."

Schulz: The striking fact is that these children that had early surgery
had a visual acuity better than 0.1 single optotypes in later years. It is
worthwhile doing an operation if the parents are motivated to go on with
treatment.

ALBINISM: AN ANOMALY OF MATURATION OF THE VISUAL PATHWAY

Patricia Apkarian, Wim van Veenendaal, Henk Spekreijse

The Netherlands Ophthalmic Research Institute, Amsterdam

INTRODUCTION

The electrophysiological pathognomonic in human albinism is visual evoked potential asymmetry following full-field monocular stimulation. Different patterning of the cortical representation of albino VEP asymmetry has been reported (Creel 1979; Carroll et al 1980; Coleman et al 1979). Examination of the related experimental procedures indicates that the reported differences are primarily due to variants in stimulus and recording conditions. The most reliable method of recording the albino "signature" is VEP pattern appearance/ disappearance (Creel et al 1981; Apkarian et al 1983, Wolf et al 1984). Under this mode, albino asymmetry, at least in the adult, is expressed as a shift in hemispheric representation of primarily the early positive component (CI) of the pattern onset response from the left hemisphere following full-field right eye stimulation to the right hemisphere following full-field left eye stimulation (see fig 1). It is worthwhile to note that this particular pattern of hemispheric lateralization is specific to albinism and should not be confused with VEP asymmetry resulting from non-associated optic pathway anomalies such as pathway lesions and tumours or asymmetries from normally occurring hemispheric response dominance (Blumhardt et al 1977; Müller-Jensen et al 1981; Maitland et al 1982).

VEP asymmetry in albinism presumably reflects the paucity of ipsilaterally destined retino-fugal projections, an anomaly of the retino-geniculo-cortical pathway termed optic pathway misrouting and observed in all albino species thus far investigated (for review, see Witkop et al 1982; Taylor 1978). Concurrent with abnormal organization of the optic pathways are disturbances at the retinal level; the genetic mutation which gives rise to albinism also severly disrupts retinal histogenesis and ganglion cell differentiation.(Murakami et al 1982; Stone et al 1978). In human albinos, this results in foveal hypoplasia (Fulton et al 1978), the predominant clinical symptom of which is reduced visual acuity (Duke-Elder 1964).

Abnormal melanin metabolism during embryogenesis has been implicated as the presumptive precursor of retinal and pathway anomalies associated with albinism. Although the pathogenesis of these disturbances is not yet fully understood, recent morphological and physiological studies in the naturally occurring albino animal model (Silver and Sapiro 1981; Strongin and Guillery 1981; Silver 1984) have demonstrated the prominent role of melanin for normal retinal neurogenesis and axonal trajectory along the immature optic cup and stalk. The deleterious effects of disturbing the delicate embryological processes involved in retinal differentiation and patterning of chiasmal decussation are evident at birth and appear to predetermine the final course of visual pathway maturation (Shatz and Kliot 1982).

The non-invasive electrophysiological correlate of the resultant optic pathway misrouting can be readily observed in human albinos. The over 100 albinos ranging in age from 2.5 to 65 years tested in our laboratory under comparable conditions, demonstrate albino VEP asymmetry with virtually a 100% detection rate. The corresponding occurrence of zero false positives in our control groups which include heterozygote family members and non-albinos evincing one or more albino symptoms (e.g. iris translucency, foveal hypoplasia, nystagmus, fundus hypopigmentation), has justified the inclusion of this test in routine ophthalmological examination when the condition of albinism is indicated. The presence or absence of VEP asymmetry can also be considered the determining factor in differential diagnosis. The high degree of reliability of evoked potential assessment in human albinism, however, does not extend, as yet, to infants and younger children under the age of about 3 years, an age range in which albino diagnosis by conventional means is most difficult.

Evoked potential testing of albinism in pediatric populations is complicated by the fact that, as described earlier, viable asymmetry is best obtained with stimulus and recording conditions which facilitate isolation of the first positive component of the PNP (positive, negative, positive) pattern onset response. The infant pattern onset response, however, lacks the adult-like triphasic waveform i.e. components CI, CII and CIII. Full maturation of these distinct components is not reached until around puberty (de Vries-Khoe and Spekreijse 1982; Spekreijse 1983). Despite the lack of adult waveform complexity, component specific or rather latency specific albino asymmetry can be observed in children even as young as 4 to 5 years (e.g. see figure 2), a period in visual system development in which the EP waveform is still immature, predominantly showing only a single positive peak. Below this age period, however, appreciable response specificity in albino asymmetry is not detected (Apkarian et al 1984). Rather, the whole response, when measurable, appears to lateralize. The major difficulty in detecting this form of response lateralization is the prerequisite of state stationary conditions not only within a given recording epoch but also from left to right eye stimulation. For it is the left eye/ right eye response comparison that establishes the misrouting correlate. If monocular responses cannot be obtained under comparable states, the determination of albino asymmetry is precluded. In an attempt to facilitate detection of the albino pathway anomaly in infants, we have investigated the possibility of recording contralateral lateralization with flash stimulation. As previously reported (Creel et al 1981; Apkarian and Spekreijse 1985) and again demonstrated in this presentation, the relative insensitivity of transient flash stimulation for detecting misrouting negates its practical application in older children and adults. However, the general non-specific immature pattern response (Spekreijse 1978) and the less complicated flash waveform (Barnet et al 1980) suggest that flash stimulation may help to extend reliable electrophysiological diagnosis to the albino infant.

METHODS

Subjects

The six oculocutaneous albinos presented in this study were selected from a larger albino subject pool (N=123 albinos tested electrophysiologically). Albino diagnosis based on genetic history and ophthalmological examination was performed at the Netherlands Ophthalmic Research Institute, Department of Ophthalmogenetics by J.W. Delleman and D. van Dorp. Review of

the reported clinical histories indicates that each of the six albinos show
fundus hypopigmentation, absence of foveal or macular reflex, nystagmus,
strabismus and high refractive error. Photophobia, iris translucency and
reduced visual acuity were also reported. Visual acuity assessment in the
two infants was performed only at a gross level; iris translucency was not
detected in the 10 month old.

Stimulus

Luminance flash stimulation was provided by a Nihon Kohden photic
stimulator positioned at a distance of 30 cm. The intensity level was set
at 0.6 Joules; rate of stimulation was 1 Hz. Pattern stimulation for figures 1,3 and 4 consisted of checkerboard patterns of 80% contrast generated
on a Philips video monitor. The stimulus mode was pattern appearance (40
msec)/ disappearance (460 msec) at a constant mean luminance level of 90
cd/m^2. Pattern size subtended 110'. Viewing distance was 100 cm for the 4
month and 10 month old albinos and 150 cm for the adult; field size was 15°
and 10°, respectively.
For data of figure 2, checkerboard patterns with element sizes of 55'
were generated on a Sony video monitor. Duration of pattern appearance was
300 msec, pattern disappearance, 500 msec. Mean luminance was kept constant
at 64 cd/m^2; field size was 20°, viewing distance 100 cm.

Recording

Visual evoked potentials were recorded with tinned copper cup electrodes attached to the scalp with collodion and positioned with equal
spacing of 3 cm in a horizontal row, 1 cm above the inion, across the left
and right occiput. The row consisted of five active electrodes with the
center electrode located at the midline. Reference for all electrodes was
linked ears in the older children and adult and linked mastoids for the two
infants; the common ground electrode was located near the vertex. Bandwidth
of the EEG amplifiers was set at 0.5 to 70 Hz. The high frequency cut-off
(70 Hz) was set by a low-pass fourth order Butterworth filter which introduced a phase shift increasing the response latencies by about 7 msec. The
reader should make this correction when estimating peak latencies from the
responses depicted. The filtered signals were averaged with an Apple II
microcomputer (figs 1,3 and 4) or an HP2100 computer(fig 2). All signals
were displayed in real time and stored on disk for further analysis. Prior
to graphic illustration, the records were digitally filtered.

Procedure

The adult and older children were tested while seated comfortably in an
electrically shielded room; infants were seated on the lap of their parent.
Recording was interrupted by automatic artifact rejection as well as by an
observer who monitored the infant's fixation. Averaging was temporarily
halted when a corneal reflex of the stimulus could not be elicited. To help
maintain fixation at the stimulus field for pattern stimulation, the checkerboard presentation and concurrent averaging procedure were intermittently
interrupted by a children's cartoon. When pure checkerboard stimulation
replaced the cartoon and recording resumed, the movie sound track input to

an amplifier attached to the back of the stimulus monitor, continued to play. This procedure drew attention to the stimulus by auditory cueing. Attempts to maintain attention were also implemented by sound producing toys. Only the latter were employed with luminance flash stimulation.

Binocular, left and right eye luminance flash and pattern appearance responses were recorded. Monocular recordings were obtained with total occlusion of the fellow eye. Duration of the test was subject dependent.

Data analysis

Our data analysis procedures for the albino test protocol have been described in full detail elsewhere (Apkarian et al 1983). VEP asymmetry for the records presented in this report are described qualitatively. That is, by the result of visual inspection of the potential distributions across the scalp within an early time period of the response for the left eye compared to the right. The difference potential from a left (L) minus right (R) hemisphere response was also used. Right hemispheric lateralization expresses itself as a negative difference potential, left as positive. A change in sign from negative to positive upon left and right eye stimulation reflects the VEP asymmetry of interest.

RESULTS AND DISCUSSION

Adult albino VEP asymmetry

An impression of the albino VEP "signature" can be obtained by inspection of the left eye (OS) and right eye (OD) pattern response profiles of adult albino, WSB, figure 1. In this and all remaining figures, traces (rows 1-5) were derived from electrodes positioned from left (upper traces) to right occiput (lower traces). The bottom most trace is the difference potential obtained from subtracting a right hemispheric response (traces, row 4) from a left hemispheric response (traces, row 2).

In figure 1 the shift in hemispheric lateralization from left to right eye stimulation is immediately apparent. The peak of the potential distribution following left eye stimulation is localized across the right hemisphere while the peak of the potential distribution following right eye stimulation is localized across the left hemisphere. The contralateral asymmetry of particularly the early response component can also be seen by inspection of the difference potential; note the reverse in sign. In these response profiles as well as those of our larger albino sample, adult albino asymmetry is primarily restricted to an early time window of the pattern appearance response (80-110 msec) which corresponds to the latency of the CI component (Apkarian et al 1983). As stated in the introduction other response components are not reliable indicants. Although the first electrophysiological evidence of misrouting in human albinos was reported with flash stimulation (Creel et al 1974), the low detection rates and high response variability rendered these studies interesting for research purposes but not practical for clinical diagnosis. In our hands, luminance flash in adult albinos also does not yield reliable asymmetry results (Apkarian and Spekreijse 1985). For ease of comparison the relative insensitivity of the flash response in this regard is illustrated in figure 1. In general, the adult luminance flash response is a complicated waveform consisting of several minor and major, negative and positive deflections

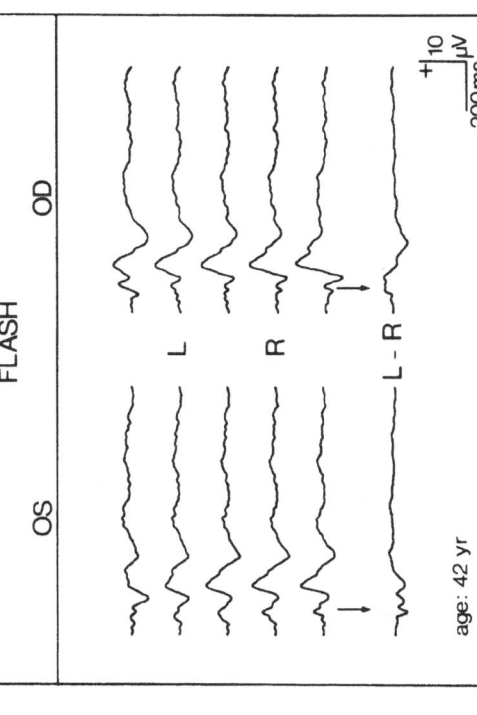

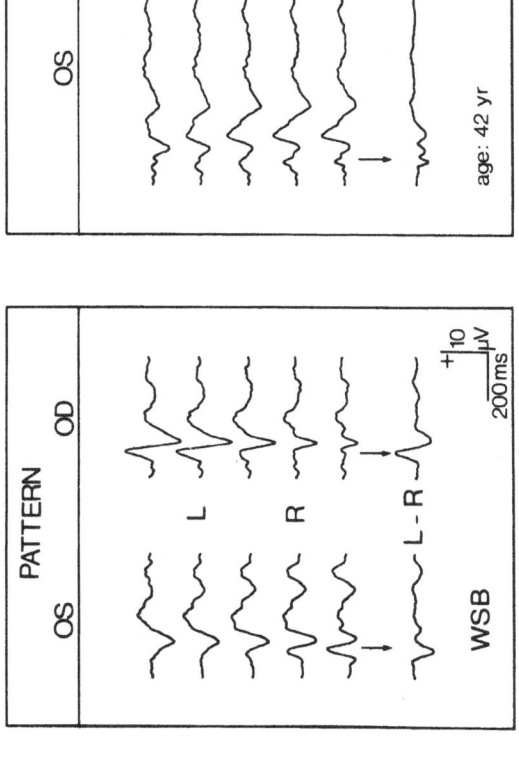

Figure 1.
Left: Left eye (OS) and right eye (OD) pattern appearance responses in adult albino, WSB. Responses depicted were derived form electrodes positioned from left (L) to right (R) occiput. The triphasic adult-like waveform is expressed by the major positive (CII), negative (CI), positive (CIII) waveform deflections. Note the dramatic change in response lateralization from left to right eye stimulation. Contralateral asymmetry occurs primarily within an early response component as seen by the difference potential. Note sign reversal (arrows).
Right: Left and right eye luminance flash responses. Presence of asymmetry is more difficult to establish. The difference potential, however, suggests contralateral lateralization.

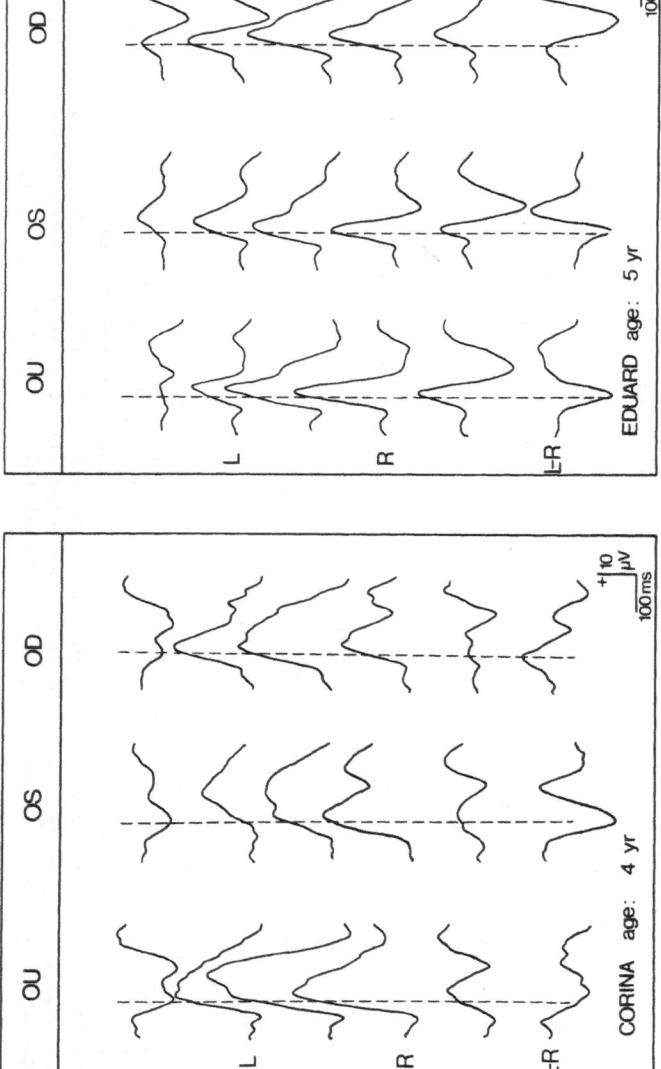

Figure 2:
Binocular (OU), left eye (OS) and right eye (OD) responses for albino, CORINA (left) and EDUARD (right). Inspection of the response profiles, particularly for the difference potential, reveals positive asymmetry around 100 msec (dashed line) for both children.

(Cigánek 1961). In the monocular luminance flash responses for WSB there is a suggestion of asymmetry for a very early response peak but its presence is somewhat obscured by the more predominant waveform deflections. To enhance the signal to noise ratio of the purported flash asymmetry component the traces depicted required over 200 averages. In contrast, the pattern responses of figure 1 were obtained with less than 100 averages. However, even with a two-fold increase in averaging time, as seen here and in our continuing studies, luminance flash asymmetry in the adult albino response is far from consistent.

Component specific asymmetry in albino children

As albino asymmetry in adults is restricted to the early CI component, what might one expect from the immature response profile which does not readily distinguish this component? To address this question, we present both the binocular (OU) as well as monocular responses (OS and OD) of two albino children, figure 2. Firstly, following binocular stimulation the response is shown to reflect an immature pattern appearance waveform. This is expressed by the presence of predominantly a single positive peak which has a latency of about 150 msec. With monocular stimulation, a curious shearing of this peak seems to occur. That is with left eye stimulation, the early portion of the response at about 100 msec (dashed line) later-alizes to the right hemisphere. With right eye stimulation, the early portion shifts to the left hemisphere. The single positive peak behaves as though two independent mechanisms were operating. Despite the absence of a clearly defined CI component, positive asymmetry is expressed at around 100 msec. The early portion of the single positive peak, corresponding to CI latency, behaves quite differently from the longer latency portion. These results imply that the immature pattern onset response, at least within this age group, reflects the upper envelope of two underlying mech-anisms, most probably the CI and CIII components, each which behaves in an independent fashion with respect to albino asymmetry.

VEP asymmetry in albino infants

The component specific asymmetry present in the responses of younger children is not readily seen in response profiles of albino infants, figures 3 and 4. The first point of interest to note is that when a mea-surable response is obtained, typically the entire positive peak appears to reflect the albino misrouting. For Martin (fig 3), tested at the age of 4 months, right eye pattern stimulation shows a single positive peak later-alized left of the midline electrode. Recordings simultaneously derived from electrodes positioned to the right of midline are surprisingly flat. Left eye pattern stimulation shows the attenuated responses now across the left hemisphere with a concomitant peak in the potential distribution localized at the right hemisphere. A similar trend is suggested in the pattern responses of Moniek, figure 4, who was tested at the age of 10 months. Though it is important to note that the variable responses obtained with the right eye of this patient precluded right to left eye comparison and consequently the determination of albino asymmetry as well. Although a viable right eye pattern response could not be elicited due to subject inattentiveness, luminance flash responses which required less subject cooperation, did yield the necessary diagnostic records. Contralateral lateralization is clearly present for the monocular flash responses for

278

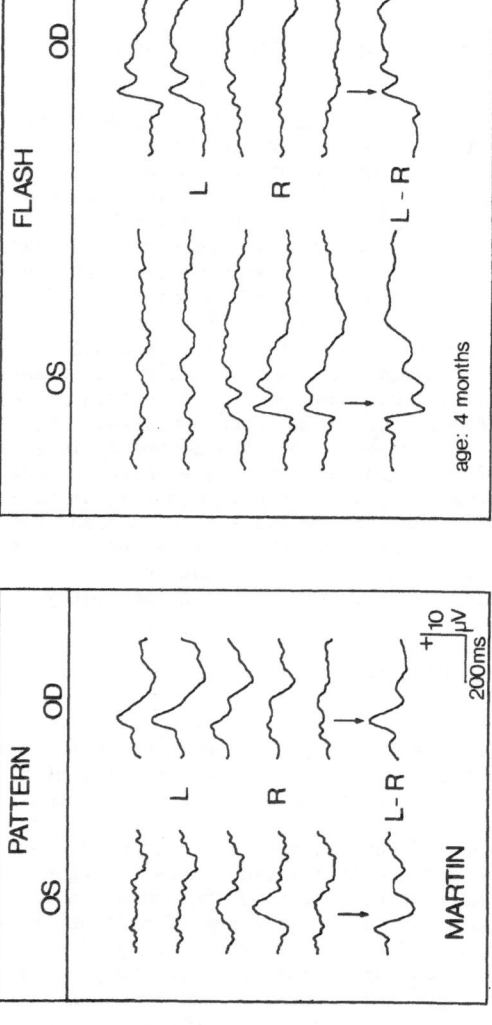

Figure 3.
Left: Left eye (OS) and right eye (OD) pattern appearance responses for albino infant, MARTIN. Contralateral albino asymmetry is present but does not show clear component specificity. Rather, the whole single positive peak appears to shift from right hemispheric lateralization to left following left and right eye stimulation, respectively.
Right: Left and right eye luminance flash response. Presence of asymmetry in the immature flash waveform is clear.

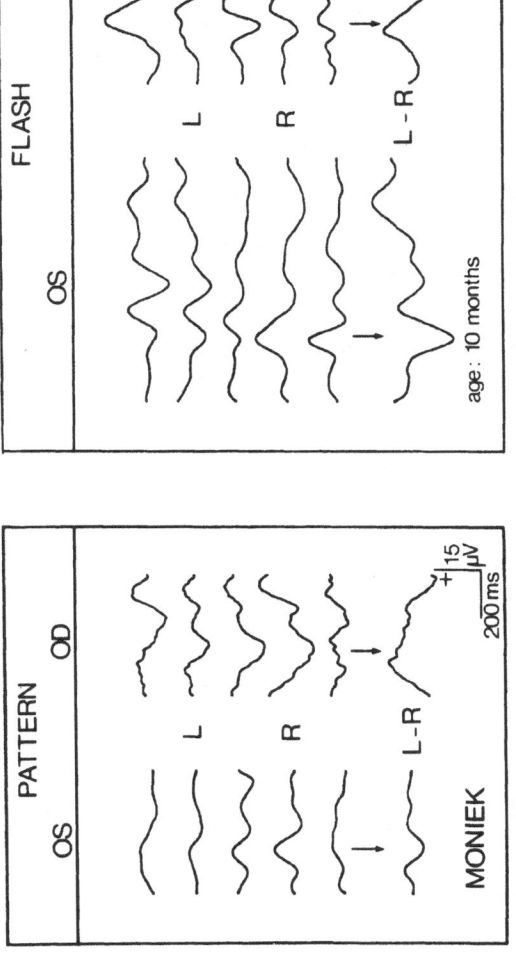

Figure 4.
Left: For details see figure 3. Note, however, that for infant MONIEK, a reliable right eye pattern response could not be elicited. Although OS shows appropriate response asymmetry, absence of a measurable response, OD negates the diagnosis of misrouting.
Right: For details see figure 3. Presence of asymmetry is clear for an early response peak but note that the flash waveform is, in general, more complicated than that of MARTIN (figure 3) who was six months younger. The difference responses show a sign reversal for the early peak.

both infants, albeit for Martin, asymmetry noted in measurable pattern responses was already a sufficient pathognomonic.

CONCLUSIONS AND SUMMARY

The normal prenatal development of the retina and optic tract is severely disrupted by the genetic mutation that gives rise to albinism (Taylor 1978; Shatz and Kliot 1982; Silver and Sapiro, 1981). At birth the substrate for impaired visual function is already well established. In contradistinction, detection of the concomitant disorder in the infant albino is not always possible and diagnosis is frequently postponed. The major impediment towards early diagnosis is the postnatal maturational process of the visual system in general. For example, foveal hypoplasia, an obligate albino symptom, is a normal condition for all neonates; a recent report indicates that full foveal development is not reached before 45 months of age (Hendrickson and Yuodelis 1984). The electrophysiological response which reflects and therefore parallels development of the distal and proximal visual processes also undergoes a rather lengthy period of maturation; a recent report indicates that full adult-like definition of the pattern onset response is not reached before the age of 100 months (Spekreijse 1984). It is therefore not surprising that the VEP test of misrouting which yields near 100% hit rates in albinos over the age of 3 years falls to near chance in the infant. On the one hand, the infant VEP pattern response is immature, lacking the full complement of response components while on the other hand, albino VEP asymmetry has been shown to be component specific (Apkarian et al 1983). Recording and stimulus conditions which enhance component isolation and thus non-invasive electrophysiological detection of optic pathway misrouting are not necessarily applicable in the albino infant. To further complicate matters is the issue of state change. The determination of asymmetry is invalidated unless left eye and right eye measures are obtained under comparable states. The nature of infant recording renders this a difficult task.

In this report we have attempted to facilitate the albino diagnosis in children under 3 years of age by introducing into our paradigm luminance flash stimulation. We justify its use based on the simplicity of the immature response profile and the positive results thus far attained. It is worth pointing out, however, that transient luminance flash stimulation in albino adults yields rather low detection rates of misrouting. The time course and transition period between the first few months of life when flash stimulation is indicated to adulthood when its usefulness is minimal must await further investigation.

REFERENCES

Apkarian P, Reits D, Spekreijse H, van Dorp D. A decisive electrophysiological test for human albinism. Electroenceph clin Neurophysiol 1983;55:513-531.

Apkarian P, Reits D, Spekreijse H. Component specificity in albino VEP asymmetry: Maturation of the visual pathway anomaly. Exp Brain Res 1984;53:285-294.

Apkarian P, Spekreijse H. The VEP and misrouted pathways in human albinism. In: Cracco RA, Bodis-Wollner I, eds. Frontiers of Clinical Neuroscience "Evoked Potentials". Baltimore: Williams and Wilkins, 1985 (in press).

Barnet, AB, Friedman, SL, Weiss IP, Ohlrich ES, Shanks B, Lodge A. VEP development in infancy and early childhood. a longitudinal study. Electroenceph clin Neurophysiol 1980;49:476-489.

Blumhardt LD, Barrett G, Halliday AM. The asymmetrical visual evoked potential to pattern reversal in one half field and its significance for the analysis of visual field defects. Br J Ophthalmol 1977;61:454-461.

Carroll WM, Jay BS, McDonald WI, Halliday AM. Pattern evoked potentials in human albinism. J Neurol Sci 1980;48:265-287.

Cigánek L. The EEG response (evoked potential) to light stimulus in man. Electroenceph clin Neurophysiol 1961;13:165-172.

Coleman J, Sydnor CF, Wolbarsht ML, Bessler M. Abnormal visual pathways in human albinos studied with visually evoked potentials. Exp Neurology 1979;65:667-679.

Creel D. Luminance-onset, pattern-onset and pattern-reversal evoked potentials in human albinos demonstrating visual system anomalies. J Biomed Eng 1979;1:100-104.

Creel D, Spekreijse H, Reits D. Evoked potentials in albinos: efficacy of pattern stimuli in detecting misrouted optic fibers. Electroenceph clin Neurophysiol 1981;52:595-603.

Creel D, Witkop Jr CJ, King R. Asymmetric visually evoked potentials in human albinos: evidence for visual system anomalies. Invest Ophtalmol 1974;13:430-440.

Duke-Elder S. System of Ophthalmology . Vol 3. Normal and Abnormal Development: Part 2, Congenital Deformities. London: Henry Kimpton, 1964.

Fulton AB, Albert DM, Craft JL. Human albinism. Arch Ophthalmol 1978;96:305-310.

Maitland CG, Aminoff MJ, Kennard C, Hoyt WF. Evoked potentials in the evaluation of visual field defects due to chiasmal or retrochiasmal lesions. Neurology 1982;32:986-991.

Müller-Jensen A, Zschocke S, Dannheim F. VER analysis of the chiasmal syndrome. J Neurol 1981;225:33-40.

Murakami D, Sesma MA, Rowe MH. Characteristics of nasal and temporal retina in Siamese and normally pigmented cats: ganglion cell composition, axon trajectory and laterality of projection. Brain Behav Evol 1982;21:67-113.

Shatz CJ, Kliot M. Prenatal misrouting of the retinogeniculate pathway in Siamese cats. Nature 1982;300:525-529

Silver J. Studies on the factors that govern directionality of axonal growth in the embryonic optic nerve and at the chiasm of mice. J Comp Neurol 1984;223:238-251.

Silver J, Sapiro J. Axonal guidance during development of the optic nerve: the role of pigmented epithelia and other extrinsic factors. J Comp Neurol 1981;202:521-538.

Spekreijse H. Comparison of acuity tests and pattern evoked potential criteria: two mechanisms underly acuity maturation in man. Behav Brain Res 1983;10:107-117.

Spekreijse H. Maturation of contrast EPs and development of visual resolution. Arch Ital Biol 1978;116:358-369.

Stone J, Rowe MH, Campion JE. Retinal abnormalities in the Siamese cat. J Comp Neurol 1978;180:773-782.

Strongin AC and Guillery RW. The distribution of melanin in the developing optic cup and stalk and its relation to cellular degeneration. J Neuroscience 1981;1:1193-1204.

Taylor WOG. Visual disabilities of oculocutaneous albinism and their alleviation. Trans Ophthal Soc UK 1978;98:423-445.

de Vries-Khoe LH, Spekreijse H. Maturation of luminance and pattern EPs in man. Docum Ophthal Proc Series 1982;31:461-475.

Witkop Jr CJ, Jay B, Creel D, Guillery RW. Optic and otic neurologic abnormalities in oculocutaneous and ocular albinism. In: Cotlier E, Maumenee IH, Berman ER, eds. Birth Defects: Original Article Series 1982;18:299-318.

Wolf BM, Simon JW, Krohel GB, Kandel GL. VER correlates of visual pathway anomalies associated with ocular albinism in patients with congenital nystagmus. Invest Ophthalmol & Vis Sci Suppl 1984;25:177.

DISCUSSION

Vital-Durand: You conclude from your evoked response asymmetry that there
is an abnormal decussation in the chiasm. Was this amount of asymmetry the
same in all patients?

Apkarian: No, the degree of asymmetry varies across patients. Our VEP
measures do not reflect the degree of misrouting, only its presence or
absence. That is, the pattern of cortical asymmetry, as determined by
response topography, yields the diagnostic indicant.

Medhorn: Since the albinotic false projection should be considered a
biological process, I wonder whether the degree of false projection does
not follow a biological scatter. Therefore I think that at least in some
albinos the type of projection should be very close to normal and the VEP
should exhibit near normal symmetry or only slight asymmetry.

Apkarian: In the over 100 albinos referred to us with different phenotypic
expression, we were able to detect the presence of contralateral asymmetry
following full-field monocular stimulation. I don't know how one answers
your question more directly except by performing morphological studies on a
large sample of normal and albino human brains.

Hache: It is not our experience. The asymmetry of the albino is difficult
to explain because we don't know which line is sick. In a misdirected
pathway the best response is on the side where there is no complex, always.
But in other occipital disease the best response can be on the side of the
good complex.

Apkarian: I agree that there are many pathological or, for that matter,
normal conditions which can lead to hemispheric asymmetry in the visual
evoked response. However, when referring to albino asymmetry, we are
referring to a particular and rather specific VEP response patterning. We
are talking about the left eye response distribution compared to the right.
In albinos, with full-field monocular stimulation of an appearing/
disappearing checkerboard pattern, the peak of the potential distribution
across the scalp shifts from right hemisphere to left following left to
right eye stimulation, respectively. It is this 'switch' in cortical
representation that reflects the albino VEP signature. pattern appearance
stimulation.

Hache: The greatest response is on the opposite side.

Harcourt: You stated that this is a pathonomic sign. One group reported
asymmetry of a similar type in infantile esotropia. There are obviously
two possible explanations, that either these patients also have increased
crossing fibres, which might explain why they have no binocular vision, but
it could also be due to the nasal preference of the eye. If there is nasal
preference then you would expect there to be asymmetry in the uniocular
VER. Do you think that some part of asymmetry may not be due to abnormal

afferent fibres, but to abnormal fixation behaviour of the eye.

Apkarian: Are you referring to a recently published article on dissociated vertical deviation? The authors claim that they have found albino asymmetry. I have also tested a patient with dissociated vertical deviation under precisely the conditions of the test that they reported. I have to say that, at least in this one patient, I could not reproduce their results. Though more patients must be tested, my preliminary results strongly suggest that patients with DVD do not show electrophysiological evidence for albino misrouting. It may well be possible that this group of patients does show a VEP anomaly of some sort. However, for albinism they test negative, for the published article also does not provide evidence for albino misrouting. I began my lecture by saying that the electro-physiological pathognomonic in albinism is contralateral asymmetry following full-field monocular stimulation of an appearing/disappearing checkerboard pattern.

Lee: There are two populations within DVD, one of which shows the response and one of which doesn't. The nystagmus of which they speak is not manifest wobbly nystagmus as albinos have, but is latent nystagmus and should be damped with both eyes open. I take your point, the one you found might have been one of the negative ones.

Apkarian: Firstly, not all albinos manifest nystagmus. In those who do, the degree and type of nystagmus varies from pure jerk to pseudocycloid with corresponding velocities of as low as about 2 deg/sec to as high as 110 deg/sec. Secondly, in the paradigm of the authors who studied DVD patients, their results are based on monocular half-field pattern reversal stimulation. In our hands, we have found that reversal stimulation fares rather poorly with patients having nystagmus. We have also found it rather difficult to obtain reliable half-field results with nystagmus patients because of their fixation difficulties. And finally, even in those albino patients (typically with less severe nystagmus) from whom a reversal response can be obtained, the final asymmetry results are frequently inconsistent and difficult to interpret. For these reasons, among others, we base our electrophysiological misrouting diagnosis on the pattern onset (appearance) response.

Jay: How I can but agree with almost all that Apkarian has said. I don't think there is any doubt now that all albinos have a very strange anatomy of their visual pathways, and this is a very interesting fundamental question. What worries me is their saying that it is a pathognomonic sign, because that is putting the onus on the investigator to have examined every other condition under the sun. I suspect there will be other conditions found where the pathways are abnormal.

Apkarian: I would like to say that our albino VEP test is now routinely used in our Amsterdam clinic laboratory as an objective aid in differential diagnosis.

OBJECTIVE EVALUATION OF BINOCULAR COOPERATION IN NORMALS AND STRABISMICS
BY MEANS OF VISUAL EVOKED RESPONSES

Emilio C. Campos, M.D.

Department of Ophthalmology
University of Modena
Modena, Italy

INTRODUCTION

Early detection of children with strabismus could reduce the severity
of sequelae to this condition. However, evaluation of the presence or
absence of normal binocular cooperation can in pre-verbal children only be
inferred in the case of a cosmetically evident strabismus. Subjects at
risk (e.g. with easily decompensating heterophoria) or patients with
microstrabismus cannot be identified.

BINOCULAR SENSORY ANOMALIES IN STRABISMUS

At this point it appears important to outline the binocular sensory
anomalies of strabismus. In childhood, and particularly in congenital and
early onset strabismus, diplopia and confusion are readily eliminated.
The two main anti-diplopic mechanisms are suppression of the deviated eye
and anomalous retinal correspondence (ARC). The former is generally found
in large angle deviations, whereas the latter prevails in small-angle
strabismus (Bagolini, 1976). ARC supports and anomalous type of binocular
vision, which develops in spite of the deviation. It is defined as
anomalous binocular vision (a.b.v.) (Bagolini, 1976; Campos, 1982).
A.b.v. is not as sophisticated as normal binocular vision: rarely is it
associated with stereopsis. Moreover, a.b.v. is easily decompensating,
and finally it does not prevent the development of amblyopia of the
deviated eye, if the strabimus is non-alternating.

BINOCULAR VER IN NORMALS

Visual Evoked Responses (VER) can be used to objectively assess the
state of binocularity in non- cooperating subjects. In normals, a pattern
VER obtained with the two eyes open is significantly larger than the
monocular recordings (Fig. 1). This phenomenon has been defined as
summation (Campos, 1979; Apkarian et al, 1981 a, b). Other parameters
have been used as well to assess binocular cooperation with VER. Among
others facilitation has been considered (Apkarian et al, 1981 a, b).
However, this phenomenon, represented by a binocular signal larger than
the sum of the two monocular ones, presents some pitfalls. It is not
always readily elicitable in normals and requires more sophisticated
equipment for its detection than summation. That summation is indeed an
expression of binocular cortical integration is supported by its absence
in both spontaneous (Fig. 2) and artificially induced diplopia (Fig. 3).

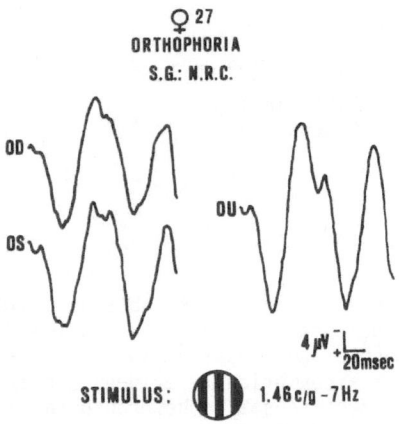

Fig 1. The binocular VER (OU) is larger than the two monocular ones (OD and OS) in normals. VER summation is present.

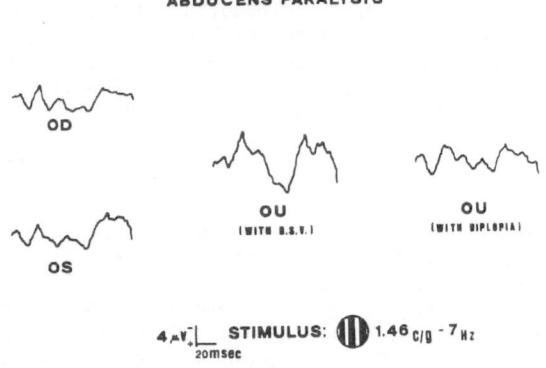

Fig 2. VER summation is absent in the position of diplopia in a case of post-traumatic abducens paralysis.

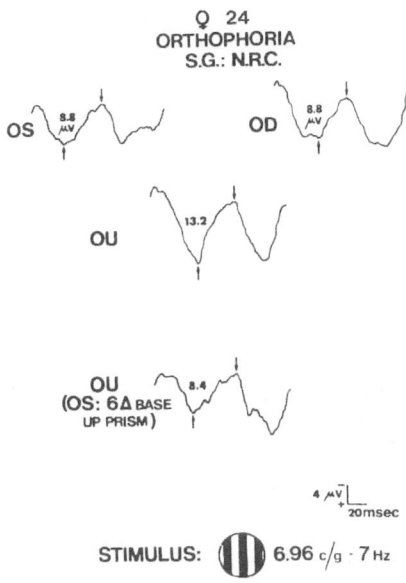

Fig 3. VER summation is absent when diplopia is artificially induced by means of vertically based prisms.

BINOCULAR VER IN STRABISMUS

In patients with strabismus, two situations are found, when binocular VER are recorded.

a. Summation is absent in the case of suppression of the deviated eye. This takes place both in large-angle and in small-angle deviations (Fig. 4).

b. Summation is present when ARC supporting anomalous binocular vision is found (Fig. 5) (Campos, 1979; Campos and Chiesi, 1983).

Therefore a differentiation between normals and strabismics on the basis of the presence or absence of summation is incorrect because summation is also found in those strabismics who exhibit ARC. It is also impossible to differentiate these two groups by judging the amount of summation found, as previously suggested (Amigo et al, 1978). In fact, there is a great variability both in normals and in strabimics regarding the entity of summation.

288

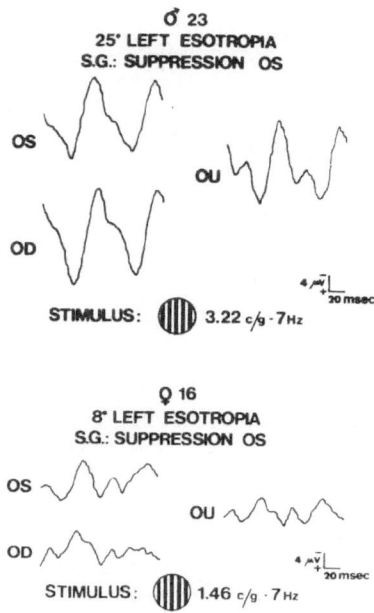

Fig 4. VER summation is absent in strabismus, when suppression of the deviated eye is found with striated glasses.

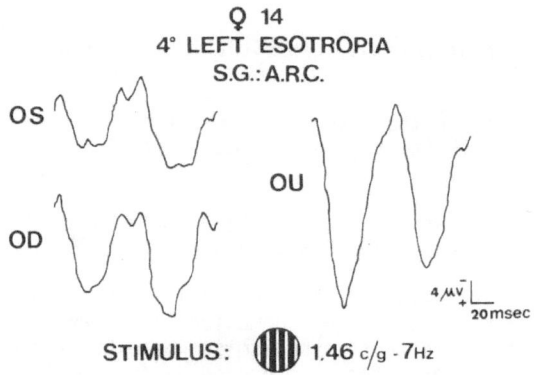

Fig 5. VER summation is present in strabismus, when anomalous retinal correspondence supporting anomalous binocular vision is found with striated glasses.

A simple method can, however, differentiate normals from strabismics when recording binocular VER. It is based on the anteposition of neutral density filters to the fixing eye. In strabismics with ARC, summation disappears as early as with a 0.4-0.5 log U filter. In normals, at least a 1.5-1.7 log U filter is necessary to interrupt summation. Interestingly, subjects with easily decompensating heterophoria behave as strabismics with ARC do (Campos and Chiesi, 1983). In summary, it is possible, by means of VER to differentiate normals from strabismics. It is also possible to detect subjects at risk, such as children with easily decompensating heterophoria.

PRACTICAL IMPLICATIONS

Recording of VER in pre-verbal children does not require either narcosis or sedation. The whole procedure lasts between 15 and 30 minutes.

From the practical viewpoint, it is advisable to associate the Irvine 4 prism diopters test to the recording of binocular VER in subjects with easily interruptable summation. The Irvine test informs on the presence of normal fusional vergences. If it is pathological in a subject with easily interruptable summation (with neutral density filters), one is dealing with a microstrabismus. If the Irvine test is normal, one can safely conclude that an easily decompensating heterophoria is present. In the first instance anti- amblyopic treatment started immediately is the only therapeutic measure. In the second case, i.e., heterophoria, cycloplegic refraction has to be performed at once. Then the baby has to be seen on a monthly basis until it is possible to establish whether one is dealing with an eso- or exophoria. In the first instance, when hyperopia has been found, glasses should be prescribed in order to possibly prevent the development of a manifest strabismus.

SUMMARY

Pattern Visual Evoked Responses (VER) can be used to objectively assess binocular cooperation. VER summation is an expression of binocular cortical integration. Summation is present in normals and in strabismics with anomalous binocular vision (ABV) supported by anomalous retinal correspondence (ARC). Summation is absent in patients with strabismus and suppression of the deviated eye. Normals and strabismics with ABV can be differentiated by recording VER with neutral density filters in front of the fixing eye: summation disappears with weaker filters in strabismics as compared to normals. Subjects with easily decompensating heterophoria behave as strabismics with ABV do. Therefore, VER allows an early detection of subjects at risk (easily decompensating heterophoria) and of patients with microstrabismus.

REFERENCES

Amigo G., Fiorentini A., Pirchio M., Spinelli D.: Binocular vision tested with evoked potentials in children and infants. Invest. Ophthalmol. Visual Sci. 1978; 17:910-915.

Apkarian P., Levi D., Tyler C.W.: Binocular Facilitation in the Visual Evoked Potential of Strabismics Amblyopes. Amer. J. Optom. & Physiol. Optics 1981; 58:820-830

Apkarian P., Nakayama K., Tyler C.W.: Binocularity in the Human Visual Evoked Potential: Facilitation, Summation and Suppression. Electroencephalogr. Clin. Neurophysiol. 1981; 51:32-48.

Bagolini B.: Part one. Sensorial anomalies in strabismus (Suppression, Anomalous Correspondence, Amblyopia). Doc. Ophthalmol. 1976; 41:1-22.

Campos E.C.: Visione binoculare anomala nell'esotropia concomitante: valutazione obiettiva con potenziali visivi evocati. Proc. Italian Ophthalmological Soc. 1979; 59:156-161

Campos E.C.: Anomalous Retinal Correspondence : Monocular and Binocular Visual Evoked Responses. Arch. Ophthalmol. 1980; 98:299-302.

Campos E.C.: Binocularity in comitant strabismus: Binocular Visual Field Studies. Doc. Ophthalmol. 1982; 53:249-281.

Campos E.C., Chiesi C.: Binocularity in comitant strabismus: II. Objective evaluation with visual evoked responses. Doc. Ophthalmol. 1983; 55:277-293.

DISCUSSION

Hyvarinen: Do you know if your patients have stereopsis?

Campos: If you test them with random dot stereograms, almost all of our patients with small angle strabismus don't show a positive result.

van Lith: You talk about summation and cortical integration. As long as you use the word summation then I am not quite sure what you mean. Then you say cortical integration. I have the same problem; I don't know whether it is a real cortical integration or that it is just an electrical summation. When you have an alternating strabismus with two eyes which have good vision, are you also seeing summation? If you measure each eye separately you have a good evoked potential pattern. When you do the two eyes then you have no addition, because the pattern in one eye is on the fovea and on the other eye outside the fovea. So that is my problem.

Campos: Let me try to answer this important question. Summation could be an expression of cortical integration. I deduce this from the the fact that in the presence of simultaneous perception, in a case diplopia both artifically induced and not artificially induced, you don't have the presence of summation. Summation is absent when stimulating an eccentric area only in the presence of suppression. In fact, independently from the amount of the deviation summation is absent in patients with suppression. If summation would be absent only in really large angles of deviation then I would agree with you that this is simply a problem of too eccentric presentation in the deviated eye. However, summation is absent also in small-angle strabismus where the presentation is not more eccentric, when there is suppression. On the contrary, there is summation in subjects in whom there is a constant strabismus with ARC. This should be proof that summation is an expression of cortical integration.

Verriest: We charted binocular visual fields with the Goldmann perimeter without any dissociation between the two eyes. We found that in all cases of strabismus there is binocularly more sensitivity than in monocular vision. We found also that the better eye is more sensitive in cases of strabismus than in the normal subject (that is, when we compare the fixating eye in strabismus with the dominant eye in a normal subject we obtain a better sensitivity in the case of strabismus). Did you find something similar from the amplitude of the evoked response?

Campos: I would like to mention that once you test the VEP, for technical reasons you are acting on information closely related to the posterior pole while you don't know what happens in the periphery. It means that something is happening in the periphery and it is impossible to collect it. I presented only qualitative measurements. I was not interested in quantitative judgement. I was interested simply in inhibition from the deviated eye acting on the fixing eye. We are interested in showing that there are differences between binocular and monocular situations.

Sireteanu: Did you use different sizes of the stimulus? Did your results vary with size?

Campos: The size of the stimulus on the screen was about 18°.

Lennerstrand: We have been looking at this and other types of visual evoked techniques for evaluating binocular vision. A correlation between stereoscopic acuity is better for binocular interaction than for summation may be a more useful tool. By the way, Did you try it on children?

Campos: Yes, with the same results. I don't have enough longitudinal data to be really sure of what is going to happen. I agree with you that summation may be a rough paradigm to look at. The problem with strabismus is that whenever you try to dissociate the two eyes in order to present them with different stimuli in order to see whether there is a co-operation, you are very readily provoking retinal rivalry which in strabismus ends up in suppression. Therefore it is a tricky situation.

Atkinson: I was going to elaborate on that and ask about the age groups. You said you did find binocular summation in newborns, normal newborns?

Campos: I am defining children who are aged more than 4 months, not newborn?

Van Lith: I will just give a warning because when you find absent summation when you stimulate both eyes it might be amblyopia, provided that other causes for an absence of response, like a tumour in the optic nerve, have been excluded.

Campos: Absolutely.

Harcourt: What do you think would be found using the method of binocular assessment described by Braddick and Atkinson?

Campos: The method that they propose does not inform on sensory fusion. The latter is the capability we have to perceive two images which are sufficiently equal and see only one. I am afraid that this technique elicits retinal rivalry because one eye had a red filter in front of it and the other one had a green filter.

Braddick: I call it stereopsis.

Campos: It is compatible with stereopsis. As far as sensory fusion is concerned it is certainly provoking retinal rivalry.

Braddick: I am not sure what that means.

Campos: With differences in colours between the two eyes, it means that you can integrate in order to achieve depth perception, but this situation is compatible with fusion.

Braddick: The difference in colour leads to rivalry in colour but there is an abundance of data that rivalry in colour can coexist with fusion of the spatial aspects, and given that fusion it can give rise to stereopsis. There is one contour perceived, and that contour is a joint contribution of the two eyes and can generate stereopsis.

Campos: I would like you to test this in a strabismic patient and you will see how labile the sensory state of the subject is, much more that a normal person. Therefore any type of situation which disturbs this may create more false pathological cases.

DARK ADAPTATION ASSESSMENT IN CHILDHOOD, ESPECIALLY EARLY
CHILDHOOD (REVIEW)

Guy Verriest

Department of Ophthalmology, Ghent University

INTRODUCTION

Recording a dark adaptation curve in children is generally assumed to be even more difficult than mapping the visual
field because the common procedure is not only long and tedious, but also because it requires a prolonged stay in
darkness which could frighten the subject, or send him to
sleep.

Moreover, most ophthalmologists consider that electroretinography is not only easier, but also more sensitive
than psycho-physical dark adaptation testing. They forget
that general anesthesia required for electroretinography in
children always includes a risk and that dark adaptation ability does not necessarily parallels ERG amplitude: e.g. it
often happens in beginning retinitis pigmentosa that dark
adaptation is still normal whereas the electrical action potential is already (seemingly) abolished. In such conditions, dark adaptation behaviour is important for diagnosis,
follow-up and rehabilitation. Moreover it cannot be missed
for the assesment of whatever kind of night blindness.

METHODS REQUIRING ACTIVE COOPERATION FROM THE SUBJECT

Conventional full assessment of the dark adaptation curve during 15-30 min, as done in adults by means of an adaptometer such as the Goldmann-Weekers apparatus, is possible
from the age of 5 or 6 years on, and even from the age of 4
years on in very cooperative children; however the examiner
has to speak continuously with them as well during light
preadaptation as during subsequent dark adaptation.

Young (1981) obtained in two five-year-old children
full 36 min dark adaptation curves for small peripheral targets in Maxwellian view : however, while the adult controls
self-adjusted a neutral density wedge until the target was
seen about half the time, child subjects "clicked" a party
noise maker in one hand when they saw the target or "squee-
ked" another noise maker in the other hand when all they saw
was darkness, the wedge being adjusted by the experimenter
until the child responded equally with both hands.

Hyvärinen and Lindstedt (1981) recommend the application
of Thornton's (1977) method in children for assessing cone
adaptation : the child is taught to sort pieces of white,

red and blue papers in piles, whereafter the procedure is repeated in reduced light. The colours of the red and blue papers being chosen as to have the same lightness in scotopic
vision, the child will confuse the red and blue papers in reduced light if cone adaptation is defective.

METHODS BASED ON PREFERENTIAL LOOKING BEHAVIOUR

Assessment of dark adaptation is one of the different
possible applications of the methods of visual function assessment in children and in (even premature) infants by the
observation of preferential looking behaviour (as in general
patterned, moving or blinking targets are preferred to unpatterned, static not changing ones). Teller's (1979) more
refined forced-choice preferential looking technique has to
be preferred. It requires an adult observer who has to state, on each trial, in which of two possible positions a stimulus is presented, this judgment being based only on his observation of the infant's eye and head movements. The observer can simultaneously hold the infant if he is provided with
a view of the infant's face, e.g. by means of a periscope
(Regal 1981 : fig. 1) or of an infrared video system (Powers,
Schneck & Teller 1981). The observer's percent correct
responses are plotted for e.g. several target luminances to
yield a psychometric function from which the infant's thresholds are inferred. The luminance of the target needed for
the adult observer to be correct on 75% or 70% of the trials

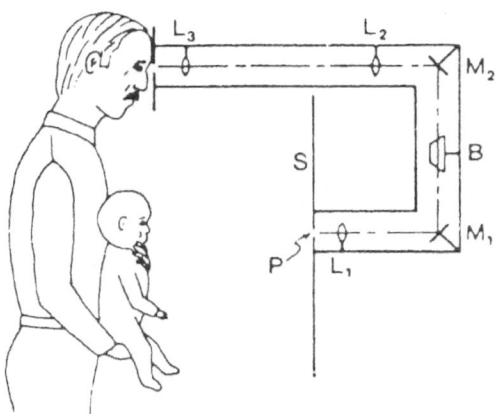

Fig. 1. — Forced-choice preferential looking technique: periscope allowing the adult
observer to observe and to hold the infant (From Regal, 1981).

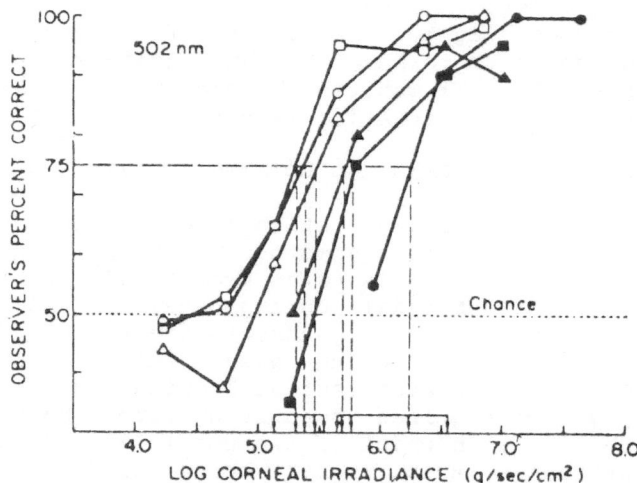

Fig. 2. — Absolute visual threshold psychometric functions for three 3-month olds (open symbols) and for three 1-month olds (filled symbols). Each threshold (75 % correct by adult observer) is indicated by an arrow on the abscissa. (From Powers, Schneck and Teller, 1981).

is taken as the estimate of the infant's threshold : figure 2. Several speakers have shown during this workshop that statistical assessment by means of a psychometric fonction can be replaced by a much more rapid staircase method. In every case the separation between the detector (the infant) and the decision maker (the adult observer) yields some information loss and so somewhat increased threshold values (Powers, Schneck and Teller 1981).

Preferential looking techniques have to be modified for children aged more than one year because of their greater mobility and the increasing gaze unsteadiness : the child is then asked to touch the chosen stimulus, and he has now to be rewarded (Gwiazda, Birch & Held 1981).

Contrarily to the visual acuity studies, in which a patterned field is offered with a blank field, in dark adaptation studies a single (preferably patterned) field is projected on either the left or the right side of the screen. Powers, Schneck and Teller (1981) noted that, if the infant is alert, judgements tooks only 1-5 sec to make, perhaps because there is nothing but the stimulus within the infant's view.

Clinical tests on dark adaptation in infants based on preferential looking behaviour were described long before Teller's papers for studies on avitaminosis. The method of Friderichsen and Edmund (1937) consisted of keeping the infant in a perfectly dark room. The infant is held by an assistant so that his face is free. The person performing

the test places himself in front of the child, finding the
child's face and forehead with his hand and holding a lamp at
a distance of 10 cm from it. The lamp emits flashes from various positions. Moreover the intensity of the light is increased by steps of .25 log units by removing Tscherning pho-
tometric glasses placed in front of the lamp. The lowest intensity of light causing certain mimic reflexes, oculomotor
refixation, head turning after the light or light catching is
considered as the threshold, or, more properly, as the "minimum reflexible". These authors added that the most reliable
results are obtained with children from 6 weeks to 6 months
of age if the greatest importance is attached to mimic reactions or to saccadic eye movements, and that the experimenter must try to obviate the sources or error implied by the
child's sleep or drowsiness (all the more he is able to go on
sleeping with his eyes wide open). They add also that, in
order that the experimenter may be able to perceive the
child's face at threshold illumination, he must be maximally
adapted to darkness.

This is in fact the weak point of Edmund's procedure.
Indeed Lewis and Haig (1939) stated that the threshold intensity could not be determined because at low illuminance levels the experimenter was unable to observe whether the baby
was responding to the light. Accordingly they improved the
method by fastening a vial containing a fluorescent radium
paint on the forehead of the baby. After 30 min dark adaptation a light was moved from side to side through an arc of
180° at about 10 cm in front of the baby's eyes and the lowest intensity of the light already eliciting a rolling of
the head in the direction of the light was considered as the
threshold. This characteristic response has to be distinguished from random movements. It is difficult to carry out
the test if babies cry or are restless.

Such reflexive jerking of the head in response to light
was also used by Peiper (1926) and by Trincker and Trincker
(1955) to demonstrate the Purkinje phenomenon in infants,
but, strangely enough, we found in the literature no recent
reference at all of clinical applications of the preferential
looking technique in adaptometry. Only Taylor (1978) recommended a very crude test used by neurologists : the infant
(in an alert but restful state) is held supine parallel to
a diffuse source of light such as a window or an X-ray box; after
a few seconds a normal infant turns his head toward the light,
and, when he is then turned 180°, he will turn his head back
toward the light.

OTHER OBJECTIVE ADAPTOMETRIC METHODS

"Objective" determination of the dark adaptation curve
by means of the observation of the appearance of an optokinetic reaction while increasing the luminance of a moving
stimulus was first described by Rieken (1941a). The detection of the optokinetic reaction can be done either by observing the illuminated fellow eye (Rieken, 1941a), or by

placing on the non tested or on the tested eye a contact lens provided with luminescent dots (Rieken, 1941b), or by electro-nystagmography (Jonkers, 1947). A same apparatus was simul-taneously used for such an objective adaptometry and for sub-jective psycho-physical adaptometry by Verriest and Haznedaroglu (1969) in normal subjects and by François, Verriest, Haznedaroglu and Van de Casteele (1972) in subjects suffering from eye diseases : fig. 3

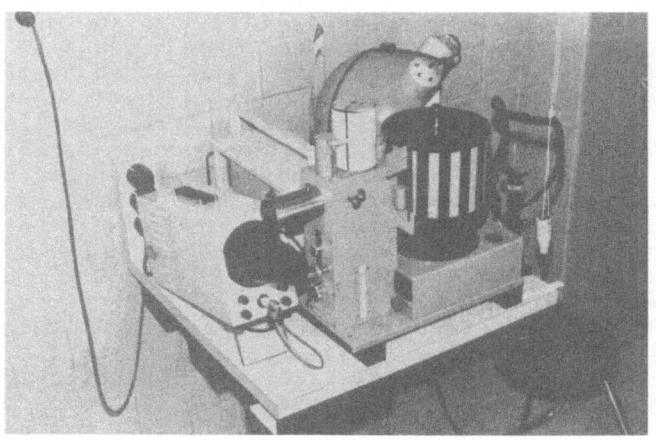

Fig. 3. — Combination of the Goldmann-Weekers adaptometer and optokinetic drum with electronystagmography. With such an apparatus dark adaptation can be measured in an objective way in younger children, and simultaneously in a psychophysical way and in the objective way in older subjects. (From Verriest and Haznedaroglu, 1969).

Rieken's method requires only one measurement for each threshold and is thus more suited than the preferential looking technique for the determination of a dark adaptation curve im-plying a continuous threshold change. The cone plateau can be assessed.

A drawback of Rieken's method is that the objective threshold is some tenths of a log unit higher than the sub-jective one, all the more the eyes are moving in darkness and as the typical opto-kinetic nystagmus is preceeded by less typical reactions (Ohm 1953, Jonkers 1947, Verriest & Haznedaroglu 1969) : fig. 4. The "objective" dark adapta-tion curve has to be determined on these first, less typical motor reactions (Verriest and Haznedaroglu 1969).

As optokinetic nystagmus is reliably present since full-term or somewhat premature birth (Forman, Cogan & Gillis 1957), Rieken's method can be used for studying dark adaptation in children (Ohm 1956). Verriest and Haznedaroglu (1969) assessed in this way dark adaptation in normals from the age of 3 years, while François, Verriest, Haznedaroglu & Van de Casteele (1972) obtained by means of the objective method results in pathologi-cal eyes of children aged from 3 to 5 years in whom the conven-tional subjective method was of no use.

It is evident that the electro-retinographic methods for assessing dark adaptation can be applied to children as well as to adults.

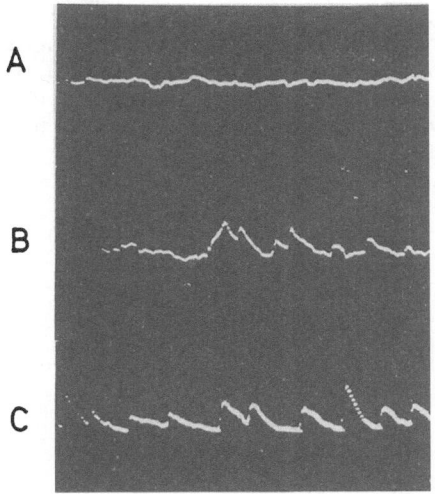

Fig. 4. — Tracing on the oscilloscope (A) when the optokinetic stimulation is sublim-
inar (B) at the first optokinetic reactions (C) when full optokinetic nystagmus is developped.
(From Verriest and Haznedaroglu, 1969).

In this connection we must cite the papers of Dobson,
Riggs & Siqueland (1974) and of Dobson, Cowett & Riggs (1975).
In order to assess the dark adaptation function of 4-year-old
children, they light-adapted one eye for 1 min (field covering 66°, retinal illuminance of 5.9 log scotopic Td). Following this bleach, the assistant who was holding the child
directed its gaze into a Ganzfeld. The light entering the
Ganzfeld was blue (thus stimulating preferentially rods over
cones) and was intercepted by a sectored disc which rotated
to produce four 100 msec flashes per second during 4 sec
every 1 to 2 minutes. The stimulus luminances necessary to
maintain a constant amplitude median response across time
were plotted as function of time in the dark and were fitted
by Alpern's function describing typical adult dark adaptation
data.
      Let us mention only to be complete objective dark adap-
tation assesment based on measurement of visual pigment concentration, pupil surface or amplitude of visual evoked
response.

DEVELOPMENTAL DARK ADAPTATION CHANGES

      Many of the authors who studied the relationship between
age and a given peripheral mean threshold after long dark
adaptation stated that such a threshold is higher in younger
children or in teenagers than in young adult age.

Concerning infants, Powers, Schneck & Teller (1981) used a forced-choice preferential looking technique and showed that 3-months olds were about 1 log unit less sensitive throughout the spectrum than adults, and that 1-month olds were about .7 log unit less sensitive than 3-month olds (in the 3 groups spectral sensitivity was scotopic) : fig. 5.

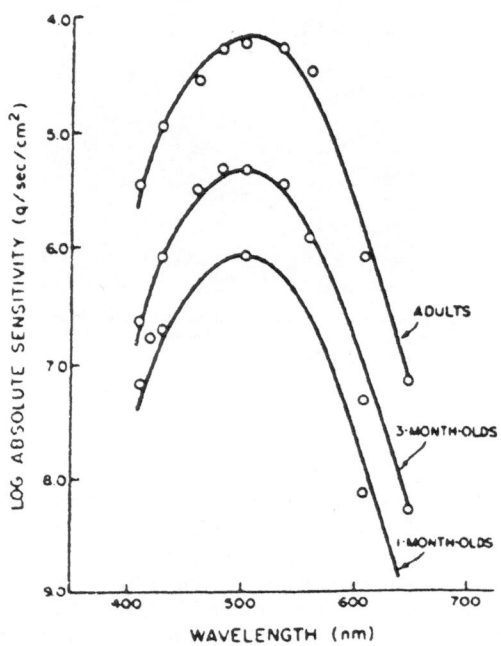

Fig. 5 . — Average spectral sensitivity on an ordinate of absolute intensity at the cornea. Solid curves: CIE standard sensitivity function for scotopic vision in adults. (From Powers, Schneck and Teller, 1981).

Concerning the dark adaptation curve, Verriest & Haznedaroglu (1969) observed that adaptation speed is slower in (3 to 12 years old) children than in adults in the photopic segment (thus before the Kohlrausch kink) but not in the scoropic segment (thus after the kink) : fig. 6. We have no data concerning infants.

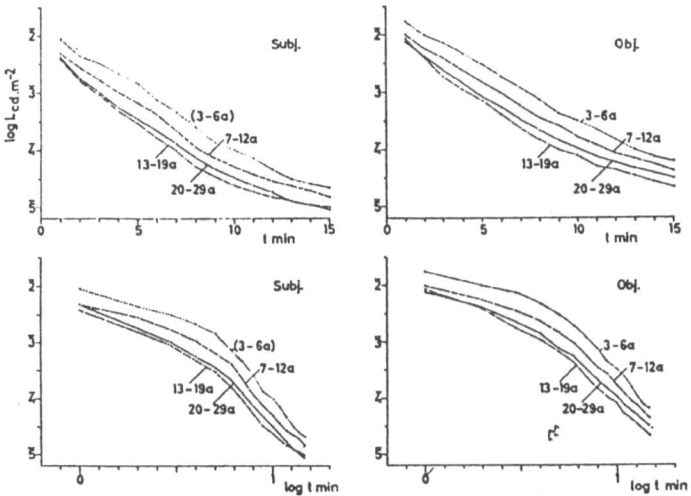

physically (left) and objectively on basis of optokinetic reactions (right). The time scale is either natural (above) or logarithmic (below). The brackets for the youngest age group (3-6-yr olds) mean that the psychophysical data have been extrapolated from the objective ones. (From Verriest and Haznedaroglu, 1969).

REFERENCES

Dobson V, Cowett RM, Riggs LA. Long-term effect of phototherapy on visual function. J Pediatrics 1975; 86 : 555-559.

Dobson V, Riggs LA, Siqueland ER. Electroretinographic determination of dark adaptation functions of children exposed to phototherapy as infants. J Pediatrics 1974; 85 : 25-29.

François J, Verriest G, Haznedaroglu G, Van de Casteele J. Application à la pathologie oculaire de la mesure subjective et objective de l'adaptation à l'obscurité à l'aide d'un même appareillage. Ann Oculist (Paris) 1972; 205 : 787-812.

Friderichsen C, Edmund C. Studies of hypovitaminosis A, II. A new method for testing the resorption of vitamin A from medicaments. Am J Dis Children 1937 ; 53 : 89-109.

Gorman JJ, Cogan DG, Felus SS. An apparatus for grading the visual acuity of infants on the basis of OKN. Peadiatrics 1957; 19 : 1008.

Gwiazda JE, Birch EE, Held R. Le développement de la vision chez l'enfant. La Recherche 1981 ; 12 : 1348-1353.

Hyvärinen L, Lindstedt E. Assessment of vision in children. Stockholm : SRF Tal & Punkt, 1981.

Jonkers GH. On objective adaptometry. Ophthalmologica 1947; 114, 397-408.

302

Lewis JM, Haig C. Vitamin requirements in infancy as determined by dark adaptation. J Pediatrics 1939; 15 : 812-823.

Ohm J. Objective Prüfung der Sehleistungen mit Hilfe der optokinetischen Augenbewegungen. Stuttgart : Ferdinand Enke, 1953.

Ohm J. Optokinetische und optostatische Reaktionen bei Kindern. Klin Mbl Augenheilk 1956; 129 : 255-258.

Peiper A. Über die Helligkeits- und Farbenempfindungen der Frühgeburten. Arch Kinderheilk 1926; 80 : 1-20.

Powers MK, Scheck M, Teller DY. Spectral sensitivity of human infants at absolute visual threshold. Vision Res 1981; 21 : 1005-1016.

Regal DM. Development of critical flicker frequency in human infants. Vision Res 1981; 21 : 549-555.

Rieken H. Objektive Adaptometrie. Klin Mbl. Augenheilk 1941a; 107 : 1-11.

Rieken H. Zur Methodik der objektiven Adaptometrie. Klin Mbl Augenheilk 1941b; 107 : 306-316.

Taylor D. The assessment of visual function in young children : An overview. Clinical Pediatrics. 1978; 17 : 226-323.

Teller D. The forced-choice preferential looking procedure. A psychophysical technique for use with human infants. Infant Behav Devel 1979; 2 : 135-153.

Thornton SP. A rapid test for dark adaptation. Ann Ophthalmol 1977; 9 : 731-734.

Trincker D, Trincker I. Die ontogenetische Entwicklung des Helligkeits- und Farbensehens beim Menschen. I. Die Entwicklung des Helligkeitssehens. v Graefes Arch Ophthalmol 1955; 156 : 519-534.

Verriest G, Haznedaroglu G. Mesure subjective et objective de l'adaptation à l'obscurité à l'aide du même appareillage et application de celui-ci à l'étude comparative de l'adaptation depuis l'enfance jusqu'à l'âge adulte. Vision Res 1969; 9 : 769-783.

Young DC. Dark adaptation in five-year-old children and adults. Vision Res 1981; 21 : 811-814.

DISCUSSION

Vital-Durand. How do you quantify the beginning of optokinetic nystagmus response? In the previous slide you said that the line in the middle is what you called atypical OKN.

Verriest: Already in darkness there is some unsteadiness of looking. Moreover, when one augments progressively the luminance of the target, the first optokinetic reactions are weak and irregular.

Vital-Durand: They are not there.

Verriest: They are there but they are not as beautiful as here. There you have to watch that you record when there are only a few responses.

Spekreijse: Then you are near the threshold sometimes. You perceive and mark it sometimes and sometimes you miss it.

Vital-Durand: Then you have to compute the gain so that you can quantify the eye position relative to stimulus displacement. What is actually the gain that you observed?

Verriest: We lose about .2 log units of sensitivity.

Vital-Durand: What I meant is that the slow components of the nystagmus can be added together and related to the amount of displacement of the target. The percentage of these two values is the gain of the response.

Verriest: Everything you do with the first reactions, the threshold you obtain by objective means, is somewhat higher than by subjective means.

Spekreijse: You use this as an indication that the subject has seen for the first time the pattern.

Verriest: Yes.

Spekreijse: But I am not convinced by what I saw in the different curves in the last slide. I think if you bring them together they are different in variability.

Verriest: You see the slope of the curve, and we found a statistical difference. Measurements were made on many cases.

Spekreisje: What do you think is the mechanism?

Verriest: I have no explanation.

De Laey: From a clinical point of view usually we are interested in the
answers. Isn't is more easy to wait for 15 minutes resting in the dark?

Verriest: Yes, and this you can do.

De Laey: You therefore look at the slope and you make a whole dark
adaptation curve and you look at the end result after 30 minutes.

Verriest: However, you can be interested in the dark adaptation curve
itself, eg, because there are some diseases in which the dark adaptation is
slow.

De Laey: But perhaps this method of first plateau is not always even a
satisfactory method in adults.

Verriest: The distinctness of the first plateau depends much on the method
that is used for recording the dark adaptation curve. When one uses a
strong preadaptation, or a more central field, one sees better the first
plateau. The method we use in Ghent is an integral one on the whole visual
field and it is not advantageous for seeing the cone plateau. I would like
to add that with the preferential looking technique one has to make several
measurements in order to have a single result; such a technique is more
difficult to apply to a changing condition like dark adaptation.
Optokinetic nystagmus is better for following dark adaptation.

VISUAL FIELD MEASUREMENTS, OPTOKINETIC NYSTAGMUS AND THE VISUAL THREATENING RESPONSE: NORMAL AND ABNORMAL DEVELOPMENT

Jackie van Hof-van Duin and Gesine Mohn

Department of Physiology I, Erasmus Universiteit Rotterdam
P.O.Box 1738, 3000 DR Rotterdam, The Netherlands

INTRODUCTION

Experimental studies in animals have shown that visual deprivation early during development may lead to electrophysiological and anatomical neuronal changes accompanied by permanent defects of several behavioral visual functions which include asymmetrical monocular optokinetic nystagmus (OKN), absence of the visual component of the threatening response, and visual field defects.
Neuronal changes have been described to be irreversible only if visual deprivation occurs during a circumscribed period of susceptibility to abnormal visual influences (Hubel and Wiesel, 1970). In humans, the existence of such a sensitive period for visual input restriction is generally accepted, but its time course is (still) unknown. Assuming that neuronal pathways retain their plasticity, i.e. remain sensitive to changing input until maturation is completed, a possible approach to obtain some insight into the time relation of the human sensitive period is a comparison of the development of several visual functions in normal human infants and in infants which are at risk of neurological abnormalities, since is known that neurological disorders in children are often accompanied or complicated by the presence of visual defects.
In the present study, results of behavioral measures of visual functions in children with neurological disorders will be discussed. Because of the high incidence of abnormal OKN, absence of the visual threatening response and visual field defects in these patients, we also studied the development of these functions in normal fullterm and in prematurely born infants with low or high risks of later neurological abnormalities.

SUBJECTS

Two groups of patients with neurological disorders accompanied by visual impairments were examined. The first group of patients (n=67), aged 1.5 month to 19 years, were permanently hospitalized with severe mental and multiple handicaps. The second group of patients (n=69), aged 2 weeks to 23 years were usually not hospitalized, visually impaired children with varying neurological disorders (congenital disorders n=41 (59%); acquired disorders n=28 (41%)). Psychomotor development ranged from normal , via children with slight retardation to severely mentally handicapped patients.

The development of visual functions was studied in 79 healthy, fullterm infants born at term (40 plus or minus 2 weeks of gestation) aged 4–65 weeks at the time of testing. The results were compared to those of 125 infants born 4–14 weeks prematurely, whose postnatal age ranged from 3–75 weeks (corrected age ranging from minus 4 to 65 weeks). For each infant, complications during the early postnatal period were assessed by means of a 10-items score based on respiratory, circulatory and alimentary problems, bilirubine levels, phototherapy, convulsions and ultrasound scans. Of the 125 preterms tested, 46 were considered at low risk for abnormalities on the basis of this score and normal early postnatal development. The other 79 were considered at high risk for abnormalities according to one or more of the following criteria: an Apgar score of < 6 after 5 minutes; complications of the postnatal development by more than 7 days mechanical ventilation or phototherapy; surgery for open ductus arteriosus and/or necrotizing enterocolitis; convulsions; persistent abnormal ultrasound scans in infants with a birthweight of < 2000 g. This high risk group was divided into neurologically normal (n=44) or neurologically abnormal (n=37) infants on the basis of initial and later neurological examinations.

METHODS

In all infants and patients, ocular motility was examined, the presence or absence of strabismic deviations and of spontaneous (binocular) and/or latent (monocular) nystagmus was noted, direct and indirect pupillary reflexes were tested, and the presence of eye contact, fixation and following eye movements to a light or object were examined.
Optokinetic nystagmus (OKN), which is the oculomotor response to movement of a large, patterned stimulus, was tested in hospitalised infants/patients by observing binocular and monocular eye movements in response to movements of a large piece of paper covered with randomly spaced dots (1 square cm), which was moved to the right and to the left at a distance of about 25 cm in front of the child's eyes. If the clinical condition of the patient allowed it, horizontal OKN was recorded electro-oculographically. In this case, OKN was stimulated by seating the child in the centre of a rotating drum (diameter 150 cm, height 120 cm) the walls of which again consisted of paper covered with random dots. OKN was tested binocularly and monocularly with both clockwise (CW) and counterclockwise (CCW) stimulus movement.

The visual threatening response was tested by observing whether closure of the eyelids was seen to a rapidly approaching object, while the infant was seated behind a piece of plexiglass which prevented tactile stimulation. Testing without plexiglass showed whether the tactile and motor (subcortical) components of this response were present.

Binocular and monocular visual fields were measured using 4cm diameter STYCAR white balls mounted on black sticks, and presented against a uniform background. While the child fixated a centrally presented ball, a second target was slowly moved from the periphery towards the fixation point. Eye or head movements towards the peripheral ball were taken to indicate the borders of the visual field. During our later examinations this method was quantified by using an arc perimeter consisting of two 4cm wide black metal strips mounted perpendicular to one another, each with a radius of 40cm. The infants' reactions were assessed by a concealed observer who was unaware of the location of the peripheral target. In patients, both horizontal and vertical dimensions of the visual field were usually measured; in infants, measurements were usually restricted to the horizontal visual field.

RESULTS

Results obtained in the two groups of patients are shown in Table I.

TABLE I
ASSESSMENT OF VISUAL FUNCTIONS IN VISUALLY IMPAIRED

MULTIPLY HANDICAPPED CHILDREN
N=67, AGED 1.5 MONTH-19 YEARS

FUNCTIONAL LEVEL	(n)	OBSERVED RESPONSES	NEGATIVE REFLEXES	POS.PUPILLARY REFLEXES	POS.OKN	POS.FOLLOWING	POS.VISUAL THREAT	RESTRICTED VISUAL FIELD	NORMAL VISUAL FIELD
NEGATIVE REFLEXES	(3)		3						
POS.PUPILLARY REFLEXES	(5)	—		5					
POS.OKN	(7)	—		7	7				
POS.FOLLOWING RESPONSES	(12)	—		12	7	12			
RESTRICTED VISUAL FIELD (POS.FIXATION)	(31)	—		31	31	31	20	31	—
NORMAL VISUAL FIELD (POS.FIXATION)	(9)	—		9	9	9	9	—	9
TOTAL	(67)		3	64	54	52	29	31	9

NEUROPEDIATRIC PATIENTS
N=69, AGED 2 WEEKS-23 YEARS

FUNCTIONAL LEVEL	(n)	OBSERVED RESPONSES	NEGATIVE REFLEXES	POS.PUPILLARY REFLEXES	POS.OKN	POS.FOLLOWING	POS.VISUAL THREAT	RESTRICTED VISUAL FIELD	NORMAL VISUAL FIELD
NEGATIVE REFLEXES	(0)	—							
POS.PUPILLARY REFLEXES	(2)	—		2					
POS.OKN	(7)	—		7	7				
POS.FOLLOWING RESPONSES	(12)	—		12	8	12	4		
RESTRICTED VISUAL FIELD (POS.FIXATION)	(39)	—		39	39	39	32	39	—
NORMAL VISUAL FIELD (POS.FIXATION)	(9)	—		9	9	9	9	—	9
TOTAL	(69)			69	61	60	45	39	9

A distinction was made between a number of different levels of visual functioning. The lowest of these was the absence of pupillary reflexes, which was encountered in respectively 3 and no patients in the two groups. Positive pupillary reflexes in the absence of any other positive visual response were found in 7.5% and 3%. in the two groups. Ten percent of the patients showed positive OKN besides pupillary reflexes, but no other sign of behavioural visual function.

The next level of visual functioning consisted of positive following responses to light which were found in 12 patients in each group. When the succeeding level, of positive and steady fixation was attained (in resp. 60% and 70% in the two groups), the visual threat was also usually found to be positive, and visual field size could be measured (43% / 65%). A normal extension of the visual field was present in only 13%, whereas restricted visual fields were measured in 60% and 57% of the patients, confirming earlier results (van Hof-van Duin and Mohn 1983).

Spontaneous and/or latent nystagmus was seen in 81% and of the patients, and interfered with OKN assessment in 7% of all patients. Binocular OKN in patients with positive visual functions was symmetrical in only 16%, asymmetrical in 67%, and could not be elicited in 10%. Monocular OKN was nearly always asymmetrical, with a superiority of the temporal-to-nasal (TN) component in patients with symmetrical binocular OKN, whereas in cases with asymmetrical binocular OKN, the same direction preference was usually seen in monocular OKN.

The development of monocular OKN in 106 healthy fullterm and 51 low risk preterm infant is shown in Fig 1.(left side). Normal fullterm infants show a strong asymmetry in monocular OKN, with a preference for temporal-to-nasal stimulation during the first 3 months after birth.

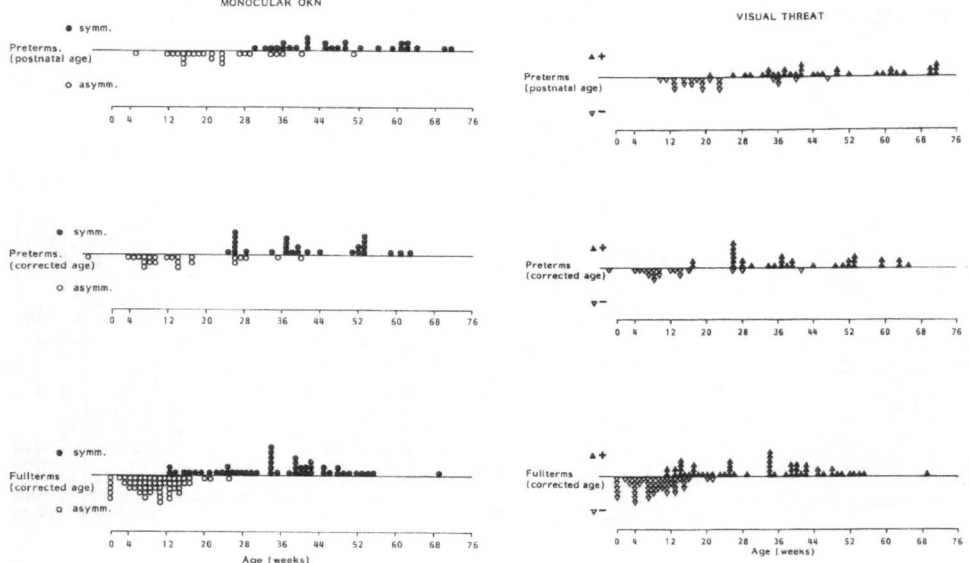

Fig.1: Development of monocular optokinetic nystagmus (mon OKN)(Fig.1a) and of the visual threat response (Fig.1b) in low risk preterm and fullterm infants. Results of preterms are plotted in terms of postnatal age (top row) and corrected age (middle row).

* In this and other Figs results of preterms plotted in terms of corrected age data seem to be grouped at 12 and 26 weeks, due to the fact that infants were always tested during outdoor clinical control sessions, which were held at comparable ages.

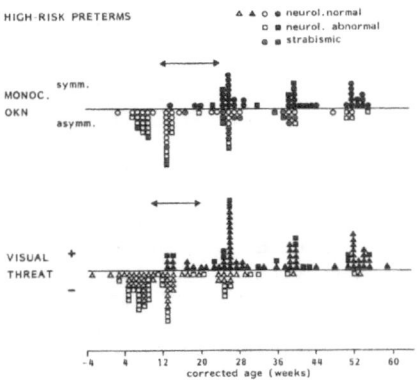

HIGH-RISK PRETERMS

Fig.2: Development of mon OKN and of visual threat response in high risk preterm infants

Symmetrical monocular OKN was first observed from 3 months onward; at 20 weeks of age, nearly all normal fullterms showed symmetrical OKN. When the results of the preterm infants are plotted in terms of postnatal age (Fig.1a, top row), the transition from asymmetrical to symmetrical OKN occurred later and over a longer period than in fullterm infants. When, on the other hand, ages were corrected for prematurity (Fig.1a, middle row) ,most infants showed symmetrical OKN at 26 weeks. High risk preterms, and particularly infants with a manifest strabismus, were often found to have no or a very late transition from asymmetrical to symmetrical OKN (Fig.2).

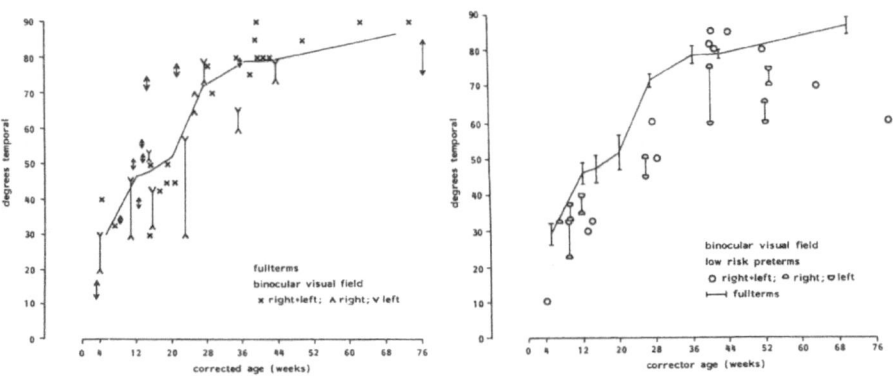

Fig.3: Binocular visual field measurements obtained in normal fullterm infants (left) and in low risk preterm infants (right).

310

The visual component of the threat response first appears around 12 weeks
in normal fullterm infants (Fig.lb, bottom row), whereas the tactile and
motor components of this reflex are present shortly after birth.   Preterm
infants showed the same maturation of this response when corrected age was
used (Fig.lb, middle row), while when age was calculated from birth, the
onset of the visual threat response appears to be later and more gradual
(Fig.lb, top row). In preterm infants at risk of abnormal development, the
appearance of the visual threat response was frequently observed at much
later ages or not at all (Fig.2).
Measurements of the horizontal visual field indicated a gradual increase of
the binocular visual field of normal fullterm (Fig.3, left side) and low
risk preterm infants (Fig.3, right side), starting at about 30 degrees on
both sides at 4 weeks of (corrected) age, and reaching near-adult size at
9-12 months. In preterm infants with a high risk of abnormalities (Fig.4),
smaller fields were often measured, with a slower, more gradual progression
than in either fullterms or low risk preterms. The neurologically abnormal
high risk preterms showed the smallest visual field sizes.

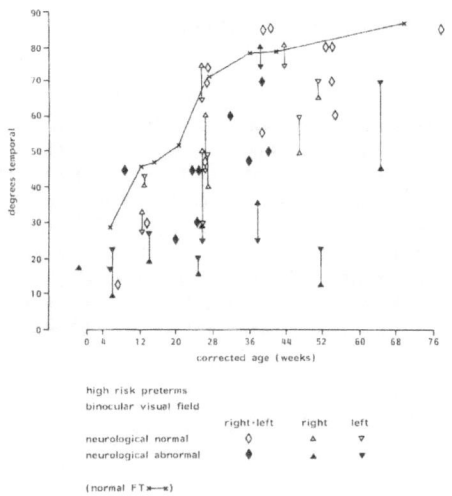

Fig 4 Binocular visual field measurements obtained
in high risk preterm infants.

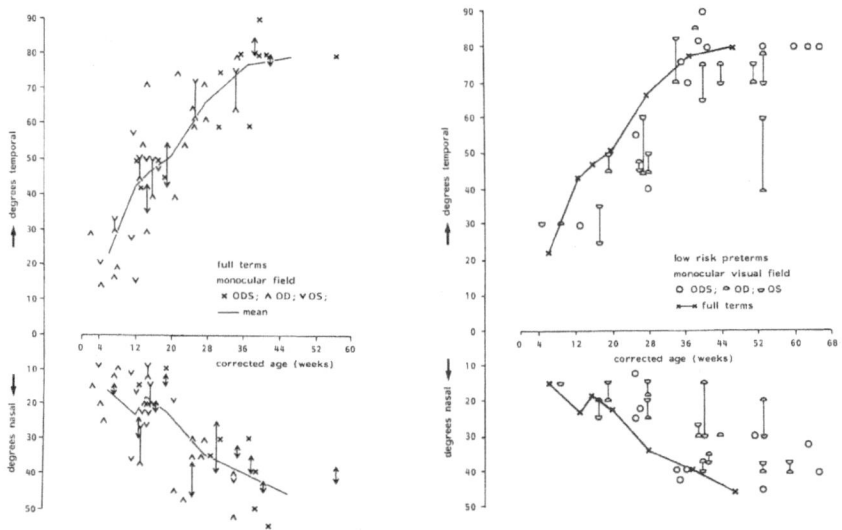

Fig.5: **Monocular visual field measurements obtained in normal fullterm infants (left) and in low risk preterms (right).**

As shown in Fig.5 (left side), the monocular temporal visual field of fullterm infants follows the same progression as is seen in binocular testing. By contrast, the nasal visual field seems to be limited to 15—20 degrees up to an age of 20 weeks, after which there is a gradual increase until values of around 45 degrees are reached between 9 to 12 months. Low risk preterm infants, if plotted according to corrected age (Fig.5, right side), show a similar development of both the temporal and the nasal field. High risk preterm infants and particularly those with neurological abnormalities, often showed lower values than low risk preterms of comparable age (Fig.6).

312

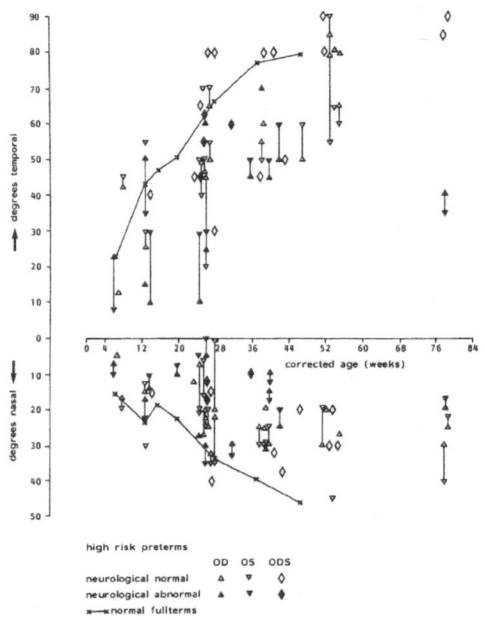

Fig.6: Monocular visual field measurements obtained in high risk preterms.

DISCUSSION

The incidence of visual impairments we observed in the two groups of
multiply handicapped children and neuropediatric patients was very high and
similar for the two groups. The severity of the impairments spanned a wide
range of functional levels, from the absence of pupillary reflexes to
measurable, though often abnormal, acuity, visual field size, etc. When
consistent fixation was present, the visual threat response was usually
also positive, and visual fields could be assessed, which, however, showed
defects in 60% of the patients. Abnormal OKN was found very frequently and
most often consisted of asymmetrical binocular OKN, which tended to also
determine the asymmetry seen in monocular OKN.
In normal fullterm infants, binocular OKN has been found to be present from
birth (Gorman 1957; Dayton et al 1964). The presence of directionally
symmetrical monocular OKN appears to depend on cortical processing of
visual information (van Hof-van Duin 1978; Atkinson 1979). In agreement
with earlier studies (Atkinson 1979; Naegele and Held 1982), symmetrical
monocular OKN was observed in normal fullterm infants from 3 months
onwards. When the postnatal age of preterm infants is used, the transition
from asymmetrical to symmetrical OKN occurs much later, but when age is
corrected for prematurity, the results overlap more closely with those of
the fullterms.
Similar results were found concerning the maturation of the visual

component of the threat response. In normal fullterm infants, this reflex appears after 10 weeks of age, confirming the findings of White (1971), and Peterson et al (1980) normal preterm infants showed the same maturation of the response only when assessed according to corrected age.

The binocular visual field of fullterm infants was found to increase gradually from birth (Fig.3), confirming and extending earlier studies (Tronick 1972; MacFarlane et al 1976; Lewis et al 1979). An adult-size of the visual field was reached by one year of age. A similar development was also found in low risk preterms of comparable corrected age, both for the binocular and the temporal monocular visual field. The nasal visual field seems to show a period of very little development up to 20 weeks of (corrected) age, and to only increase after this age.

These results on the development of monocular OKN, the visual threat response and the visual fields in preterm infants all fail to provide any evidence for a possible accelerating influence of the extra visual experience available to these infants in the period up to the expected date of term. Similar findings have been described for the development of visual acuity (Van Hof-van Duin et al, 1983; Van Hof-van Duin and Mohn , 1983,1984; Mohn and van Hof-van Duin 1985, this volume). Our results indicate that preterms with a high risk of neurological abnormalities showed smaller visual field sizes and delays in the development of monocular OKN and the visual threat response, as well as lower acuities (Mohn and van Hof-van Duin, this volume). Follow-up examinations of these infants are needed to determine whether the early visual deficits are predictive of later neurological outcome, as suggested by earlier studies (Miranda et al 1977; Harmant et al 1983).

In conclusion, development of a wide range of visual functions seems to be related to conceptional or corrected rather than postnatal age in preterm infants. There is no indication of an acceleration of development in low risk preterm infants due to the extra visual experience. In preterm infants at high risk of neurological abnormalities, particularly those showing neurological abnormalities, a slow development of several visual functions is often found. Further studies are needed to determine whether this slow development only represents a delay, or whether the deficits are permanent.

SUMMARY

Neuropediatric patients showed a high incidence of visual impairments such as abnormal OKN, absence of the visual threatening response, and visual field defects.

The development of visual field size, monocular OKN and the visual component of the threat response was compared in 79 normal fullterms and in 46 low risk and 79 high risk preterm infants.

No significant differences in maturation of visual responses were seen between fullterm and low risk preterm infants of the same conceptional age. This is of clinical importance for the detection of possible abnormalities of visual function, particularly since it seems likely that deficits may become permanent if treatment is delayed beyond a certain age. Preterm infants with a high risk of neurological abnormalities more often showed small visual field sizes and delayed development of monocular OKN and the visual threat than low risk preterms of comparable corrected age.

314

ACKNOWLEDGEMENTS

We are grateful to the staff of the Department of Pediatrics, Subdivision Neonatology, Sophia Children's University Hospital, Rotterdam , the staff of the Beatrix-Irene Children's Clinic, Rotterdam and the staffs of the Well-Baby Clinics "Schuilenburg", Dordrecht and Zoetermeer, for their support and cooperation. We would like to thank A.Gispen-van Dobbenburgh, A.Evenhuis-van Leunen, H.Frenkel and F.Groenendaal for their help in testing the infants as well as administrative assistance.

REFERENCES

Atkinson J. Development of optokinetic nystagmus in the human infant and monkey infant:an analogue to development in kittens.In Freeman RD, ed. Developmental Neurobiology of Vision. New York: Plenum Press, 1979:277-88.

Dayton GO Jr, Jones MH, Aiu P, Rawson RA, Steele B, Rose M. Developmental study of coordinated eyemovements in the human infant. Arch Ophthalmol 1964;71:865-70.

Dubowitz LMS. A study of visual function in the premature infant. Child: care health and development 1979;5:399-404.

Gorman JJ, Cogan DG, Gellis SS. An apparatus for grading the visual acuity of infants on the basis of optokinetic nystagmus. Pediatrics 1957;19:1088-92.

Harmant K, Roucoux M, Culee C, Lyon G. Visual attention and discrimination in infants at risk and neurological outcome. Behav Brain Res 1983;10:203-07.

Hubel DH, Wiesel TN. The period of susceptibility to the physiological effects of unilateral eyeclosure in kittens. J Physiol (Lond) 1970;206:419-36.

Lewis T, Maurer D, Milewski A. The development of nasal detection in young infants. Invest Ophthamol Vis Sci Suppl 1979;271.

MacFarlaine A, Harris P, Barnes J. Central and peripheral vision in early infancy. J Exp Child Psychol 1976;21:532-38.

Miranda SB, Hack M, Fantz RL, Fanaroff AA, Klaus MH. Neonatal pattern vision:a predictor of future mental performance? J Pediat. 1977;91:642-47.

Mohn G, Van Hof-van Duin J. Preferential looking acuity in normal and neurologically abnormal infants and pediatric patients. This issue.

Mohn G, Van Hof-van Duin J. Behavioural and electrophysiological measures of visual functions in children with neurological disorders. Behav Brain Res 1983;10:177-89.

Morante A, Dubowitz LMS, Levene M, Dubowitz V. The development of visual function in normal and neurologically abnormal preterm and fullterm infants. Develop Med Child Neurol 1982;24:771-84.

Naegele JR, Held R. The postnatal development of monocular optokinetic nystagmus in infants. Vision Res 1982;22:341-46.

Peterson L, Yonas A, Fisch RO. The development of blinking in response to impending collision in preterm, fullterm, and postterm infants. Infant Behav Develop 1980;3:155-65.

Tronick E. Stimulus control and the growth of the infant's effective visual field. Perception and the Psychophysics 1972;11:373-75.

Van Hof-van Duin J. Direction preference of optokinetic responses in monocularly tested normal kittens. Arch Ital Biol 1978;116:471-77.

Van Hof-van Duin J, Mohn G. Optokinetic and spontaneous nystagmus in children with neurological disorders. Behav Brain Res 1983;10:163-77.

Van Hof-van Duin J, Mohn G, Fetter WPF, Mettau JW, Baerts W. Preferential looking acuity in preterm infants. Behav Brain Res 1983;10:47-50.

Van Hof-van Duin J, Mohn G. Vision in the preterm infant. In: Prechtl WFR, ed. Continuity of Neural Functions from Pre- to Postnatal Life. Spastics Int Med Publications, Oxford, England: Blackwell Scientific Publications Ltd, 1984: Clinics in Developmental Medicine 94:93-115.

White BL. Human infants: Experience and Psychological Development. Englewood Cliffs NJ: Prentice-Hall 1971.

DISCUSSION

Fielder: I am interested when you are doing your visual field, how do you know that you are measuring visual field and not attention characteristics?

van Hof-van Duin: That is one of the most difficult things and is dependent on the age of the infants. A baby of 6 months old, if tested once, anticipates and starts looking for the second ball. Secondly, there is the problem of spontaneous eye movements. We try to use statistics to evaluate spontaneous eye movements. The observer is blind as to where the stimulus is; all eye movements are scored, when the baby is fixating, and when the baby looks away from the centre ball. It is possible that, for a baby with many spontaneous eye movements, our records indicate that the baby's visual field is between 60° and 75°. Other babies' visual fields may be defined more precisely.

Campos: Are the restrictions not determined by the size of the ball you have chosen?

van Hof-van Duin: No, because we do visual acuity measurements.

Campos: We have seen the acuity development, so it is possible that the visual field looks restricted because of that.

van Hof-van Duin: That would be possible, but we use a ball of 1.5 inches (4 cm) diameter. Besides, the identical field sizes are measured when using larger balls.

Campos: At what distance?

van Hof-van Duin: Thirty six cm for the baby, so it is really quite large.

Verriest: We have started a programme of visual field determination. At first we performed electro-oculography at the same time and we checked that interest response was correct by means of the deflections of the electro-oculogram. This can be made automatically. Secondly, we would avoid the fixation problem by using only one light. The child looks at the one light and we then present the second light relative to the first one, and so we have no more the problems with fixation.

van Hof-van Duin: At what age did you do that?

Verriest: This we did on all kinds of patients.

van Hof-van Duin: I mean in babies.

Verriest: No, in babies refixation occurs when the usual visual field response occurs.

van Hof-van Duin: But we now try to measure visual fields in babies.

Verriest: You can do it with a child of 2 or 3 years. But babies have no experience. But I think that this method of going from one point to the other is good.

van Hof-van Duin: But it is too difficult for babies, we have tried that.

Campos: As far as OKN is concerned, it is a problem to use it for quantitative assessment, because we don't know about the maturation of the mechanism. Dealing with it quantitatively and looking only at symmetry it is all right, but if you look at the presence or absence of response then you may be unable to judge whether the response is originating from the periphery which has nothing to do with the centre. In fact, you may have a macula which is completely nonfunctional and still have an OKN. Also you may have a lack of OKN just because the patient's attention was not there.

van Hof-van Duin: No, in children you don't have that problem. It is absolutely impossible to use OKN for acuity measurement, because in blind children positive OKN can be obtained. On the other hand, negative OKN may be found in cases of spontaneous nystagmus or latent nystagmus. For acuity measurements OKN cannot be used, so it is not important whether one stimulates the fovea, the extra-foveal region or the peripheral retina.

Atkinson: I think someone ought to support van Hof-van Duin in this business of OKN. Clinicians have asked us whether OKN can be suppressed if you are using whole drum stimulation or a full field rather than a small drum. The way we have tested this is to get an adult sitting in front of the screen for half a minute or so. If they can't suppress OKN in that time we take that as good enough evidence that the field is large enough to make it unlikely that any baby could suppress it. There is nothing to fixate in this situation and the field is 120° across. Now if you use a small field any baby or child will be able to suppress OKN. We have compared EOG recordings with direct observation. There is the possibility that if you have recording electrodes on the face, you may alter the child's eye movements and so may get different results from EOG recordings that you get from direct observation of eye movements. That should always be remembered, particularly with babies because if the head is held to ease the EOG recording, you may be suppressing the head movements that would otherwise be made. It is important to recognise that possibility, because your technique may be affecting the eye movements that are made.

NASAL FIELD DEFECTS IN STRABISMIC AMBLYOPIA

Ekkehard Mehdorn

University Eye Clinic, Lübeck (FRG)

INTRODUCTION

The postnatal development of the visual field in human infants is less well understood than that of visual acuity. Recent studies indicate that the visual field is not yet fully expanded at birth. Especially the nasal field appears to be rather constricted or even blind as compared to the temporal field, and its development lags behind (Maurer et al 1983). Similar findings have been obtained in kittens (Sireteanu & Maurer 1982). Experiments in kittens have further shown that the normal development of the visual field depends on a normal visual stimulation as does the development of visual acuity. Monocular deprivation and strabismus hamper the normal expansion of the visual field, especially that of the nasal field (Gordon et al 1979; Ikeda & Jacobson 1977; Peck et al 1980; Sherman 1973; Tumosa et al 1982; Van Hof-Van Duin 1977; Zablocka & Van Hof-Van Duin 1980).

In the ophthalmological literature amblyopia is usually equated with reduced central acuity and the assumption is made that the peripheral field of amblyopic eyes is more or less normal (Duke-Elder & Wybar 1973). The present investi-gation, however, shows that nasal field defects similar to those found in experimental animals do exist in human ambly-opes although they are less frequently associated with central amblyopia than in deprived animals.

PATIENTS

Strabismic and non-strabismic amblyopes as well as non-amblyopic strabismus patients were included in the study (Table 1). Especially amblyopes with a deep amblyopia (visual acuity 0.1 or less) were selected for perimetry since it was assumed that peripheral field defects might be more frequently detected in this group of patients. The majority of patients were adolescents or adults, the youngest child was 10 years old. All patients underwent an intense ophthalmological and orthoptic examination. Patients with organic abnormalities of eyes or visual pathways that could have been responsible for visual field defects were excluded. If possible, the onset of strabismus was docu-mented by earlier photographs. Only a few of the patients had received some sort of amblyopia therapy during their childhood. To enhance their cooperation the patients were informed that perimetry was done for "scientific purposes".

They were not informed, however, that the aim of perimetry was to look for nasal field defects.

PERIMETRY

Static perimetry was performed with the computer assisted perimeter "Octopus" using program no.21. This program allows relatively rapid screening of the entire field with slightly suprathreshold stimuli (6dB above the threshold of the age group) presented randomly at locations separated horizontally and vertically at a distance of 15 degrees. At any location of the field where no normal sensitivity is found, the exact threshold is determined by means of a staircase procedure. The print-out gives the numeric difference between the normal threshold of the age group and the patient's threshold. To better visualize the defects a kind of grey scale print-out is also available (cf. Fig. 2). The size of the target corresponds to Goldmann target III which minimizes refraction-specific artefacts. Presentation time is 100 msec.

To exclude refraction scotomas retinoscopy was always performed and the central 30 degrees of the field were tested with the appropiate near correction. Patients with retinoscopic abnormalities and fundus ectasias were excluded. Special attention was paid to the control of fixation. Perimetry was temporarily stopped when the patient turned his head and the eye had drifted towards nose or lateral canthus. A few number of patients could only be tested at the Goldmann perimeter, but their responses to kinetic stimuli were checked with static stimulus presentations. There was no major discrepancy between kinetic and static fields.

RESULTS

Nine out of 39 patients with deep strabismic amblyopia showed a marked constriction of the nasal field or even a complete nasal hemianopia in the amblyopic eye (Fig.1 and 2). The visual fields of the non-amblyopic eyes were normal. Central scotomas were not always detected by the Octopus, probably due to the patients eccentric fixation and the small number of central stimuli generated by program no.21 which is not particularly designed to pick up small central scotomas. Three additional cases of deep strabismic amblyopia exhibited a general depression of the visual field in the amblyopic eyes .

In strabismic patients with moderate or slight amblyopia (visual acuity 0.2 or more) and in those without any amblyopia no visual field defects were found.

Four amblyopic patients without strabismus showed only a general depression and concentric constriction of their visual fields. Two of these patients had an anisometropic amblyopia with visual acuities of 0.1 and 0.2. The third

case had an ametropic amblyopia (visual acuity 0.2) due to a
bilateral uncorrected astigmatismus of 5 dpt. The fourth
case had been operated 20 years ago on a bilateral cataract
at the age of 3. The cataracts had first been noticed at the
end of the first year and had become denser during the next
months. One of his eyes had been lost after an unsuccessful
operation for retinal detachment.

Not included in Table 1 are 3 cases with an unoperated
monocular congenital cataract, strabismus and slight
microphthalmus. All three cases showed a loss of the central
and nasal fields. Only a residual island of sensitivity
could be detected in the temporal field. Although their
cataracts did not allow an inspection of the fundus, an
organic retinal or optic nerve abnormality seemed improbable
(but not definitely excluded) since the swinging flashlight
test revealed no or only a slight afferent pupillary defect.
The gross nasal and central defects of these cases may thus
be attributed to their very deep amblyopia (hand movements
in the temporal field).

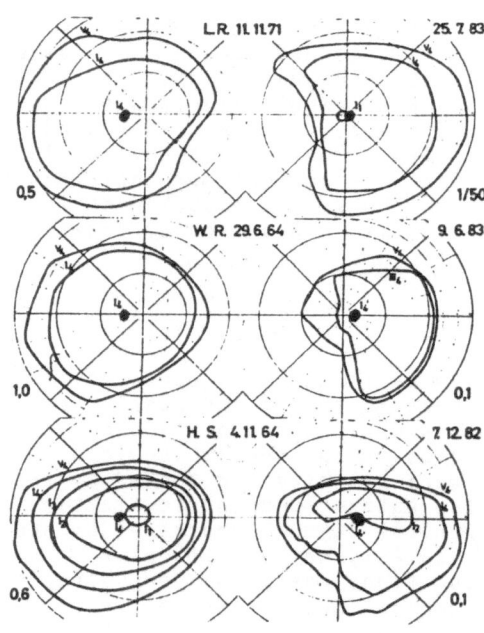

Fig.1: Nasal field defects in 3 cases with deep strabismic
amblyopia. Kinetic perimetry (Goldmann).

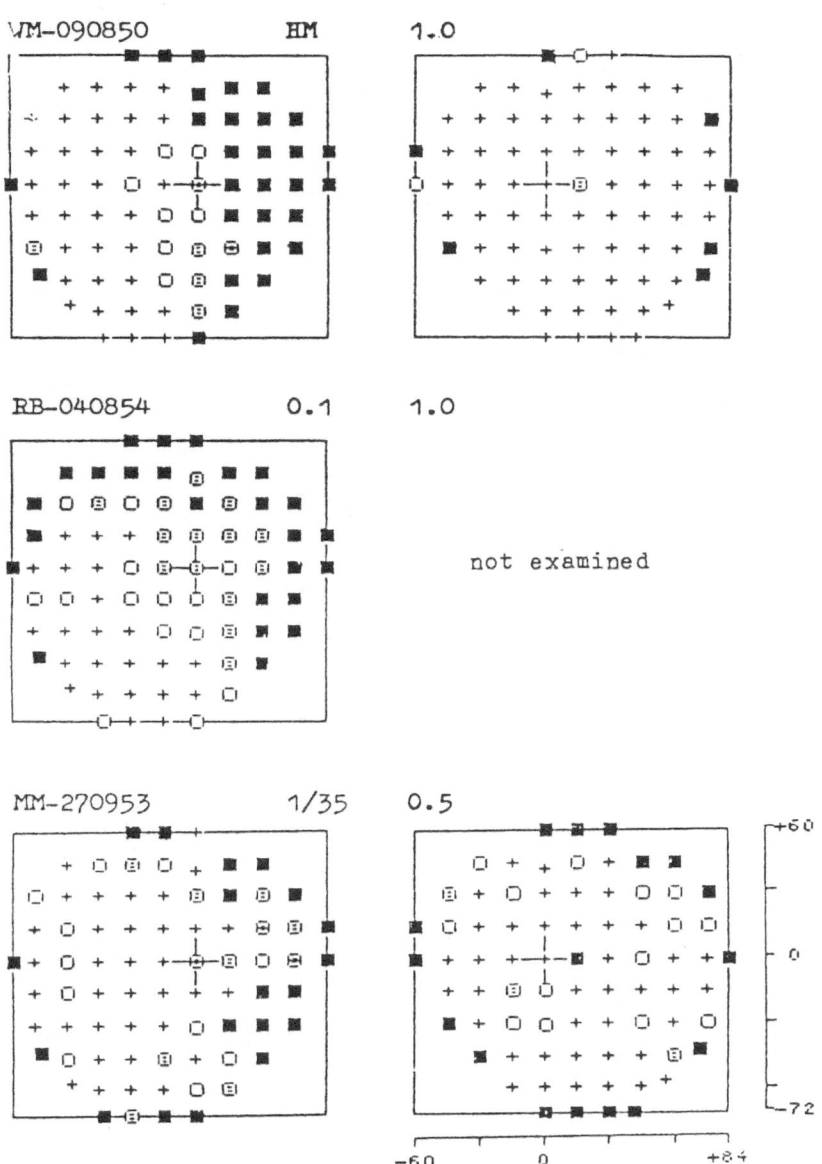

Fig. 2a & 2b:
Nasal field defects in 6 cases with deep strabismic
amblyopia. Static perimetry (Octopus). Visual field of the
left eye =left side. Black squares indicate absolute
defects, + =normal sensitivity. Other symbols = relative
defects.

322

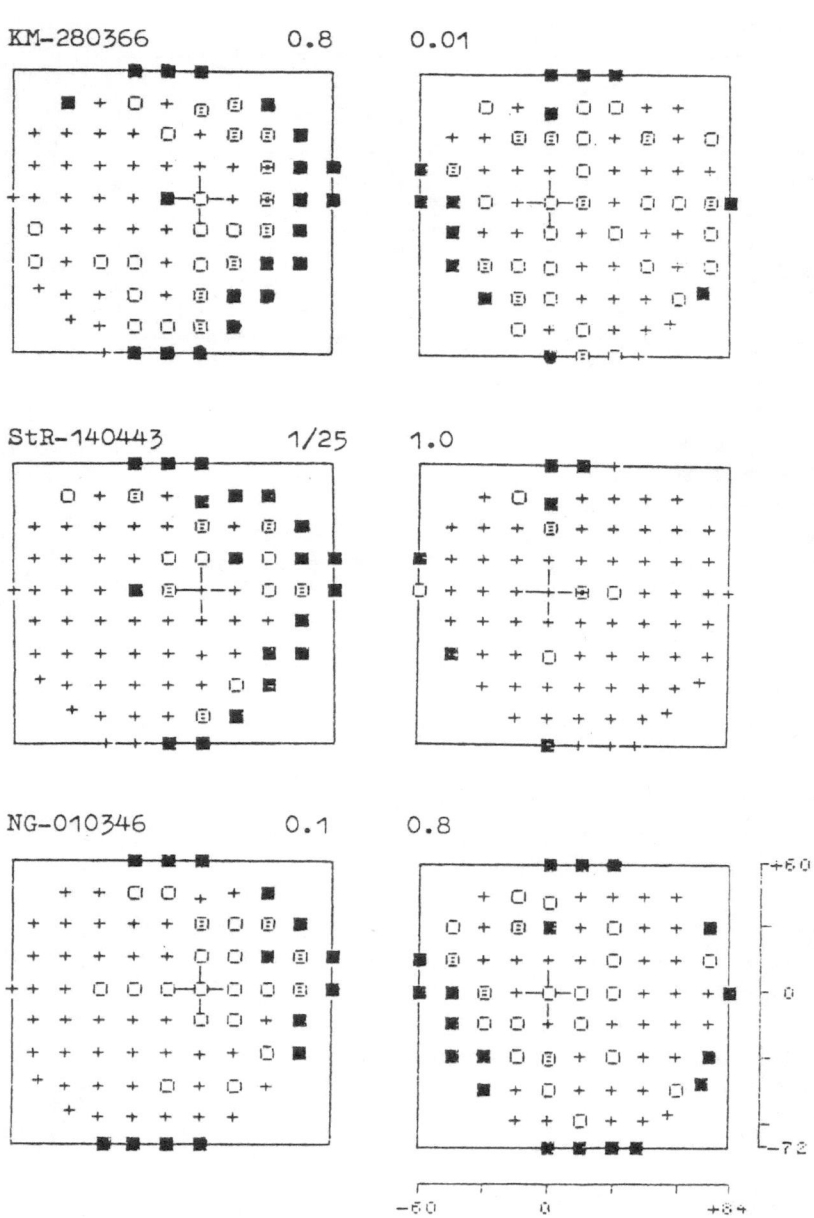

Fig. 2b

Fig. 2b

Table 1

	Deep strabismic amblyopia	Strabismus with moderate or no amblyopia	Amblyopia without strabismus
Nasal field defects	9	-	-
General depression	3	-	4
Central defects only	27	11	-
Total	39	11	4

DISCUSSION

All patients included in Table 1 underwent a thorough ophthalmological examination to exclude any organic abnormality of the fundus or of the visual pathway that could have been responsible for any kind of field defects. The normal appearance of the non-amblyopic eyes' visual fields is further evidence against an organic visual pathway lesion. The swinging flashlight test revealed no or only a slight afferent pupillary defect that was not correlated with the extent of the visual field defect or the depth of amblyopia. Organic lesions, especially in those cases with a complete nasal hemianopia should have led to very impressive afferent pupillary defects. Perimetric artefacts caused by poor fixation, head turn or uncorrected ametropia were excluded as far as possible. The dense nasal defects were reproducible with confrontation visual field testing. Thus we may conclude that the field defects discussed here are related to the deep amblyopia.

Three types of field defects were associated with amblyopia: central scotoma, nasal hemianopia or nasal constriction, and general depression of the whole field. Central field defects are a well known aspect of strabismic and non-strabismic amblyopia of all degrees and need not to be discussed here in detail. Nasal field defects and a general depression of the whole field were only found in cases with deep amblyopia. It is interesting that nasal field defects were only encountered in the 9 patients with strabismic amblyopia (less than 25% of the cases with deep strabismic amblyopia) but not in patients with non-strabismic amblyopia, while a general depression of the field occurred in both groups. This observation raises the suspicion that strabismus may play a crucial role in producing nasal field defects and that form deprivation per se may not be sufficient. On the other hand, strabismus without amblyopia was not found to be accompanied by nasal field defects. The publications dealing with field defects after monocular deprivation in kittens do not help in the decision whether nasal field defects develop only if deprivation is accompanied by strabismus since the authors did not ensure that their kittens had not become strabismic after monocular lid suture.

Until the present it is not possible to explain conclusively why some cases had nasal field defects and others had not. It has been argued that the shadow of the nose is responsible for the physiological limitation of the nasal field (Schmidt et al 1971). Starting from this hypothesis one could argue that in the case of strong convergent strabismus the shadow of the nose limits the nasal field much more than normal and thus exaggerates the physiological nasal constriction of the field. The partial occlusion of the eye in strong unilateral esotropia may contribute to the development of nasal field defects in these cases but it is certainly not the only mechanism that is responsible for the development of these defects. At least in one of the cases with a complete nasal hemianopia (case W.M., Fig. 2) it was documented by photographs that he had never had more than a few degrees of esotropia but mainly a hypertropia.

The nasal field defects cannot be the consequence of longstanding suppression scotomas of the deviated eye as one might suspect at first glance. The suppression scotomas one can easily detect in esotropia by means of striated glasses, at the synoptophore or with other haploscopic devices are located in the temporal field. But my patients who were all more or less esotropic had nasal field defects. This obvious contradiction between the location of the suppression scotomas and the location of the field defects observed in deep strabismic amblyopia casts some doubt onto the classical suppression theory of amblyopia as it is expressed in the ophthalmological literature (Duke-Elder & Wybar 1973).

If one follows the idea that amblyopia is caused by an inhibition of those parts of the visual system which develop after birth one could conceive why some patients with strabismic amblyopia show nasal field defects and others do not. It has been shown in kittens (Sireteanu & Maurer 1982) and in human infants (Maurer et al. 1983) that the nasal field is more or less blind at birth and reaches its full extension about the third month. These data are in agreement with the clinical observation that the temporal retina is relatively immature at birth. If amblyopia develops during the first months of life it could affect the development of the nasal field. If it occurs later, say at about the end of the first year or even later, the development of the nasal field is completed and can no longer be disturbed. The development of the central vision, however, still continues until puberty (Hohmann & Haase 1982) and central amblyopia may develop after the first year of life. It is difficult to substantiate this hypothesis in a clinical study, since adult patients often do not know about the exact onset of their strabismus. If possible, it was tried to document the onset of strabismus by means of photographs. So far no case was found which contradicts the hypothesis outlined here. Why some patients with deep strabismic amblyopia do not develop nasal field defects but rather a general depression of their field as do patients with non-strabismic amblyopia remains open to speculation.

SUMMARY AND CONCLUSIONS

9 out of 39 patients with deep strabismic amblyopia (visual acuity 0.1 or less) showed nasal constrictions or nasal hemianopias in the visual field of the amblyopic eye. The nasal field defects are regarded as nasal amblyopias and may be explained by an inhibition of the postnatal development of the nasal field.

REFERENCES

Duke-Elder St, Wybar K. Ocular motility and strabismus. In: Duke-Elder St, ed. System of Ophthalmology, Vol VI. London: Kimpton. 1973.

Gordon B, Moran J, Presson J. Visual fields of cats reared with one eye intorted. Brain Res 1979; 174:167.

Heitländer H, Hoffmann K-P. The visual field of monocularly deprived cats after late closure or enucleation of the non-deprived eye. Brain Res 1978; 145:145.

Ikeda H, Jacobson SG. Nasal field loss in cats reared with convergent squint. Behavioural studies. J Physiol 1977; 270:367.

Maurer D, Lewis TL, Brent HP. Peripheral vision and optokinetic nystagmus in children with unilateral congenital cataract. Behav Brain Res 1983; 10:151.

Peck CK, Barber G, Pilsecker CE, Wark RC. Visual field defects in cats reared with cyclodeviations of the eyes. Exp Brain Res 1980; 41:61.

Schmidt D, Reuscher A, Kommerell G. Über das nasale Gesichtsfeld bei Strabismus fixus divergens. Graefes Arch klin exp Ophthalmol 1971; 183:97

Sherman SM. Visual field defects in monocularly and binocularly deprived cats. Brain Res 1973; 49:25

Sireteanu R, Maurer D. The development of the kittens visual field. Vision Res 1982; 22:1105

Tumosa N, Tieman SB, Hirsch HVB. Visual deficits in cats reared with unequal alternating monocular exposure. Exp Brain Res 1982; 47:119.

Van Hof-Van Duin J. Visual field measurements in monocularly deprived and normal cats. Exp Brain Res 1977; 30:353.

Zablocka T, Van Hof-Van Duin J. Perimetry in binocularly deprived cats . Neurosci Lett Suppl 1980; 5:138.

DISCUSSION

Sireteanu: We did a very similar study on 25 patients and did not see any nasal loss although we looked for it.

Mehdorn: What was the visual acuity of the amblyopes you tested?

Sireteanu: Some of our subjects had a visual acuity of 0.1 or less and even those did not show a nasal field defect. So it is interesting to see what the differences are between those who show a defect and those who don't.

Mehdorn: I can only repeat that 25% of my patients with deep strabismic amblyopia did show nasal field defects.

Sireteanu: We had 8 very deep amblyopes and 2 of them should have shown this defect, but they didn't.

Mehdorn: A sample of 8 is certainly not sufficient for statistics. I am the first to have systematically looked for nasal field defects in amblyopes but I am not the first to have discovered these defects. If you look through the literature you can find several short remarks concerning visual perception in the peripheral temporal field of deep amblyopes. Further evidence for the real existence of these defects is the fact that some of my patients knew about their nasal defects as long as they could remember. And finally, with the Octopus perimeter you cannot influence the performance of the patient. You cannot produce nasal defects as you can on the Goldmann perimeter. With the Goldmann perimeter you can produce any defect you want, with the Octopus perimeter you are sure that it is not an artefact introduced by yourself just because you are looking for nasal field defects.

Hache: Do you use kinetic and static measurements on the same patient?

Mehdorn: Yes, I did this several times, but I could not find a substantial difference.

van Hof-van Duin: In our preterm babies who are at high risk of abnormalities, many are strabismic and their nasal field develops later. You were mentioning central defects, what do you mean by that?

Mehdorn: I mean defects in the centre of the visual field.

van Hof-van Duin: Is that something that is found by others too?

Mehdorn: Yes, until recently it was a generally held belief that amblyopia is accompanied by central visual field defects only.

van Hof–van Duin: In answer to Sireteanu's question, if (deep) amblyopia
starts at a later age, say after the first year of life, one probably will
not find a nasal defect.

Mehdorn: It is certainly difficult in a retrospective study to confirm my
hypothesis that nasal field defects occur only if the amblyopia had
developed during the first year of life. If possible, the patients bring
early photographs to document the onset of their squint. So far I have no
case that contradicts my hypothesis.

Verriest: In alternating hyperphoria we also found (with Rosa Fusco)
statistically significant lower sensitivity in the inferonasal quadrant.

Fiorentini: Development in animals might be relevant to these findings.
Different evoked potential responses from the nasal and temporal portions
of the amblyopic eye have been reported, and there are behavioural
experiments which show a complete loss of nasal field with spared temporal
field in the deprived eye of monocularly deprived kittens.

APPARENT BLINDNESS DUE TO SACCADIC PARALYSIS OR DELAY

by P. Fells, R.B. Jones, B. McCarry and J. Hungerford

Moorfields Eye Hospital, London

This may seem a perverse choice of topic for discussion at a meeting devoted to the detection and assessment of visual impairment in pre-verbal children but I hope that its relevance will become apparent. Some of the tests used in objective assessment of visual acuity, such as the preferential looking method, assume that the infant has normal control of its eye and head movements. Four infants have been brought to me because their mothers had thought them to be blind. Clinical observation showed that the normal ocular motor results of visual stimulation were missing and were later replaced by distinctive thrusting movements of the head on attempting to change fixation.

Before describing these patients a brief review of the normal pattern of eye and head movements in infancy is required. Five week old infants use a series of hypometric saccades to fixate a peripheral target with little head rotation (fig. 1) (ref. 1). By eight weeks fewer saccades are needed, but notice that alternative eye and head movements may appear with hypermetric displacement of gaze (fig.2). The number of saccades increases with target eccentricity but progressively decreases with age (fig. 3). By three months of age infants may use different combinations of eye and head movements to capture a peripheral visual target (fig. 4) (ref. 2). Note particularly that in some infants the head movement precedes the eye movement, but this combination is rarely seen in adults whose typical response is a single saccade onto target followed by head rotation during which a compensatory eye movement in the opposite direction is required to maintain fixation.

Smooth pursuit movements are seen at four weeks of age provided

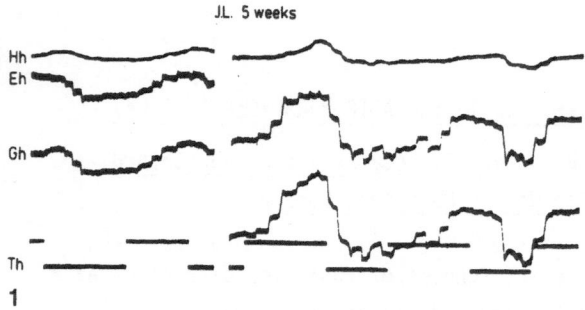

JL. 5 weeks

1

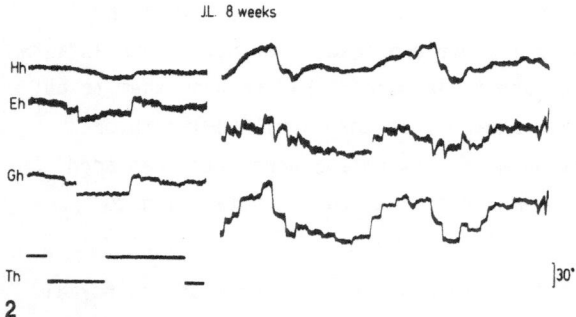

JL. 8 weeks

]30°

2

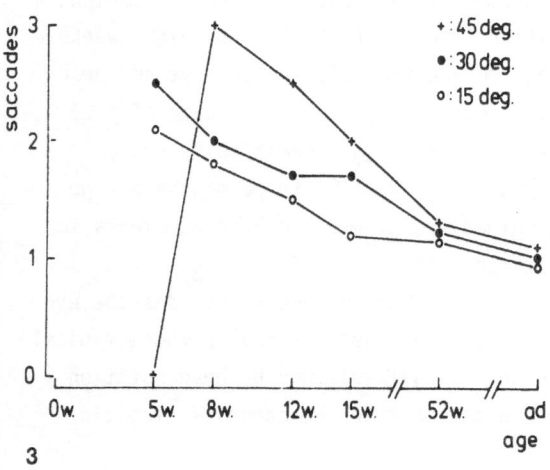

+ : 45 deg.
• : 30 deg.
○ : 15 deg.

3

CAPTIONS

Fig. 1   Co-ordinated eye and head movements made by the same baby
and   at five weeks (fig. 1) and at eight weeks (fig. 2). The
Fig. 2   left traces show the most common behaviour of several
          hypometric saccades. The right traces show larger,
          hypermetric responses.

          Key: Hh = horizontal head position
                Eh = horizontal eye position
                Gh = horizontal gaze position
                Th = target position

Fig. 3   The evolution with age of the mean number of saccades made
          to fixate targets lying at 15°, 30° and 45° of eccentricity.
          At five weeks the 45° target is never fixated.

          Key: The age is in weeks
                ad = adult

Fig. 4   Typical patterns of co-ordinated eye and head movements
          used to capture peripheral visual stimuli. Time is along the
          horizontal axis. The arrows represent the time at which the
          peripheral stimuli are presented. Stimulus size and direction
          are indicated. Upward represents movement to the left, and
          downward to the right for both eye and head movement traces.
          The responses shown are for three month old infants.

Fig. 5   Representative VOR responses. Eye movement records show
          responses to externally imposed head movements. Gaze
          records are the summation of eye and head movements and
          represent visual fixation. Time is along the horizontal
          axis. Upward represents movement to left, and downwards to
          the right.

Acknowledgments: Figures 1, 2, 3 are from the paper by Roucoux, Culee
and Roucoux: Development of fixation and pursuit eye movements in human
infants; and figures 4 and 5 are from the paper by Regal, Ashmead and
Salapatek: The co-ordination of eye and head movements during early
infancy: a selective review, both published by permission of Behavioural
Brain Research.

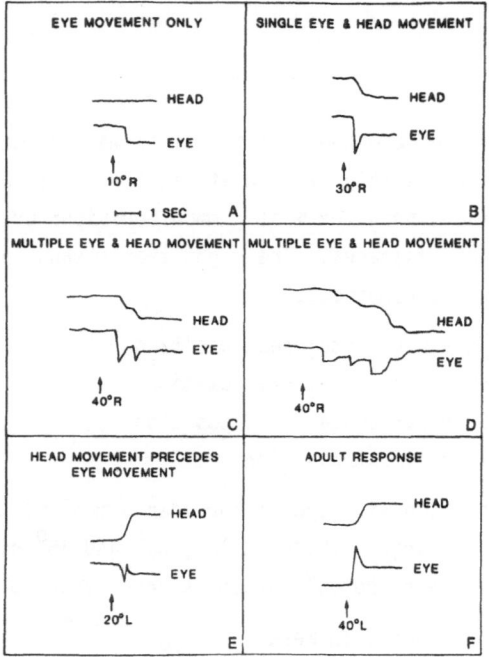

4

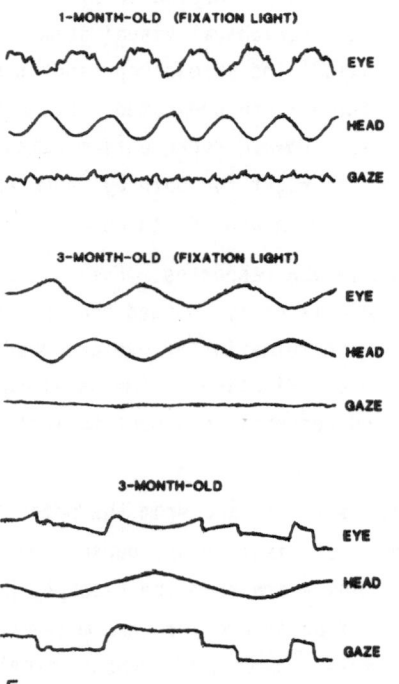

5

For legends
see page 331.

that target velocity is low enough, about 10 degrees per second.
By four months of age pursuit is smooth at 28 degrees per second
but with some saccades at 40 degrees per second.

The vestibulo-ocular reflex (VOR) also demonstrates eye
movements, this time in response to externally imposed head rotations
(fig. 5). The compensatory eye movements that maintain gaze direction
have become much smoother by three months of age. Furthermore, some
infants can do two things at once as shown here with slow compensatory
eye movements cancelling out the head rotations with superimposed
saccadic gaze shifts. The normal three month old infant exhibits a
remarkably full repertoire of co-ordinated eye and head movements with
reflex control.

Case Reports

Details are given below of the four apparently blind from birth
infants:

Case 1

R.B., male, was born normally at forty weeks after a pregnancy
interrupted by recurrent bleeding. His mother was convinced that he
was blind from birth until at four months old he reacted to a fluorescent
light that flickered when it was switched on. Head thrusts were
noticed at that age, mainly to infant's left. When seen at Moorfields
at twelve months he had head thrusts to either side but was reluctant
to follow targets to the left. No convergence was elicitable. In
his general development he was slow in sitting up and in crawling. By
fifteen months rather jerky following movements to right and left were
present with occasional large saccades. Convergence was normal, as
was his CT scan.

Case 2

A.H., male, after a normal pregnancy was born by elective
Caesarean section at thirty eight weeks. A pneumothorax quickly healed.

His parents considered his fixation was very poor and by seven weeks
old he smiled only to sounds but not to visual stimulation. Intermittent
exotropia was seen from three months with head thrusts to the right
and later to the left. When examined at Moorfields at thirteen months
there was left exotropia with head thrusts to either side. Full eye
movements were produced by doll's head rotations and on whole body
rotation saccades were just beginning. His general development was
normal. By eighteen months the head thrusts were fewer with saccades
to right and left, and vertically. He was reluctant to follow targets
horizontally, especially to the left (table 1).

PATIENT	ONSET AND PRESENTING SIGN	STRABISMUS	ONSET HEAD THRUSTS	ONSET SACCADES	GENERAL DEVELOPMENT
RB male 30.12.83.	blind from birth	------	4 months	12 months	slow
AH male 9.3.83.	?blind from birth	int. L-XT	3 months	13 months	n.a.d.
LB female 28.1.82.	poor eye contact from birth	int. L-ET	3 months	26 months	slow
BB male 10.19.83.	not seeing properly	?R-ET	7 months	17 months	n.a.d.

Case 3

L.B., the only female in the series, had her birth induced at
forty-two weeks. Her mother had taken Ancoloxan for morning sickness
in the first trimester. Her parents were aware of poor eye contact
from birth but by ten weeks she smiled in response to a face one metre
away. Head thrusts were seen bilaterally at three months. When checked
at Moorfields at six months, the occasional left esotropia from early
weeks had become an alternating esotropia. No saccades could be
produced. By eighteen months her general development was assessed as
being three months behind. Saccades could be elicited by the OKN drum
at twenty-six months and by three years the head thrusts were fewer with
following present bilaterally and vertically. Because of increasing

drinking a CT scan was performed, revealing dysgenesis of the corpus callosum with an intra-sellar arachnoid hernia.

Case 4

B.B., male, had a normal birth but was thought not to be seeing properly from that time. Right esotropia was queried at three months but this was not confirmed when seen at Moorfields at seven months. Head thrusts but no saccades were seen and his general development was normal. By seventeen months the head thrusts were fewer, following was better to the left and saccades were present to the left more often than to the right. Doll's head rotation was normal.

DISCUSSION

These children exhibit the features of ocular motor apraxia, a condition described by Cogan in 1952 (ref. 3, 4), but in whom the initial complaint by parents was that the child appeared blind or unable to see properly. Later examination showed that voluntary horizontal ocular movements were absent and change of gaze direction to allow re-fixation was achieved by means of lateral rotational head thrusts. Head movement to one side causes the eyes to deviate to the opposite side by the vestibulo-ocular reflex. The head is then rotated even further in its original direction beyond the line of intended fixation until the laterally deviated eyes are able to take up the new object of fixation. Then the head and eyes return towards the straight ahead position as the new fixation point is held.

In the pre-verbal child inferences about sensory input are often based on the motor responses. Infants with saccadic paralysis who have not yet developed the typical head thrusts would be considered blind on forced choice preferential looking tests. Doll's head rotations producing the vestibulo-ocular reflex are effective in the dark by one month of age in normal infants so this manoeuvre provides no evidence of vision. The whole body rotation test looking for prolonged <u>post</u>-rotational nystagmus in the blind infant is similarly nullified by the absence of saccades. The OKN drum elicits no fast phase, and the Catford drum result is similarly difficult to interpret.

It is worth recalling that one of the normal infant's strategies to fixate a peripheral target is by head turn first and later ocular movement. The four infants described here have developed this method preferentially at 3-7 months of age to the exclusion of saccades until 12-26 months old. At least one child in this series, and four out of eight in another (ref. 5), have partial agenesis of the corpus callosum. Perhaps minor forms of the agenesis are too subtle for detection by present methods of investigation. It has been postulated that interhemispheric connections may be important in the development of voluntary eye movements and that, once learned, commisural pathways may not be needed for voluntary horizontal gaze. It is proposed that these infants are obliged to use the head movement exclusively to change ocular fixation at first and that the development of normal saccadic movements is delayed.

These cases emphasise the dangers of making categorical pronouncements about an infant's visual prognosis from early clinical observations alone. Other methods of objective assessment must be used and time allowed for the central nervous system to display its versatility in providing alternative tactics to change fixation.

REFERENCES

1. Roucoux, A., Culee, C. and Roucoux, M. Development of fixation and pursuit eye movements in human infants. Behavioural Brain Research, 10, 133 (1983)

2. Regal D.M., Ashmead, D.H. and Salapatek, P. The co-ordination of eye and head movements during early infancy: a selective review. Behavioural Brain Research, 10, 125 (1983)

3. Cogan, D.G. A type of congenital ocular motor apraxia presenting jerky head movements. Trans. Amer. Acad. Ophthal. and Otolaryng., 56, 853 (1952)

4. Cogan, D.G. Congenital ocular motor apraxia. Canad. J. Ophthal., 1, 253 (1966)

5. Orrison, W.W. and Robertson, W.C. Congenital ocular motor apraxia: a possible disconnection syndrome. Arch. Neurol., 36, 29 (1979)

DISCUSSION

Vital-Durand: We have not been paying enough attention to head movement in the process of visual function. I am most surprised by the fact that you would involve the corpus callosum. What you saw on the scan of the corpus callosum on one of these children was normal, but what in the corpus callosum could be involved in ocular abnormalities of this kind? The parts of the brain which organise stabilisation of eye movement are pretty small and would not be seen on CT scan except if affected by huge abnormalities. Why did you emphasise the CT scan?

Fells: Because of the paper that was mentioned by Arensen and Robertson. They find it in half their cases and their suggestion is that it may be that this interhemispheric connection is something that is important in the development of the initiation of saccades. Once you have got them then you have learnt, then it gets built into your motor repertoire and hence they were saying that this was why when you have injuries or section of the corpus collosum later on, you don't find that they have to resort to these types of head thrusts. That was the reason why I brought it out and this is the reason why I would like to have more information about what is going on in the brain. These tests only show us very gross changes.

Vital-Durand: The group of people with agenesis of the corpus collosum is a large one described in Quebec, and they were showing anomalies of eye movements.

Mehdorn: They had squints.

Braddick: These patients will not look straight as adults.

Fells: They learn control of their eye and head movements and as adults you don't find abnormalities unless you are especially looking for them.

Fielder: I have just had brain tissue examined of such a baby who presented to me and subsequently died. The cerebellum was abnormally large. How do you assess saccadic movement? I have observed, rather anecdotally, in congenital ocuolmotor apraxia that even quite late on, say at 3 years of age, when you rotate such a child he still cannot generate saccadic movements.

Fells: What sort of rotation?

Fielder: Upright at arm's length. As you rotate the child to the right the eyes go over to the right. As vision develops the deviation is less and the eyes remain more fixated on the rotator. In congenital oculomotor apraxia the ocular motor mechanism seems unable to control this deviation and the eyes swing towards the edge of the orbit with no fast phase.

Fells: I haven't tried swinging children of that size!

Taylor: CT scanning has shown that abnormalities of the corpus callosum are present in one degree or another in 5% of the population, and I would guess in a neurological population it is probably a lot higher. I am not aware of any cases, in spite of it being a relatively common condition in a children's hospital, or in the literature, of patients who had any serious progressive disorder with ocular motor apraxia that is not clinically detectable. There have been cases of hydrocephalus but they have been detectable by other means and I really don't think it is necessary routinely to do a CT scan which involves heavy sedation or a anaesthetic plus the x-rays. We published a couple of years ago 3 patients with a saccadic palsy in addition to Leber's amaurosis with relatively good vision but with an extinguished ERG. Subsequently we found cases of that also in various cerebellar degenerations. So I think it is worthwhile in all these cases to do an ERG if you are suspicious and if you find that they have saccadic palsy.

Fells: When you do your NMR examinations, up to what age can you do them?

Dubowitz: Up to any age. The point is that we started them 4 years ago and so we have the older children who have been followed 2 or more years. It is done on adults to diagnose tumours all the time. Agenesis of the corpus collosum is very easily diagnosed. It is quite a common condition. We see about one a month.

Fells: And your ultrasound on the children is up to what age?

Dubowitz: You can do the ultrasound as long as the fontanelle is open. In normal children, if you have a good machine, this is imperative, you can do it until 6 months, but it depends on your machine.

Boergen: We do routine ultrscans and found a lot of midline defects.

EXPERIENCE WITH OUR PRESENT SCREENING PROGRAM

Lea Hyvärinen

City of Helsinki, Department of Health

INTRODUCTION

Vision screening of the $3\frac{1}{2}$-4 year olds at the children's health care centres has long traditions in all Nordic countries (Kaivonen and Koskenoja 1963, Köhler and Stigmar 1973, 1978). In Finland vision screening of pre-school children is included in the assessment of development at 3-4 years of age and at $5\frac{1}{2}$-6 years of age. It should include all children but in big cities, like Helsinki, it covers only 70-80% of children. Vision screening of the preverbal children is more effective because more than 90% of all infants attend to their regular visits at the health care centres during their first year of life.

PERSONNEL INVOLVED IN VISION SCREENING

Vision screening is shared by the public health nurse and the physician. Helsinki is a university city and its health centres are used for training of physicians. If the physician in the children's health care centre is inexperienced, then more of the follow-up of development is taken care by the public health nurses than is usual. Some physicians work permanently and know the families and their life situations better.

The Finnish public health nurse (PHN) is competent worker who first has had a $2\frac{1}{2}$ years' nursing education. After that she often has worked for several years in different hospitals, after which she has had one year of special training in health care.

In Finland we have so few orthoptists that they cannot be used for vision screening.

PRESENT PRACTISES IN VISION SCREENING IN HELSINKI

Screening for visual defects has been a part of developmental screening since 1962 and the present screening techniques for screening of the $3\frac{1}{2}$-4 year olds and the $5\frac{1}{2}$-6 year olds were developed in the late 1970s. The screening of the verbal children is based on measurement of visual acuity as line acuity and rough assessment of deviations in motor functions using Hirschberg's test, i.e. observation of location of the pupillary light reflexes, cover-uncover-test and observing monocular and binocular fixation and tracking of a small target.

LH-line acuity chart for testing at 3 meter distance (Fig.1) has been in use since 1981 (Hyvärinen et al 1980). Recently the LH-near vision card has been added to the test methods.

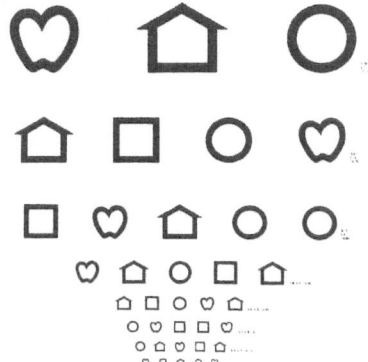

Fig.1. LH-line acuity chart is usually used at a distance of 3 meters.
It can be used at any distance but then the visual acuity values must be
calculated accordingly.

The chart used for testing of the $3\frac{1}{2}$-4 year olds is too easy for testing
of many $5\frac{1}{2}$-6 year olds. For them there is a more difficult line acuity
chart with symbols between sizes 0.1 - 2.0 (6/60 - 6/3). The chart has 3
sets of the smaller symbols, thus memorising is impossible.

Vision screening of the preverbal children is not a single examination but
consists of observations on the developmental steps. If there is delay in
maturation of visual functions the child is referred to the ophthalmologist.
Often no deviation from the normal development can be detected at the health
centre but the parents are worried about the vision of the infant. Suspicion
of deviation is accepted as a cause for referral. Infant whose parent or
sibling has or has had either squint or amblyopia, is referred to ophthalmologist at the age of 6-8 months for assessmnet and for planning of further
follow-up.

The techniques used in observation of visual development during the first
year of life have undergone thorough re-evaluation during last year. A
group of public health nurses discussed the contents of each visit of the
infant and the observations on visual development as a part of the visit.
A detailed manual (Hyvärinen et al 1984) was written and the instruments
to be used by all nurses were specified. The instruments are now: small
flashlight, 2 fixation targets (Fig.2), and a red ball mounted on a pin.

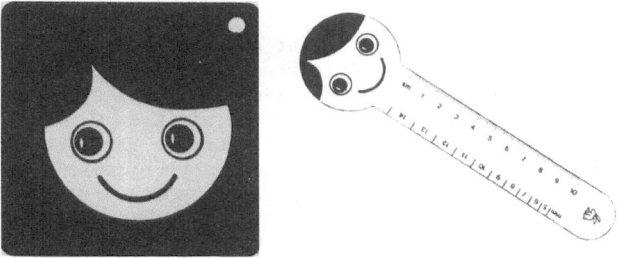

Fig.2. Two fixation targets used to assess fixation and following at 3
months and 5 months of age.

Table 1.

VISION SCREENING FOR PRE-SCHOOL CHILDREN

AGE	OBSERVATION & TESTS	DEVIATIONS TO BE RECOGNIZED
Newborn	Pupillary reaction, media clear	Coloboma of iris, cataract, squint
0-3 months	Development of ocular movements, eye contact, social smile	Roving eye movements, squint
4-6 months	Hand regard, hands to the midline, observes keenly, recognizes distant objects	Cataract may become denser and decrease vision, squint may be related to RLF or tumour
7-10 months	Peripheral vision symmetric, notices small crumbs, pincer grasp. Tests: Hischberg, tracking,visual field	Children with high hyperopia may not develop squint but are not interested in small objects
1-2 years	Recognizes people at a distance, interested in books and pictures	Squint, lack of interest in learning through vision
3-4 years	Names pictures and test symbols near and at distance, visual acuity symmetric	Night vision affected in some hereditary diseases
5-6 years	Adult like vision but difficulties with crowded visual information	Decrease in visual acuity in several hereditary diseases

(RLF=retrolental fibroplasia, disease of retina in premature infants, Coloboma of iris= part of iris missing, usually in the lower part.)

Table 1 is taken from a small booklet "Vision in Children- normal and abnormal" written for the health centre personnel and the parents of visually impaired children (Hyvärinen 1983, 1984 and in preparation). It is a short review of the well known developmental steps which should be recorded during the regular visits needed for immunization and follow-up of general development.

Since the visual development of an infant and a child is checked during regular visits and the time spent for screening of vision is short, no extra expenses are needed. The only check-up requiring slightly more time than usually for examination of vision is the visit at 9 months when both vision and hearing tests are made. The structure of this screening situation is still a matter of further discussions because BOEL-test is currently under evaluation. Vision screening of BOEL-test is insufficient for screening of the possible deviations requiring treatment and therefore it is suggested that even if BOEL-test is used, it should be preceded by examination of visual fields using mounted balls and examination of symmetry of monocular fixation and tracking.

CONTINIOUS TRAINING OF PUBLIC HEALTH NURSES

Frequent changes in the concepts related to early visual development
during last ten years necessitate continious training of personnel. This
is done in groups of approximately 20 PHNs 1 to 2 times a year. These
sessions are necessary for passing of information and for motivation of
all persons involved. A possibility of consultation by phone is also
found important.

VISION SCREENING IN HELSINKI - A MODEL?

Finland has been nominated WHO´s "pioneer country" of primary health care.
In Finland high standard of primary health care has been reached without
great total costs of health expenditure. Visual screening is an example of
follow-up of development without extra costs because it is a part of
regular visits of the infant and child to the health centre. This kind of
organization requires well trained public health nurses and good cooperation between the PHNs, the health centre physicians and the ophthalmologists.

The social structure in the Nordic countries has features that make
organization of primary health care less problematic than in many other
countries: differences between the social and ethnic groups are small, the
population as a whole is aware of the importance of health and its
attitudes are positive.

Because of the differences in the organization of primary health care and
in the structure of the society in different countries, visual screening
practices typical to Helsinki or other Nordic cities or rural communes
cannot be copied as such by most European countries. They may, however,
give new ideas to persons involved in development of screening practices
and follow-up of visual development during pre-school years.

REFERENCES:

Hyvärinen L, Näsänen R, Laurinen P. New visual acuity test for pre-school
children. Acta Ophthalmol (Copenh) 1980;58:507-511.

Hyvärinen L. Vision in Children - normal and abnormal. English edition to
be published. Swedish edition. Helsinki. Finlands svenska synskadade.1983.
Finnish edition. Helsinki. Publications of the National Board of Health in
Finland, 48. 1984.

Hyvärinen L, Kamppi H, Kinnaslampi T, Vuorenpää EK, Kettula L, Göranson P,
Ellonen R, Koniczek MR. Näön seurantatutkimus neuvolassa (Vision screening
in the children´s health care centre), manual. 1984.

Kaivonen M, Koskenoja M. Visual screening for children aged four years and
preliminary experiences from its application in practice. Acta Ophthalmol
(Copenh) 1963;41:785-786.

Köhler L, Stigmar G. Visual screening of four year old children. Acta
Paediatr Scand 1973;62:17-27.

Köhler L, Stigmar G. Visual disorders in 7-year-old children with and
without previous vision screening. Acta Paediatr Scand 1978;67:373-377.

EARLY DETECTION OF VISUAL DISORDERS IN HEALTH CENTRES IN YOUNG CHILDREN

D H Loewer-Sieger and V K Lantau

The Netherlands Ophthalmic Research Institute, Department
of Ophthalmogenetics

In the Netherlands a small team started in 1974 with a system for
early identification of visual disorders, being challenged by audiologists
who had at that time introduced into the program of Health Centres a method
of early detection of hearing defects by the Ewing method. Through this
method children of the age of 9 months are screened by specially educated
teams. Nearly 90% of the Dutch children are being examined: they regularly
visit the Health Centres and when they have reached the age of 9 months
they are summoned to come to the Centre for a special sitting.

As is to be expected, some of the children are not in the right mood to
cooperate at that moment and other have a transient deafness due to an
ordinary cold.

To avoid a too great amount of children being referred to the
specialist, the failing children have a second check-up after 4-6 weeks.

The results are:
first screening	19% with positive findings (that is children who fail the test)
second screening	5% with positive findings These children are referred to the audiologist
diagnostic examination	2% have definite defects $1^o/oo$ have permanent serious defects

For the introduction of early detection of visual disorders we had to
choose a method as cheap as possible, that is to say: a method

a) performed in the Health Centres, where already most children have
   their regular medical examinations.
b) performed by the available doctors as examiners.
c) with a fixed program that is standardized.
d) and as time is money, the sessions should be as short as possible.
e) and last but not least, feasible and reproducible in the situation
   of the Health Centres.

We chose for the simple and classic method of examination of
strabismus by Hirschberg corneal reflex lights and cover-uncover test,
furthermore binocular and monocular pursuit movements, corneal brightness,
pupillary reaction to light and the form of the pupil (6 items in the
program).

The instruments needed are only a fixation light and a small, but
interesting toy.

For a trained person the whole sitting costs in time for each child

On purpose we did not concentrate on visual acuity and refraction. By close observation of pursuit movements and comparison of the movements of one eye with those of the other eye, it is possible to get a certain impression of the fixation ability.

Visual acuity less than 0,5 to 0,2 is not noticeable, but a child with a visual acuity of about 0,1 can be identified; children with a better visual acuity but with latent or manifest nystagmus, as well.

Comparable to the screening on hearing defects a second examination is performed for the children who do not cooperate in the first session. In this way the amount of referrals, and especially the false positive referrals, is reduced.

In the organisation of the Health Centre this second examination is not so complicated, as the children of this age are coming back regularly in a period of about 6-8 weeks.

The main financial problem of the method is that the doctors need a special education, given by an orthoptist, in a course of 4 lessons, a film, a written instruction and guidance during their first year.

The family doctors and ophthalmologists should also be informed. All this acitivity costs the salary of the orthoptist.

Ideal would be if every doctor, working at the Health Centre, would be trained so well during the medical study that the task of the orthoptist in this would be superfluous.

Propagating a screening on infants at the age of 8-9 months, we do not neglect the necessity to examine the eyes of all newborns by checking the cornea and fundus reflex. Of course all children younger than 8-9 months suspected of eye trouble, should be sent to the ophthalmologist.

Indeed, through instruction of the Health Centre personnel for the screening-method attention is drawn to the visual problems of children of all ages, younger or older.

Of course we expected that with our chosen program strabismus would be the most frequent finding. In the population in the Netherlands we expect 5% squint. At the early age of 9 months, we expect less than 2,5%. Only 50% of all strabismic children start with their squint before the age of one year.

However, the children who have a squint due to cerebral lesions – and in this group strabismus is much more frequent than 5% – start squinting in their first year with a 80% prevalence instead of 50% of all squinting children. In other words: early identification of squint will reveal children with other complications than just ordinary squint.

The smallest but most important group in view of early identification is the group of children with organic eye disorders. Frequently they have in their first year an impaired optomotor eye balance.

The prevalence in this group is only approximately $1^o/oo$. The urge for early genetic advice and early habitation of these children, although such a small group, makes early discovery worthwhile.

In a program of the Health Centres, it is of course to be recommended to repeat the same screening at the age of 1 1/2 year, 3 years and 5 years, with addition of assessing visual acuity from the age of 3 years.

In 1978 we started a pilot-study in Amsterdam concerning 1200 children, during two years.

In the first examination was found:	19,3% positives
In the second examination was found:	4,4% positives
diagnostic examination	1,9% disorders

These results closely resemble the findings at the Ewing test for hearing defects.

The percentage of over-referrals (children who showed no abnormalities at the diagnostic examination) is 40. This is quite acceptable in the opinion of epidemiologists.

We made an estimation on our findings that, working with this program, every ophthalmologist in the Netherlands will see 2 or 3 infants every month, and of these 2 or 3 children one child will have no abnormalities. We think that is indeed acceptable in an ordinary practice. In our group of disorders, most of the children were squinting, some had a high degree of hyperopia (without squint), and 2 children (1,7°/oo) had an organic disease: one with cataracts, not yet discovered and one with a neurologic degeneration, also not discovered earlier.

In another group of 116 children we studied the amount of false negatives; how many children will there be with disorders, not detected by the screening method?

The 116 children were first examined in the standard program, and then, all of them - negatives and positives - had directly afterwards an extensive ophthalmological investigation (retinoscopy and fundoscopy in mydriasis). In this group we found no false negatives; the other results were conform the results of the group of 1200 children.

As the first results of the study were satisfying, we started last year our program in the east of the Netherlands.

The aim is not to examine, as a feasibility study, 6000 children, not living in a town like Amsterdam with Health Centres easy to visit by every mother, but in a region with more widely spread small Health Centres and, for instance, situated in an area where families live rather isolated.

Up till now, 900 children are involved in the study - the results are quite comparable to those of the study of the 1200 Amsterdam children. So this gives us courage to continue and strive for the ultimate: not a special screening, but incorporation of the examination in the routine program of all the Health Centres in The Netherlands, but to reach that, it probably will take some more years.

DISCUSSION

Atkinson: Did you say you thought your cerebral lesions were about 1%? Was that your estimate in the population?

Loewer-Sieger: No, I did't talk about percentage of the frequency of cerebral lesions. I talked about the prevalence of squint in the group of children with these lesions.

Atkinson: Do you have any estimates of the prevalence of cerebral lesions in the population from any of your data?

Loewer-Sieger: Yes, about 1%.

Atkinson: No, I am asking about the children with severe disability?

Loewer-Sieger: No.

Atkinson: If we take cerebral palsy as the measure. What is the size of the group that have both cerebral palsy and a visual problem which you will be picking up in your screening? Is it half your 2% cerebral palsy cases?

Loewer-Sieger: No. They don't all have cerebral palsy, and I don't talk about prevalence of cerebral palsy. I know the number of visual disorders is about 2% in all the children.

Atkinson: If it is 2% of the children, and if half of that population have a squint or visual problem, that is 1%. Do your cerebral palsy cases or severe cerebral lesion cases make up half your series in the population?

Loewer-Sieger: No, I don't think so.

Atkinson: Then I have misinterpreted your figures.

Harcourt: This comes down to whether you are dealing with whole population screening or whether these have been extracted from those who are already known to have physical and mental defects.

Loewer-Sieger: The very seriously handicapped children will not visit the health centre.

Atkinson: Thank you, that is what I wanted to find out because I wanted to know what that percentage was relative to.

Fells: You mentioned the first and the second screening that was carried out at the age of 9 months. Does this mean that all mothers and children are attending twice?

Loewer-Sieger: Not all mothers. When the children are negative in the first screening they don't need to come back. Only if there is doubt are they asked to come back. If they have obvious squints they are referred· after the first session.

Fells: And the 18 months screen. Do you find that is worthwhile? They are so difficult to test.

Loewer-Sieger: When the person is trained in this way of assessment it works.

Kommerell: I think it is the percentage of children in whom the parents have already had some suspicion that there might be something wrong.

Loewer-Sieger: We are not quite sure, but our purpose is not to concentrate on children at risk, because it is known that otherwise you can miss a lot of children, but I can't give an exact answer to that.

Kommerell: Would it be an alternative to advertise on television that parents should consult an eye doctor as soon as they suspect a strabismus in their child?

Loewer-Sieger: But I think the eye doctor will be overloaded with pseudo-strabismus, and our programme is also directed at the prevention of overloading the ophthalmologist.

Hyvarinen: It is the same thing in Finland. If we ask people to come whenever they think that their child has something wrong, we may make people aware of possibilities and have too many patients at their doctor's offices. In Finland ophthalmologists are not very willing to see small children. We get about 40% normals among these referrals and there are several of my colleagues who feel that we should get those out. They don't understand screening, and that we always get some normals.

Warburg: You say that you have no false negatives among the 116. Doesn't that mean that your method is not sensitive enough? Wouldn't you have preferred to have some false negatives? Aren't the 4% that you found too little?

Loewer-Sieger: It is only a rather small group. We don't know the value of the percentage. The epidemiologists told us we could use the figures.

van Lith: It might be from a statistical point of view that the group is too small, because you had 116 children referred to the ophthalmologist, and you had disorder in 1.9% of more than 1000 children, so that a group of 116 is too small. A second point is that you refer everything to the ophthalmologist.

Loewer-Sieger: Perhaps you misunderstood. In the 116 children we found no false negatives. We found 4 or 5 children with squint and one child with hyperopia but we didn't find false negatives. It was so that the orthoptist did not miss anything that I found afterwards on fundoscopy or retinoscopy.

van Lith: Then the group is too small.

Schulz: I should like to know about the ophthalmological investigation afterwards in the 116 cases. Did you do retinoscopy. Our findings in 204 preschool and kindergarten children were that about 5% had a squint or other ocular motility problem. With the same investigations in the kindergarten children we found, including refractive errors, up to 10% of affected children, so if you include refractive errors in the investigation it will be more than that. You don't have the investigation of refractive errors?

Loewer-Sieger: We didn't count refractive errors of less than 2 diopters in this group of 116 children. We found astigmatism and a slight hyperopia but we didn't think that was abnormal.

De Laey: When you have your screening programme, is it associated with your questionnaire? Sometimes we have a form which the parents fill in. I have experience in Belgium and I also have experience as a parent and I find it always very difficult to give good answers to the questions. One of the difficulties, and it might be of importance in a screening programme, is good written questions to parents of children who are to be examined. This is an essential part of the programme. Some information, like the history, might be important, as would the notion of intermittent squints which you will not necessarily pick up by your programme.

Loewer-Sieger: Yes, we asked those questions, but I didn't include these data in this short talk. We have a paper with the questions: are there any doubts about the eyes, is there a family history of eye problems such as squint?

Harcourt: In discussing the false negatives, at what stage is the decision about no false negatives raised? When was the total re-examined?

Loewer-Sieger: We didn't re-examine.

Harcourt: How did you conclude about the complete absence of false negatives?

Loewer-Sieger: We did not perform an ERG or other tests like that. We only performed routine ophthalmological examination the same afternoon.

Harcourt: I think that in clinical practice in children under a year with strabismus, some do have a strabismus with varying angles, but a lot of children of that age have strabismus, and extremely obvious strabismus, and the other group have extremely unobvious strabismus. How do you know that there were no false negatives if the whole group was not re-examined at a later stage? The whole problem about diagnosis of strabismus in this early age group is that there is this group of small angle strabismus, the effects of which may be quite severe. When they are seen later they are often supposed to have been of later onset, but really they have been of very early onset, but were just missed. I think the great problem is to know whether you did have false negatives.

Loewer-Sieger: I think with this screening programme we can detect a small angle of squint and we detect some degree of amblyopia.

Harcourt: With great respect it is open to debate. There are a distressing number of children who are passed as having pseudostrabismus and who eventually turn out to have real strabismus when they are older.

Loewer-Sieger: I won't say that our false negatives are really absolute.

PROBLEMS OF SCREENING AND ITS IMPLICATIONS TO THE ORTHOPTIC SERVICE IN WEST BERKSHIRE

Pauline Bagley

Royal Berkshire Hospital, Reading

INTRODUCTION

An expanding vision screening programme has been developing in West Berkshire, as in many other Health Districts in Great Britain, with the support of Ophthalmologists and other Medical Practitioners. This programme is aimed at children, aged 3½ years, concentrating on orthoptic assessment and acuity testing, usually by single optotypes.

Other assessments occur at 9 months and 18 months, undertaken by Health Visitors, and School Nurses continue the process at varying intervals throughout a child's schooldays.

Parts of the District's population are not receiving the 3½ year screening, although the demand exists. The reasons for not providing total cover are simple, in that the equivalent of 7.8 Orthoptists also have to cover the Orthoptic Training School, Orthoptic Service in four hospitals, and Visual Fields. As a result the present system is being reviewed, to determine whether reorganisation or changing the orthoptic establishment is the solution. This paper is an initial comment on the problems that arise when trying to examine the subject of screening; hence producing questions and no answers.

The projected population in the age group 0-4 for 1985 is 28,800 (6.7% of the population), rising to 32,600 in 1987 (7.4% of the population). At present an average of 18 hours per week are spent screening, excluding travelling time, which is considerable. The Health Authority funds the Orthoptists' time and travelling costs and some of the equipment. The Community funds the organisation of appointments and provides the venues, which are usually Health Centres, although some occur in General Practitioners' practices, which may have cost implications to the G.P.s.

On examination of the system the following questions have arisen:-

1) Is screening necessary?

2) What are the long-term implications of our present
   system in relation to -
   i. The achieved level of visual acuity.
   ii. Orthoptic status (e.g. cosmetic/functional)
   iii. How the V.A. or orthoptic status is achieved.
   iv. How the number of false referrals to the hospital
       are affected.

3) At what age should screening be undertaken?

4) Who should screen?

5) What investigations should be used during the
   assesement, and what are the criteria for referral?

The answer to the first question must be dependent on
resolving aspects of the other questions and ultimately
producing statistically viable information to prove a case.

The long-term implications of screening, especially in
relation to the ultimate levels of visual acuity, may be
confused with the increased awareness of the consequences of
strabismus and anisometropia on visual acuity.   Orthoptists
in West Berkshire, as in many other Health Districts in Great
Britain, participate in teaching programmes for those involved
in child assessment/health, thus resulting in more prompt and
sometimes over referral.   Fewer children with eccentric
fixation are seen other than those with microtropia.   Another
factor to consider if analysing the level of V.A. achieved on
discharge from the Orthoptic/Ophthalmic Department is the cooperation of the child and/or parents with the treatment,
especially in relation to occlusion and the wearing of
glasses.   This is a very difficult aspect to quantify.

The orthoptic status is also a term open to various
interpretations.   What is a good cosmetic appearance?   What
is a functional result?   Retrospective studies on the state
of binocular vision prove to be extremely difficult, due to
different interpretations on what are the most significant
tests.   The criteria for each category needs to be stated, to
ensure the information will be available for future analysis.

Obtaining the V.A. and orthoptic status involves various
factors such as patient/parent co-operation with the
recommended management.   Also, if trying to examine whether
early referral affects the need for surgery, the age at which
surgery is undertaken and the number of operations, then again
the individual Ophthalmologist's, Orthoptist's and parents'
criteria for a "good" cosmetic appearance, and their attitude
to the prescribing and wearing of low to moderate
hypermetropic corrections must be considered.   The various
reasons for further surgery would also have to be taken into
account for a reasonable analysis to be made.

The number of false referrals to the hospital can easily

be quantified (see table 1).   The reduction in numbers have
also occurred in the pre-screened age group;   this may partly
be due to additional "filter" clinics.   Because of our
present inability to provide assessments on all children at
3½, those considered at risk (perhaps because of a strong
family history) or with suspected strabismus are screened
regardless of age.

The age for screening, 3½ years, has been used as the age
at which a visual acuity by single optotypes is visually
obtainable and other orthoptic investigations are possible
(Cameron and Cameron 1978;   MacLellan and Harker 1979).   This
reduces the need for recall.   Any assessment at a younger age
will have its limitations.   The absence of strabismus and an
unobtainable visual acuity without a fundus examination or
refraction produces insufficient evidence to diagnose the
child as ocularly normal.   Therefore, to consider screening
at a younger age will involve other techniques/professionals/
teaching orthoptists new skills.   It will also involve a
large amount of reorganisation within the Community and
financial implications.

The natural history of refractive errors, family history
and other aetiological factors of strabismus will obviously
affect the age at onset (Ingram 1979).   The increase in
referral from the age of 2 years (see table 2) does not
necessarily indicate it is the age from which the defects
develop.   The waiting list for appointments would have to be
taken into account and the age at which the parents first
noticed a defect (often a vague subject).   The older children
are referred frequently because of asymmetry of visual acuity.
Again, a careful analysis of factors needs to be considered to
enable the correct interpretation.

Who should undertake screening?   This is dependent on
the age at which it occurs.   If 3½ years is suitable, then
the ability to undertake rapid and accurate orthoptic
assessments and visual acuity indicate the Orthoptist as the
ideal professional to be involved in Great Britain.   Costs of
such programmes also need to be considered, and Orthoptists'
time is relatively less costly than other professionals' time!

If a younger age is considered, refraction is likely to
be considered as a necessary part of the assessment.   The
practicalities of finding sufficient professionals to
undertake the task, the time and expense of such a programme
would make it unlikely to be accepted in our present economic
climate.   Photo-refraction allows a large number of children
to be assessed in a short space of time, and is probably the
only practical method of implementing such a programme
(Atkinson 1984).

The actual investigations involved in the present
programme include the single optotype Sheridan Gardiner test.
The disadvantages of single optotype tests have been discussed

at length over a period of time, and the availability of
linear matching tests does not totally solve the problem;
many children are confused and lose concentration when
presented with a selection of symbols.   The cover test,
ocular movements, convergence, a stereotest, and overcoming a
base-out 20 dioptre prism are used for orthoptic assessment,
and prove to be sufficient for the purpose and practical for
the age group.   Referral at present occurs if there is an
orthoptic anomaly and difference in acuity of one or more
lines, or defective vision in both eyes.   If the child's cooperation is thought to be a factor in the results, they are
recalled to the screening programme for re-assessment before
hospital referral.   These investigations would have to be
adapted to the capabilities of another age group.

In conclusion, on attempting to review a screening
programme, a number of queries have arisen.   To analyse the
subject correctly, a considerable amount of data needs to be
carefully collected and correctly interpreted;   this is the
next stage to be undertaken.

REFERENCES

Atkinson J, Braddick OJ, Durden K, Watson PG, Atkinson S. Screening for refractive errors in 6-9 month old infants by photorefraction.   Br Orthoptic J 1984;68:105-112.

Cameron JH, Cameron M.   Visual screening of pre-school children.   Br Med J 1978;2:1693-1694.

Ingram RM, Walker C.   Refraction as a means of predicting squint or amblyopia in pre-school siblings of children known to have these defects.   Br J Ophthalmol 1979;63:238-242.

MacLellan AV, Harker P.   Mobile orthoptic service for primary screening of visual disorder in young children.   Br Med J 1979;1:994-995.

DISCUSSION

Harcourt: I think we all have to accept that there is a certain amount of
money available in a country like ours with a National Health Service, out
of which everything has to be done, and money which is used for screening
whole populations of children cannot be used for some other purpose and
therefore the sharing out of the money is a very real problem. There are
obviously pressure groups in every subject who feel that they have a better
case than everybody else. Somewhere there have to be people who make the
hard decisions that the money is used in one direction or another, and it
is no use for a group as mature as this trying to dodge that ultimate
issue. What we have to do is to assess the real significance of what whole
population visual screening of children really can be expected to do, and
that requires hard looking at. For instance, so many per cent of children
have strabismus at age so and so, how much of that (if you excluded the
severely handicapped) would be reduced by screening. How much difference
to the final outcome of strabismus and anisometropic amblyopia if the
disorder is not discovered until a later age when additional screening or
other methods are available? So I think it is a highly complicated thing
that we are talking about. In terms of using orthoptists, the money which
is used is going to be used for that purpose rather than for some other
purpose. Are we going to say that the use of orthoptists is appropriate?
I believe that what Bagley said is perfectly true. They are the people
with the most appropriate skills to do these procedures. They are very
well trained in this country in terms of spotting ocular motility problems,
in terms of doing visual testing in children, so that if you want to use
people of the highest skills, orthoptists are the people to do it. There
are in this country something like 800 orthoptists in practice altogether,
and you have each year about 400,000 children, which means that each
orthoptist would have to be looking at something like 500 children a year
as their part of the work, which is quite a lot of work. What gains we can
see from doing this, and what is going to happen with the sloppy system we
have at the moment? We have to make the best use of the money that is
available.

Dubowitz: I think you are absolutely right, and what I would like to point
out, and what is forgotten is that screening for gross defects can be done
very easily and should be done. It is much easier to do early in the
neonatal period, and that is when it should be done, and should be done by
the houseman in charge of the baby from the neonatal unit. He can use a
red ball and a rattle and will pick up gross defects.

Taylor: You asked the question, is screening necessary? I think you could
take it further and ask what are we screening for? The big question is: do
we really care less about unilateral defects or is it necessary to screen
for unilateral visual defects whether they be amblyopia or cataract or any
other unilateral defect. Now it is very difficult to get any statistics
and we were helped by Tarkkanen from Finland who published in the BJO last
year a paper showing the incidence of disease in the good eye when the bad
eye is amblyopic. They pointed out that in Helsinki they had 35 such cases
in 20 years, 35 in 20 years in a population of 4.5 million when they
reckoned that the number of amblyopes born in those 20 years was 22,000.
Now a uniocular visual disorder, I think you would probably agree, is not a
socially significant disease. It may be irritating for the parents and it
is extremely unfortunate if you lose one eye, but I don't think that we

should be looking at uniocular disease. We should think of the money which is exactly what Harcourt said. It is entirely an economic problem and at the moment I am afraid I know nothing about other European countries; I know a little about America. In the UK the basic structure is badly trained and badly used but it is all there and it costs nothing extra, only needing better training. The neonatal test is the worst eye test of the lot.

Dubowitz: That's right, for hearing all you need is a rattle.

Atkinson: Are you including strabismus in uniocular disease?

Taylor: Yes.

Atkinson: It is important, because the incidence of strabismus is very high. If you are including it, it makes a lot of difference to what you are saying.

Taylor: I think that the social significance of amblyopia, whatever the cause, is that of a uniocular disease.

Braddick: You are not arguing against squints?

Taylor: No, that is another issue altogether.

Warburg: How many retinoblastomas would you lose if you didn't look for monocular visual defects?

Taylor: I am not saying that you should ignore squints.

Warburg: No, you are talking about screening.

Taylor: I would have thought that you would lose very little more than in the situation at the moment.

Jay: Hardly any retinoblastomas are picked up by screening.

Fielder: Retinoblastoma is rare; I have yet to see a case as a primary referral. Screening must be terribly boring. Orthoptists are going to have to do this, but if they have to screen large numbers, is there any way in which 'at risk' groups could be identified, eg retarded children, etc? Also the rather higher prevalence in the lower social classes who are less likely to present at your van. Is there any way you can pick up those at risk by breaking down into cerebral, ex-prematures and those with a family history?

Hyvarinen: I did the very same screening work that nurses do on 220 children last spring and did not find it boring. Many nurses find it interesting because they learn so much more about the children.

Spekreijse: To go back to Fielder's point, there has been preselection in the neonatal period. You get first selection, and how many children, was the question you were asking, had been selected already in the past 9 months. What is left is not much, and is it worthwhile still to go on and do the screening if you have possibilities of selection?

Warburg: If there is a COMAC action on screening it would be quite simple and not very expensive to put in a few visual screening items.

Taylor: And that would be at the right time too.

Warburg: It would be quite sensible to take the screening programme we have heard about for those at risk. But there again we come to economical questions. We might not want to screen all those at risk but only those who are most vulnerable.

Bagley: Where I am working, because we can provide total three and a half year old screening, there is actually a system whereby the health visitors are allowed to refer children at risk in the sense that 'at risk', as far as the parents are concerned, is a family history, and GPs have approved this. The orthoptist goes to the health clinic and she will have 25 or 30 children who are there because the health visitor or the mother suspects. That is far more constructive in terms of referral than going to a normal population and if you talk to the orthoptist she actually feels that is a worthwhile use of her time. If you have restricted facilities, it is the ideal way of trying to get that population. In this country, and in every other, the cost of every visit to the hospital is great. Health visitors get terribly nervous over referring. What is the hospital going to say if she refers a child and it is only an epicanthus? They are vulnerable because they are not trained. They are not going to upset the ophthalmologist but they don't mind upsetting the orthoptist.

Atkinson: When considering the cost of this, the cost that has to be subtracted is every false referral to a hospital clinic that occupies the orthoptists and somebody doing retinoscopy on that child. I don't know whether any of the Europeans here have any estimates of the false referral rate of children who have been referred to hospital at 3 to 5 years and never been found to have a problem, so are true false referrals. One estimate of this cost on a very small sample is that 40% of the under one-year-olds referred to hospital by health visitors, Gps or self referral were pseudostrabismus and have therefore cost the health service about £50 on the first visit, about £80 on the second, and then slightly less for each subsequent visit until that child is discharged at between 3 and 5 years. So it is a very significant cost to the Health Service.

Bagley: We had 52 false referrals in 1984 out of a new case population of 1000 and that has reduced dramatically in the last 10 years. We have done it by the orthoptist teaching the health visitors and the GPs. So if you have GP training, health visitor training, whether by the ophthalmologist or the orthoptist, that is not in this debate. If you educate the people who are seeing these children you will reduce false referrals.

Fells: If you are going to screen, then you must be sure that you are doing it effectively. At present there is a legal case of a child who is now 9 years of age with hopeless amblyopia in one eye who had his eyesight test over a period of two years during which the parents are claiming it was not discovered. So there is now a legal case, which may prove extremely costly, and if you are going to have screening programmes you have got to have them carried out accurately and you have got to be able to give appropriate treatment to the people failing the test.

Warburg: That is not logical because within a screening programme there is the possibility that the screening has not been precise. Otherwise it would be an examination and not a screening, so we expect a screening to have false negatives. If people don't understand that, it is their education that is wrong.

Fells: The children who come to me with late discovered amblyopia, 9 times out of 10, the right eye was tested first at the screening centre. When the screening is done at school at a late stage, the child expects to give right answers, because he knows that right answers please teachers. So you are testing his vision. You test his right eye first. Children at the school screening programme remember the whole list of letters. You cover the right eye. He knows his eyesight in the left eye has been poor since about 4, but he will recite the list of letters which he has remembered because he is trying to give the right answer to please the tester, because that is what you do in school.

Bagley: Again we respond by teaching the school nurses to have at least 5 Snellen charts under their arms, and it works wonders.

Hyvarinen: We do the same thing by having 3 sets of symbols on the VA charts, so we know that the children cannot memorise.

Fielder: There is predeliction for the left eye to be more amblyopic than the right.

Taylor: Can I come back again to the point of the age at which it is done. I put to you that your three and a half year old screening is going to give you a whole bunch of uniocular amblyopes and you try and justify that in economic terms. If you improve the screening of children in the first 6 months of life at least you are achieving much more.

Spekreijse: Yes, I think screening at three and half is silly.

Bagley: So do I, but that is how it is.

Loewer-Sieger: In the Netherlands the orthoptists are much too expensive.
We have the situation where 90% of the children are seen by health doctors,
and they are the people who have the level of intelligence to do it. You
need a few orthoptists to given them instructions and the work is done by
people who are already there.

Spekreijse: That is the kind of practical and economical aspect of it that
has to fit in if it exists.

van Lith: We have not enough orthoptists in Holland anyway.

Louly: At an EEC meeting between ophthalmologists and orthoptists, it was
strongly recommended to include screening programmes in the orthoptists'
field of activity.

Lennerstrand: We have very extensive screening in Sweden. It is done at
the age of 4 years but the age is coming down a bit. It is done in health
care centres by nurses and as a part of testing of other senses and also
other abilities of the child. Visual acuity is tested with Snellen E or an
equivalent to the Sheridan-Gardiner test. The results of visual screening
at 4 years were published a couple of years ago (Kohler L, Stigmar G. Acta
Pediatr Scand 1973; 62 :17 and 1978; 67: 373) and was followed up with the
results from the testing at 7 years in the first school year. The 4 year
screening covers a very high percentage of the children, perhaps 95-100%,
so it is very comprehensive. It is part of the follow-up for children at
the health care centres starting already in the first months of life. Of
course, a test at 4 years of life is late. If the child has a severe
refractive error it can be discovered, and can be treated with some
success.

Spekreijse: If I tried to summarise the different programmes that have
been presented today, I have a feeling the packages are about the same.
But I am surprised how the age at which the package is being presented
differs. We have heard 3 months, 9 months, 3-4 years. What is the basis
for these differences? Is it because it is packages which are also testing
for other senses and therefore vision is only a small part of it?

Lennerstrand: For Sweden that was the starting point.

Bagley: In England it has arisen almost by accident. It was the earliest
age at which orthoptists could get a reasonably complete assessment. You
are having it at 9 or 18 months, but it is done by health visitors as part
of a general assessment of the child's development. It is just that you are
not having anybody who is trained.

Taylor: I think we could learn a lot from people who have taken part in
screening for hearing defects. They seem to have got it right. They
couldn't care less about minor hearing defects, or at least not very much.
They are looking for things that are educationally significant at an early
age.

Dubowitz: There is a bit of controversy about age, 9 months is probably better than 6 months, but hearing is different because it comes and goes, perhaps with respiratory infection. It is not quite a comparable problem.

Atkinson: Can I refer you to the epidemiologist who would say that there is good evidence for stopping the hearing screening from 6 to 9 months because of the false referral rate. So before we start to go into line with the hearing tests that have arisen like Topsy, I think we ought to consider the follow-ups of the hearing test and how valuable it is. It has recently been suggested that it is not a good test or a very sensitive test.

Spekreijse: But the statistics I have seen about the hearing test in Holland have the same false referral figures as for the visual test. That seems to be the number you have to accept and that is not so high.

Loewer-Sieger: Our estimate is that once a month an ophthalmologist will see a child who is quite normal.

Spekreijse: I wouldn't be surprised if it is impossible in a screening programme, with all the restrictions of time and numbers, to get the false referral rate down.

Lee: Taylor has analysed what the risk to the individual person is who has had a unilateral visual defect left alone. They may or may not lose their other eye and it is probably a very small risk. I think it would be interesting from the EEC point of view to know what the risk to everybody else is of one-eyed people running around on the loose. I know that we always say to them, fine you can drive and do all these things. There was a letter in the American Journal of Ophthalmology about 3 years ago suggesting that there was a small trend for one eyed people to be in more serious road traffic accidents. Now they didn't say how they got one eyed, which is the interesting question. Maybe they lost the other eye in a previous road traffic accident. I do think it is a consideration. I happily pat people on the head and tell them to go away. But I don't know for sure, and that is a relevant sociological question within the boundaries of the EEC. Are they actually more dangerous?

Spekreijse: This certainly should be included if you really want to look only at the economical aspects of it.

Harcourt: Taylor left one of the bits out about the statistics, which is that the incidence of injury in the amblyopic population is significantly higher than in the general population. Part of that, as Lee says, is whether amblyopia goes with some sort of neurological defect which may make people slower in co-ordinating.

Taylor: I think what we should be screening for, in the same way as they do for hearing, visual defects which are treatable.

Harcourt: You are quite right. We are not coning down in a pure sensory way, in the way that people who are screening for hearing are. It is a much wider field. And the figures don't really say what percentage of the children who were referred had visual defects proven and what percentage had eyes that just looked in different directions.

Dubowitz: One is a remedial defect. What do we know in vision about minor defects related to education? I think this could be a study, a completely different issue.

van Lith: Concerning amblyopia, years ago in the post office there were people with amblyopia who were not allowed to work. They said that amblyopic people made more mistakes than others.

Taylor: The American Academy has decided definitely no. There is no relationship between amblyopia and dyslexia, or specific learning problems.

RAPID ASSESSMENT OF VISUAL ACUITY IN INFANTS AND CHILDREN IN A CLINICAL SETTING, USING ACUITY CARDS

Gesine Mohn and Jackie van Hof-van Duin

Department of Physiology I, Erasmus Universiteit Rotterdam
P.O.Box 1738, 3000 DR Rotterdam, The Netherlands

INTRODUCTION

The preferential looking technique for assessing visual acuity in infants has over the last ten years produced very consistent results in normal infants across different laboratories, different apparatus and different methods (Teller et al 1974; Dobson and Teller 1978; Mohn and Van Hof-van Duin, this issue). The potential clinical usefulness of the technique for detecting impairments of visual development has been demonstrated by studies of infants with ophthalmological disorders (Jacobson et al 1983; Mohindra et al 1983; Mayer 1985), and infants and also older children with neurological disorders and developmental retardation (Mayer et al 1983; Lennerstrand et al 1983; Mohn and Van Hof-van Duin 1983). Up till now, however, it has not been widely adopted for clinical use. One of the main reasons for this has been the large number of trials and thus time required for a statistically reliable acuity estimate with the standard two-alternative forced-choice (FPL) method employed.

Recently, a more rapid procedure, using so-called acuity cards, was developed by McDonald et al(1985). In this procedure the observer, instead of merely judging the position of the test grating as before, makes a subjective, integrated judgement as to whether the test grating is easy or difficult to see for the infant, or not seen at all. This arose from the observation that infants very often show quite different reactions to gratings of different stripe width. Thus a grating of wide stripes well below the infant's acuity threshold, for example, will often evoke a very clear and prolonged fixation, while near threshold, infants may scan back and forth between test grating and blank, and show a much slighter preference for the grating. Although this sort of information about an infant's reactions is, of course, available to the observer also with the two-alternative forced-choice method, it cannot actually be used in the position judgement made. By explicitly incorporating these cues into the observer's response, and also placing the rate of progression from wide to fine stripes under the observer's control, a subjective estimate of acuity can be reached in three to five minutes with the acuity cards. Binocular acuity estimates obtained by this method in normal infants between 1 and 6 months of age showed very good agreement with those found by standard FPL procedures (McDonald et al 1985).

In this report, we describe our findings and experience with the acuity card procedure in normal and neurologically abnormal infants and children examined in a variety of clinical settings.

SUBJECTS AND METHODS

Binocular and/or monocular acuity was assessed in a total of 218 infants and children divided for clarity into the following categories:

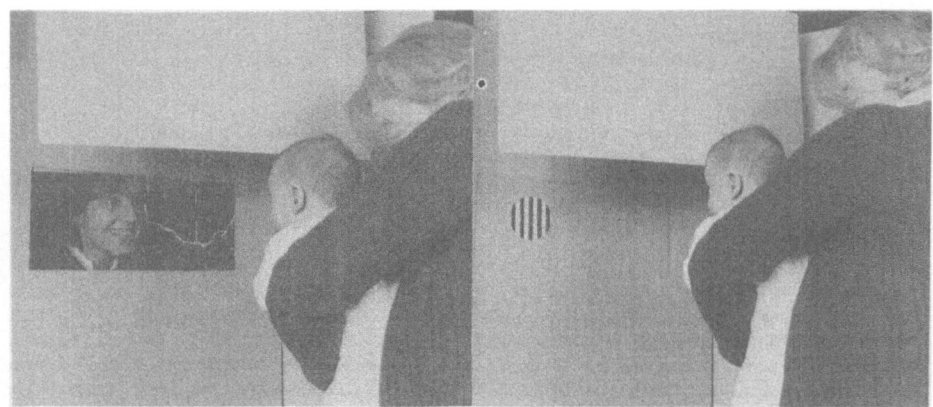

Fig.1:In the acuity card procedure, the observer attracts the infant's attention to the centre of the aperture and then presents one of the acuity cards.

1. Fullterm (n=69) and preterm (n=50) infants with no or only mild perinatal complications and normal neuromotor development, aged between − 3 weeks and 17 months post-term ("corrected age").
2. Fullterm (n=40) and preterm (n=16) infants considered at risk of neurological abnormalities due to perinatal problems such as asphyxia or intracranial hemorrhages, with normal or abnormal neuromotor development, aged between 2 weeks and 20 months from term.
3. Pediatric neurological patients (n=24) with a variety of neurological disorders and usually clear developmental delay, aged between 21 months and 12 years.
4. Severely multiply handicapped patients (n=19) living in a home, aged 16 months to 22 years.

Testing took place in outpatient clinics at the Sophia Children's University Hospital and the Zuiderziekenhuis, Rotterdam, where preterm and fullterm infants came for regular developmental check-ups; at the Department of Physiology I, Erasmus Universiteit Rotterdam, and at the Beatrix-Irene Clinic for multiply handicapped children.

The apparatus used was identical to that of McDonald et al(1985), and consisted of a grey cardboard screen with a large rectangular aperture through which the acuity cards, made from the same cardboard, were presented to the infant at a distance of 40 or 57 cm (Fig.1). The acuity cards are similar in design to those first described by Dubowitz (1980). Each card contained a high-contrast test grating and a "blank" target of very fine, unresolvable stripes, matched to the test grating in colour and mean luminance, with a peephole for the observer in the centre between the two targets. The stripe width of the test gratings could vary between 2.5 degrees and 1.25' (0.2 to 24 cycles/degree) in approximately half-octave steps. In each trial, the infant's attention was first attracted to the centre of the aperture by the observer (Fig.1), and then the card was presented, lending a peek-a-boo game character to the procedure. Starting with a grating well below the normal acuity age norm of the infant, cards with gratings of decreasing stripe width were presented in rapid succession, often using 1-octave steps initially, until the region of the acuity threshold appeared to be reached. At this point, the infant was shown a grating near or at threshold in alternation with a grating 0.5 octaves finer, and judged to be above threshold, at least 6 times each. During these trials, the observer usually presented the cards without knowing the test grating's position, and then reversed the card on the second presentation to check if the infant's fixation changed accordingly, thus incorporating a position judgement into the procedure.

Acuity was assessed binocularly in 210 infants and children; monocular acuity estimates for both eyes were obtained in 50 infants and children. In 19 children, both the acuity cards and a standard FPL procedure described previously (Mohn and Van Hof-van Duin 1983) were used to assess acuity in the same test session.

RESULTS

The results of binocular acuity assessments in the normal fullterm and preterm infants are shown in Fig. 2, in comparison to the mean acuity we obtained in similar groups of infants with the FPL procedure (Mohn and Van Hof-van Duin, this volume). In both preterm and fullterm infants there is clearly very good agreement between the results of the two procedures, with a tendency, particularly in fullterm infants, for acuity card estimates to lie above the mean FPL acuity from 4-6 months onward.

Direct comparisons of acuity estimates obtained in infants tested with both procedures are shown in Fig.3. Again, the close agreement between acuity cards and FPL is evident. The difference was never more than one octave and usually half an octave or less, which is no more than the normal variability found within the standard FPL procedure. No consistent trend for acuity card estimates to be higher than FPL values was seen in these direct comparisons. However, the acuity card procedure did seem to increase testability. Of 7 further children in whom testing with both FPL and the card procedure was attempted, five could not be interested in FPL, which was always tried first, but could be tested successfully with the acuity cards. The peek-a-boo aspect of the acuity card procedure also proved very successful with children of the notoriously difficult age of 1-2 years. Of 50 children in this age group in whom testing was attempted, 47 could be tested successfully, with the results either within the normal acuity range, or lower in children with neurological or ophthalmological disorders. The remaining three children were all neurologically abnormal; two showed no fixation even of the widest stripe width presented.

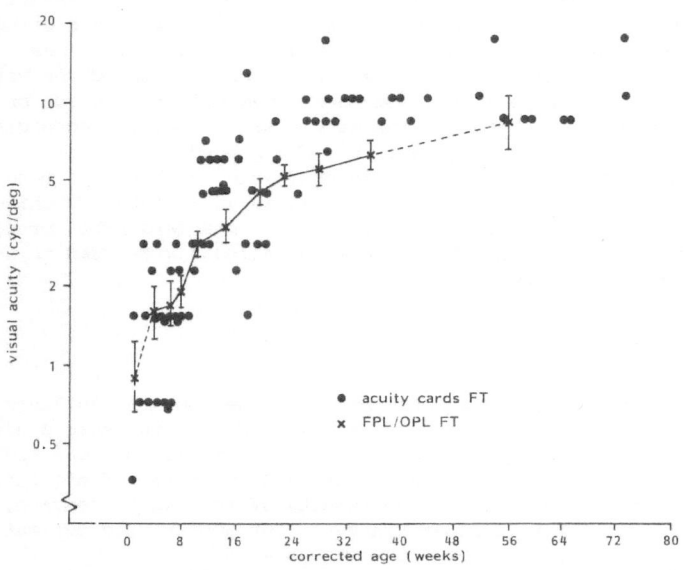

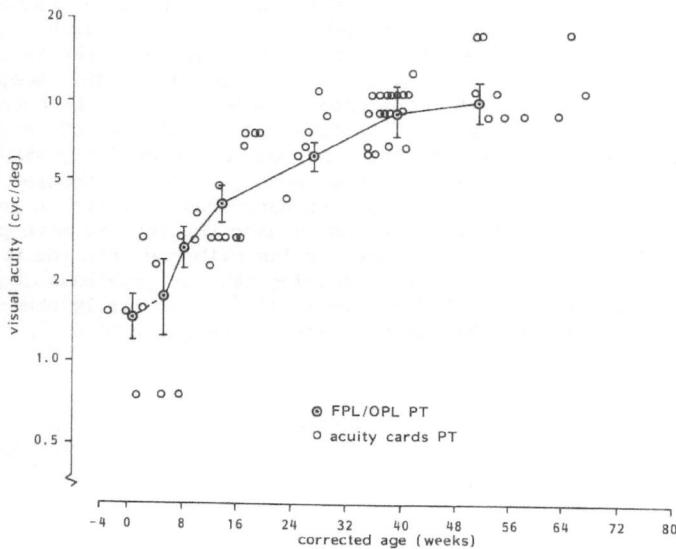

Fig.2: Individual acuity estimates obtained with acuity card procedure in normal fullterm (above) and preterm (below) infants, compared to the mean FPL-acuity found for similar groups of infants in our laboratory.

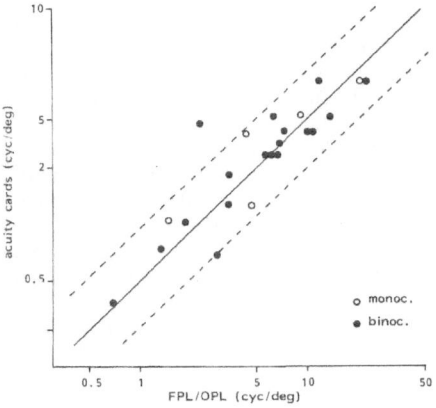

Fig.3 Relation between acuity esti-mates obtained with the acuity cards and an FPL procedure in infants tested with both methods. Points falling on the solid diago-nal line would show perfect agree-ment between the 2 procedures; the stippled lines indicate one octave (factor 2) difference in acuity estimates.

Fig.4: Relation between acuity esti-mates in the right and left eyes of 50 infants and children. Identical values fall on the solid diagonal line; the stippled lines indicate an interocular acuity difference of one octave.

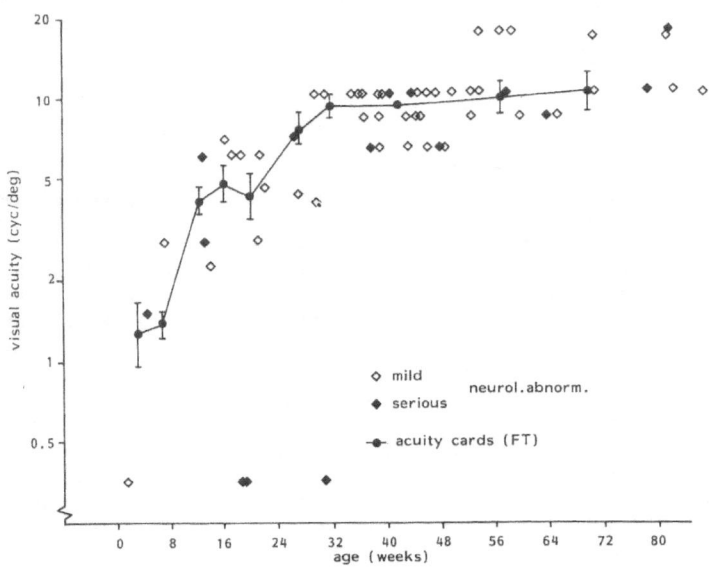

Fig.5: Acuity estimates obtained in infants at risk of abnormal development due to perinatal complications, with normal or abnormal neurological development at the time of testing. The line gives the mean acuity of normal fullterm infants tested with the acuity card procedure.

Monocular acuity estimates in infants and children with no ophthalmological disorder or alternating convergent stabismus were very similar to binocular estimates, both in normal and neurologically abnormal children. The relation between acuity of the right and the left eye in the 50 children tested is shown in Fig.4. Children with no ophthalmological disorder or alternating strabismus usually had equal or very similar acuities in the two eyes; interocular differences of more than 0.5 octave were seen in one normal infant, 5 children with alternating strabismus and a fixation preference for the eye with better acuity, and one child with psychomotor retardation. In children with ocular disorders like albinism, a corneal opacity, coloboma etc., the interocular acuity difference was always in the expected direction except in an albino infant with no diagnosed cause of the interocular difference.

Results obtained in the infants at risk of abnormal neurological development are shown in Fig.5.

The infants were divided into those with normal or mildly abnormal neuromotor development, and those with serious neurological disorders like hydrocephalus, hemi- or quadriplegia, or clear developmental retardation. The great majority of these infants had normal acuities, including 6 infants with hydocephalus of whom 4 had received a ventriculo-peritoneal drain. Very poor acuity was found in an infant with severe pneumobronchial dysplasia and an infant with clear developmental delay.

Of the 24 patients with neurological disorders and 19 severely multiply handicapped patients, only one could not be tested successfully due to insufficient cooperation. Four children did not fixate even the widest stripes. In the remaining children, acuity varied clearly with the severity of the neurological disorder and psychomotor retardation, as well as occasional ophthalmological defects, with normal or near-normal acuities only in children with mild neurological symptoms.

DISCUSSION

The acuity card procedure used in the present study differed in three aspects from that described by McDonald et al (1985). Firstly, the minimum difference in stripe width between test gratings was decreased to half an octave, as opposed to the octave steps originally used. This was felt to considerably increase the sensitivity of the acuity estimates, and may also have reduced the variability of the results. Secondly, gratings with very fine stripes rather than grey cardboard were used for the blank targets, which reduced the possibility that the children might react to differences in colour rather than stripewidth between the test grating and blank. Initial observations with cardboard blanks suggested that the danger of colour differences being used was particularly great in older children eager to do well in the test, but the possibility obviously cannot be excluded also in younger children. Thirdly, in the study by McDonald et al (1985), the observer was blind to the stripewidth of the test grating, knowing only that stripewidth decreased with successive cards, while in the present study the observer was allowed to know the stripwidth, although in practice this was often neglected for time-serving reasons. The good agreement in the acuity estimates obtained in normal infants in the present and the earlier study suggests that this procedural difference had little effect on the results. Finally, several neurological patients were tested without the large screen by holding up the cards alone at the appropriate distance. In general, however, the screen was felt to be useful for preventing the child from being distracted from the test.

The results of the present study indicate that acuity estimates obtained in normal infants with the acuity card procedure are in close agreement with those found with standard FPL/OPL procedures, confirming and extending the find ings of McDonald et al(1985). Binocular acuity in normal fullterm and preterm infants up to 1.5 years was very similar to that of infants of similar ages tested with FPL procedures in our and other laboratories (Atkinson et al 1977; Allen 1979;Gwiazda et al 1980; Mayer and Dobson 1982; Birch et al 1983; Mohn and van Hof-van Duin, this volume). The finding that between the ages of 4-12 month s, estimates obtained with acuity cards often lay above the mean FPL acuity of this age range might suggest a motivating effect of the peek-a-boo game of the card procedure, but more data are needed to confirm this trend. Direct comparisons of acuity card and FPL/OPL acuity estimates in individual infants showed no consistent advantage of the acuity cards, but again indicated very close agreement between the resulst obtained with the two procedures. The peek-a-boo game did increase testability, although not necessarily the acuity estimate found, in infants between one and two years of age, who are notoriously difficult to test even with operant preferential looking techniques (OPL) (Mayer et al 1982; Birch et al 1983).

Interocular acuity differences seen with monocular testing were little more than 0.5 octave in normal children and many children with alternating strabismus, suggesting that a difference of one octave in acuity estimates between the two eyes may be an indication of a true interocular difference. More data will need to be collected, however, before such a limit , which can also vary with age, can be set with any certainty. The variability of the results was on the whole similar to that of other studies of monocular acuity using acuity cards or FPL procedures (McDonald, personal communication; Atkinson et al 1982; Dobson 1983).

The results obtained in the high risk infants and neurological patients indicate that the acuity card procedure can be used as successfully in patients as in normal infants. Both in normal and in neurologically abnormal infants and children, the success rate of testing was practically 100%. Out of the total of 218 children tested, only one severely retarded patient could not be tested successfully due to lack of cooperation.

The great majority of the infants at risk or with evident neurological disorders, showed normal visual acuity for age. Observations in high-risk preterm infants, using FPL for acuity assessment, suggest that acuity is often below normal in these infants up to the corrected age of approximately 4 months, even when neurological development is normal (Mohn and van Hof-van Duin, this volume). Not enough patients below 4 months of age were tested with acuity cards to allow a comparison; however, from 4 months onward, acuity was normal as in the preterm infants tested by FPL.

In the older neurological patients, acuity was very often below normal or very poor, and varied with ophthalmological disorders and the severity of psychomotor retardation, as previously described in FPL/OPL studies of similar patient populations (Lennerstrand et al 1983; Mayer et al 1983; Mohn and van Hof-van Duin 1983). Testing patients with severe psychomotor retardation often took somewhat longer than the 3-5 minutes usual in normal infants, but generally did not exceed 10 minutes. In addition, because such patients' gaze and fixation patterns are very often unclear and difficult to judge due to spontaneous nystagmus or strabismus, the observers' confidence in the accuracy of the acuity estimate was frequently lower than with normal children. In such cases,the grating position judgement of the FPL procedure was often used more extensively than with normal children as a means of reassuring the observer about her/his assessment of the patients's reaction; if position could not be judged reliably, the grating was asssumed to be unresolvable to the child. Even though the true acuity threshold may not have been reached in some of these patients, the estimate obtained was nevertheless felt to give a useful indication of the child's visual capacity, which often could not have been assessed in any other way.

In conclusion, we found the acuity card procedure to yield results wholly comparable to those of standard FPL procedures in normal infants, while test duration was shorter and testability often better. The findings in infants and children with neurological disorders indicate that the procedure is equally successful in these patients, and a very promising tool for use in clinical conditions.

ACKNOWLEDGEMENTS

We are grateful to the staff and their coworkers at the Infant Vision Laboratory, Univ. of Washington, for providing the acuity cards, and initial experience with the procedure in their laboratory. We thank F.Groenendaal, H.Frenkel and A.Evenhuis- van Leunen, who assisted with testing of the infants. Our thanks also go to the staff of the Dept. of Neonatology, Sophia Children's University Hospital, the Dept. of Pediatrics, Zuiderziekenhuis, and the Beatrix-Irene Clinic, Rotterdam, for their friendly cooperation. B.Weijers built several testing screens and A.Gispen-van Dobbenburgh typed the manuscript.

REFERENCES

Allen JL. The development of visual acuity in human infants during the early postnatal weeks. PhD Dissertation, Univ.Washington, Seattle 1979.

Atkinson J, Braddick O, Moar K. Development of contrast sensitivity over the first 3 months of life in the human infant. Vision Res 1977b;17:1037-44.

Atkinson J, Braddick O, Pimm-Smith E. "Preferential looking" for monocular and binocular acuity testing of infants. Br J Ophthalmol 1982b;66:264-68.

Birch EE, Gwiazda J, Bauer JAJr, Naegele J, Held R. Visual acuity and its meridional variations in children aged 7 to 60 months. Vision Res 1983;23:1019-24.

Dobson V. Clinical applications of preferential looking measures of visual acuity. Behav Brain Res 1983;10:25-39.

Dobson V, Teller DY. Visual acuity in human infants: A review and comparison of behavioural and electrophysiological studies. Vision Res 1978;18:1469-83.

Dobson V, McDonald MA, Teller DY. Visual acuity of infants and young children: Forced -choice Preferential Looking procedures. Am Orthoptic J

1985;in press

Dubowitz D. Portable version of Fantz box for assessment of visual function. The Lancet 1980;1:1279-80.

Gwiazda J, Brill S, Mohindra I, Held R. Preferential looking acuity in infants from two to fifty-eight weeks of age. Am J Optomet Physiol Opt 1980;57:428-32.

Jacobson SG, Mohindra I, Held R. Age of onset of amblyopia in infants with esotropia. Doc Ophthalmol Proc Ser 1981;30:210-16.

Jacobson SG, Mohindra I,Held R. Monocular visual form deprivation in human infants. Doc Ophthalmol 1983;55:199-211.

Lennerstrand G, Axelsson A, Andersson G. Visual testing with "preferential looking" in mentally retarded children. Behav Brain Res 1983;10:199-203.

Mayer DL, Dobson V. Visual acuity development in infants and young children as assessed by operant preferential looking. Vision Res 1982;22:1141-52.

Mayer DL, Fulton AB, Hansen RM. Preferential looking acuity obtained with a staircase procedure in pediatric patients. Invest Ophthalmol Vis Sci 1982;23:538-43.

Mayer DL, Fulton AB, Sossen PL. Preferential looking acuity of pediatric patients with developmental disabilities. Behav Brain Res 1983;10:189-99.

Mayer DL, Fulton AB, Hansen RM. Visual acuity of infants and children with retinal degenerations. Ophthal Ped Gen 1985; in press.

McDonald MA, Dobson V, Sebris L, Baitch L, Varner D, Teller DY. The acuity card procedure: a rapid test of infant acuity. Invest Ophthalmol Vis Sci 1985; in press.

Mohindra I, Jacobson SG, Held R. Binocular visual form deprivation in human infants. Doc Ophthalmol 1983;55:237-49.

Mohn G, Van Hof-van Duin J. Behavioural and electrophysiological measures of visual functions in children with neurological disorders. Behav Brain Res 1983;10:177-89.

Mohn G, Van Hof-van Duin J. Preferential looking acuity in normal and neurologically abnormal infants and pediatric patients. 1985; this volume.

Teller DY, Morse R, Borton R, Regal D. Visual acuity for vertical and diagonal gratings in human infants. Vision Res 1974;14:1433-39.

Van Hof-van Duin J, Mohn G. Visual field measurements, optokinetic nystagmus and the visual threatening response: normal and abnormal development. 1985; this volume.

Van Hof-van Duin J, Mohn G, Fetter WPF, Mettau JW and Baerts W. Preferential looking acuity in preterm infants. Behav Brain Res 1983;10:47-51.

TO WHAT EXTENT IS IT POSSIBLE TO QUANTIFY MONOCULAR OR BINOCULAR VISUAL
IMPAIRMENT IN PRE-VERBAL CHILDREN? ROLE OF CLINICAL SIGNS AND OF
ELECTROPHYSIOLOGICAL AND PSYCHOPHYSICAL TESTING TECHNIQUES

Emilio C. Campos, M.D.

Department of Ophthalmology
University of Modena
Modena, Italy

INTRODUCTION

In the last decade or so there has been a growing interest to set up
techniques evaluating visual function in pre-verbal children.
Essentially, visual evoked responses (VER), preferential looking (PL)
techniques, and optokinetic nystagmus (OKN) have been used to obtain
quantitative information. All these techniques have been instrumental in
obtaining data on the development and the process of plasticity of the
visual system. The information obtained in this manner is of utmost
importance for establishing the functional prognosis for certain
conditions, e.g., congenital cataracts, strabismic amblyopia.

Clinical signs, whose observations provide inference on visual
function, can be easily employed as well. From the practical viewpoint,
the question arises of when the information provided by clinical signs is
sufficient or when more sophisticated testing techniques of visual
function should be utilized.

CLINICAL SIGNS

Clinical signs will be briefly reviewed first.

1. Strabismus. If a manifest non-alternating strabismus is present, one
can safely infer that the deviated eye is amblyopic. If the strabismus is
alternating, almost equal visual acuity in the two eyes should be
expected. In the presence of congenital strabismus, normal binocular
vision is absent. The same happens for early onset strabismus (before age
one) or for those types of strabismus which take place later in life
(between 1 and 5 years of age) which are not treated immediately.

Sometimes a manifest strabismus is not cosmetically evident. In this
case some information can be gained by: (a) observing the symmetry of
corneal light reflexes; in strabismus the corneal reflex of the deviated
eye is shifted nasalward (exotropia) or temporalward (esotropia). (b) If
a cover-test elicits refixation movements, ocular misalignement is
present. (c) The Irvine 4 prism diopters test is particularly applicable
in the case of microstrabismus. However, this test requires that the baby
is able to maintain fixation for a few seconds. A 4 diopters base-out
prism is put in front of one eye. A saccadic movement in the direction
opposite to the base of the prism takes place in the two eyes if the
subject has central fixation in the eye with the prism in front of it. In

the presence of normal fusional vergences, i.e., normal binocular vision, a vergence movement in the opposite direction follows the saccade. If this vergence movement is absent, the test is pathological and a strabismus can be inferred. However, the 4 diopters test occasionally provides false normals and false pathological responses (de Decker et al, 1984). (d) Obviously ocular motility should be tested. (e) Fixation with the visuscope can be examined as early as 3 months of age. If it is central, a good functional prognosis can be expected. (f) Finally, covering the only seeing eye provokes an immediate crying reaction in the baby. No reaction is elicited by covering the non-seeing eye.

2. Presence of amblyogenic conditions. They include monolateral ptosis, corneal opacities, monolateral and bilateral cataracts, vitreous pathologies. These conditions can be detected by simple observation or with ophthalmoscopy (a cataract is amblyogenic when it is impossible to observe the macula with an ophthalmoscope).

3. Presence of causes of organic amblyopia. These include macular and optic nerve pathologies. Obviously, ophthalmoscopy is the appropriate way for their detection. An abnormal (Marcuss Gunn phenomenon) or lacking pupillary light reflex should direct towards more thorough examination.

4. Nystagmus. The presence of nystagmus itself is a cause of bilateral amblyopia when there is no position of rest. Ocular nystagmus can be neuro-muscular or sensory in origin. The first one is generally jerky, whereas the second one is pendular, although mixed forms can be found. Any condition which prevents the development of visual acuity higher than 6/30 bilaterally, causes a sensory nystagmus, if the cause is effective before the second year of life. In fact the fixation reflex does not develop. Although no definite data are available from the literature, we have observed that sensory nystagmus does not develop before five months of age. Typically, sensory nystagmus is due to bilateral congenital cataracts (treatable condition) or to bilateral optic atrophy (untreatable condition).

Summarizing, clinical signs qualitatively detect visual acuity differences between the two eyes and allow the decision to be made of whether a visual acuity is higher or lower than 6/30. They also provide information on the presence or absence of normal binocular vision.

ELECTROPHYSIOLOGICAL AND PSYCHOLOGICAL TECHNIQUES

Turning our attention to the more sophisticated testing techniques, i.e., VER, PL and OKN, their primary importance rests on the insite they provide on development of visual functions. Essentially, through them we know that:

I. Visual acuity develops in the first 6-8 months of life from 6/600 to 6/6. It can decrease and not be restored if the cause of its reduction is not immediately eliminated, until 6-7 years of age.

II. Binocular vision is present as early as 3-4 months of age. In fact depth perception can be detected by means of VER and PL. The plastic period for binocular vision lasts until 8-10 years of age.

VER, PL, OKN can provide quantitative information on visual function that is impossible to obtain with the use of clinical signs. Some drawbacks in the clinical application of the above mentioned techniques should be considered.

VER: Although the results are easily repeatable, no narcosis is necessary, and technicians can perform the examination, the instrumentation is quite expensive both in selling price and the maintenance. Also, a VER does not always correspond to visual acuity, as found with psychophysical investigations (typically with an optotype). In fact, it tells us only that the visual system is <u>potentially</u> able to resolve details corresponding to given characteristics of the stiumulus. Higher and more complex cortical association functions which provide the end-result of visual acuity are untested with VER. Finally, VER have been found to be present in cortical blindness.

PL: The instrumentation is not expensive. However, well-trained technicians have to be employed and examinations are quite time-consuming. Monocular testing is often technically very difficult in newborn children. It is also not clear whether PL strictly corresponds to visual acuity. In short, PL has not entered into the armamentarium of testing techniques for visual function in clinical set-ups.

OKN: This is the easiest and cheapest technique. It can be performed in an office or in a nursery. If an OKN is elicited, a given visual resolution threshold can be safely inferred. The OKN can be absent because the attention of the child is not maintained on the drum or because the OKN mechanism maturation is not completed. Besides, low resolution values may not be necessarily foveal but peripheral retinal responses. The OKN is most useful for comparing the visual function of the two eyes during the course of treatment (e.g. of amblyopia).

Generally speaking, aside from some pitfalls, VER is the most reliable and clinically acceptable technique for obtaining refined quantitative information on visual function. OKN also provides quantitative information, which is, nevertheless, less refined and accurate. It can therefore be used as a first approximation for routine clinical evaluations.

The last question to be addressed is when is it clinically useful to have quantitative information on visual function, which can only be obtained with VER (or PL)? I have been using, mainly for research purposes, all the above mentioned techniques. My judgement is therefore not biased by incompetence or lack of knowledge, and I can safely state that in the vast majority of cases clinical signs will suffice for deciding whether a child sees or whether function differences exist between the two eyes. In essence, this is what is needed for making the diagnosis and giving the appropriate information to the parents.

VER are most useful for assessing differences in visual function between the two eyes, when the clinical signs give dubious responses. They are also of great importance for following in time improvement (due to treatment) and deterioration (e.g., in case of macular dystrophies) of visual function. Finally, used in the flash mode, VER can provide <u>qualitative</u> information on the function of the visual pathway in children with opaque media, which may need surgery (corneal opacities, cataracts, vitreous alterationS). The fact that visual function is not accurately quantitized does not generally negatively influence our diagnosis or

treatment capabilities: as often happens, certain types of investigations
are "a la page," and if you did not perform or order them, you may be
underestimated by colleagues and patients alike. Too often, when a VER is
requested, the specific question is put on the level of visual acuity.

The VER response, as said, can be compatible with a given acuity, but
cannot be considered to correspond to it! I strongly believe that refined
testing in a clinical environment should be performed only if the benefit
for the patient is clearly demonstrable. Obviously, this should not
interfere with the need of using sophisticated techniques for research
purpose. The ophthalmologist involved in this type of research must play
a double role and see himself on one side as a researcher and on the other
as a a physician.

SUMMARY

Clinical signs suggesting impaired visual function in pre-verbal
children are discussed. They include observation of the eye alignment and
of nystagmus, occlusion test, cover-test, Irvine 4 prism diopter test,
ophthalmoscopy and refraction. Qualitative judgements are normally
possible in this way. Visual Evoked Responses (VER), Preferential Looking
techniques (PL) and Optokinetic Nystagmus (OKN) provide quantitative
information. Advantages and pitfalls of these methods for clinical use
are considered. VER is the technique which is advisable for clinical
puroposes.

Finally, an attempt is made to answer the question of the necessity
of quantitative information on visual function for clinical judgements.

REFERENCES

Campos E.C.: Some thoughts on visual function testing in newborn babies.
In: Francois J., Maione M. eds. Pediatric Ophthalmology. Chichester: John
Wiley and Sons, 1982:333-335.

Campos E.C., Chiesi C.: Critical analysis of visual function evaluating
techniques in newborn babies. Int. Ophthal. 1985. In press.

de Decker W., Bagolini B., Campos E.C., Dannheim E., Haase W., Noorden von
G.K.: What do we investigate by the four prism diopter test. In: Gregersen
E. ed. Trans European Strabismological Association 14th Meeting.
Copenhagen; 1984:215-227.

POPULATION VISION SCREENING AND INDIVIDUAL VISUAL ASSESSMENT

Janette Atkinson, Oliver Braddick

Visual Development Unit, Department of Experimental Psychology,
University of Cambridge

INTRODUCTION

Testing of vision in early childhood may be undertaken for two rather
different reasons. In vision screening, a large group of the population,
in whom vision problems have not yet been identified or suspected, are
tested to pick up the subgroup who either have a manifest vision problem,
or who show precursors which place them at risk of developing such a
problem. In visual assessment, tests are conducted with a relatively
small number of children who have already come to the attention of the
medical services. An assessment of their visual function is needed either
to guide diagnosis and treatment, or to assess the implications of a
visual disorder for the child's development and capabilities. Of course,
assessment and screening should be considered as an integrated service in
the sense that children who fail a screening test will require follow-up
with a fuller visual assessment. However, screening and assessment lead
to very different requirements for the tests to be used.

Because a screening test has to be applied to large numbers of
children, it is not economically practical to use a test which requires
highly skilled personnel, or even more than a few minutes of the time of
paramedical staff. Furthermore, since the great majority of children will
yield negative results, parents cannot be expected to make large invest-
ments of time and effort to participate; in particular, they will not
generally be willing to travel far, so tests must be excluded which depend
on expensive specialized equipment that can only be installed at a few
centres. Acceptability to families is important since, ethical issues
aside, anything which dimishes participation in a screening programme
reduces its value.

A screening test must be inexpensive and simple, but the follow-up of
positive or doubtful cases is likely to be more elaborate and time
consuming. It is therefore important that the screening test should yield
clear cut rather than 'doubtful' results in the vast majority of cases,
and that the number of 'false positives' should be small. False positives
incur not only the costs to the service of follow up, but also unnecessary
anxiety and inconvenience to the patient's family.

In our group we have experience of a variety of behavioural and
electrophysiological tests which can give information on acuity and binocular function in infancy. However, none of these have the simplicity,
portability, or ease for general health care personnel which have been
described above as criteria for a screening test. Furthermore, it is our
view that under the likely conditions of a screening programme they would
not yield a satisfactorily low proportion of doubtful, false positive, or
false negative results. Therefore, with presently available techniques we

are sceptical that there is any value in using acuity or binocular vision testing as a screening procedure in the first 3 years of life. This view is reinforced by the fact that many impairments one might wish to detect are monocular and that monocular acuity testing in infancy is more than twice as arduous as binocular.

In contrast, the technique of isotropic photorefraction (Atkinson et al, 1981a) allows refractive errors to be detected by orthoptic staff operating readily portable equipment after a modest period of training. We have therefore been using this instrument in a trial programme of population refractive screening for 6-9 month infants. This screening programme, and its evaluation in terms of diagnostic and predictive utility, are discussed below.

Compared to screening, visual assessment is required for a very much smaller number of children, in all of whom there are good grounds for suspecting visual impairment. A much greater investment of effort in each case is therefore feasible and justified. Diagnosis, decisions on treatment, and advice on education or rehabilitation all require a global picture of the child's visual capabilities, and so a range of tests is needed, related to distinct visual functions. Patients can come to a central assessment unit and so sophisticated equipment and specialist personnel can be used if necessary. While a screening test must end in a categorical decision (to refer or not), the outcome of assessment is a much fuller quantitative and qualitative description. The issue of 'false positives' does not arise in the same form: the aim of assessment is to provide the best estimate available of the child's visual function, with any uncertainties that may be present explicitly stated.

In assessment, therefore, tests of monocular and binocular acuity, accommodation, refraction, oculomotor function, binocularity, and central visual function may all be appropriate, the exact combination depending on the reasons why the child has been referred. Quite separately from our screening programme, we have undertaken visual assessment on a range of infants and young children referred because of paediatric or ophthalmological problems; our procedures and goals in such assessments are outlined in a later section.

INFANT REFRACTIVE SCREENING PROGRAMME

One goal of a screening programme is to detect conditions that are manifest but have not otherwise come to the attention of health services. Another goal may be to identify children who, although they may not have a problem which impairs vision at the time of screening, are 'at risk' of developing such a problem. The screening will have its greatest value if it is possible to provide treatment for the 'at risk' group to prevent the later onset of a visual problem.

In the context of refractive screening, a group which may be at risk are infants having a moderate to high degree of hypermetropia. Such hypermetropia in infancy has been found to have a high correlation with later onset of strabismus and amblyopia (Ingram et al, 1979). The existence of a correlation does not answer whether this link is causal, with the excessive accommodation needed to overcome hypermetropia leading to overconvergence and thereby strabismus, or whether hypermetropia and strabismus are associated for some other reason. If the strabismus is of accommodative origin, then the detection of hypermetropia in refractive screening could allow prescription of a spectacle correction to reduce accommodation and thus prevent development of strabismus. Our refractive screening programme therefore includes a randomised controlled trial of partial refractive correction of infant hypermetropia as a preventive measure for preschool strabismus and amblyopia.

The photorefractive screening programme for 6-9 month infants, currently underway in Cambridge and Bristol, has a number of aims:

1. Early identification of refractive errors and strabismus.
2. Investigation of the predictive value of refractive screning for later visual disorders.
3. Study of the natural history of development of refraction.
4. Test of prevention of strabismus and amblyopia by spectacle correction in a randomised controlled trial.
5. Evaluation of the acceptability of photorefraction in the context of community screening.

The procedure for the screening and follow-up has been described in some detail in Atkinson et al (1984), as have some of the early results, so only a brief summary, under the above headings, will be presented here.

1. Early detection of refractive errors and strabismus

Figure 1 shows the refractive errors identified in Cambridge and Bristol in the initial period of the screening. The two populations look very similar: 5% have a significant degree of hypermetropia while myopes and anisometropes are each 1-2%. Partial analysis of a longer period of screening in Cambridge generally confirms the incidence of hypermetropia (4% of 3141 infants now screened) and of other refractive errors. The orthoptic examination carried out alongside photorefraction found a very small incidence of manifest strabismus in this age group, representing strabismus of early onset in considerably less than 1% of the population. We presume that in the majority of preschool children with strabismus the onset must be after one year of age.

2. Predictive value of refractive screening

The regular follow-up examinations of children identified with abnormal refractions at 6-9 months have been described in detail by Atkinson et al (1984). All those followed up have an examination of the fundus when first referred, and an orthoptic examination on every visit. We monitor acuity (using preferential looking on younger children) and accommodation (using noncycloplegic photorefraction). A child who at any stage is found to be strabismic or amblyopic is referred for the appropriate ophthalmological care immediately.

As well as the children with refractive errors, one control infant with normal refraction is selected for every hypermetrope detected. This control group is also followed up, in order that the incidence of later visual problems may be compared between infants who have refractive errors at 6-9 months and those who do not.

At the end point of our programme at 3 1/2 years of age each child who has been followed up is assessed to see whether vision is normal or abnormal. We use the Sheridan Gardiner single optotype test and a development using the same letters in a 'crowded' form (Atkinson et al, in prep.). From studies of visually normal children at this age we take a single optotype acuity of 6/6, and 6/9 on our crowded test, as acceptable performance. If any child fails to show these levels of acuity initially their refraction is rechecked, and the child retested with any new spectacle correction that may be required. Any child who fails to show 'normal acuity' on two such tests is considered amblyopic. We also test for normal binocularity using the TNO stereo test.

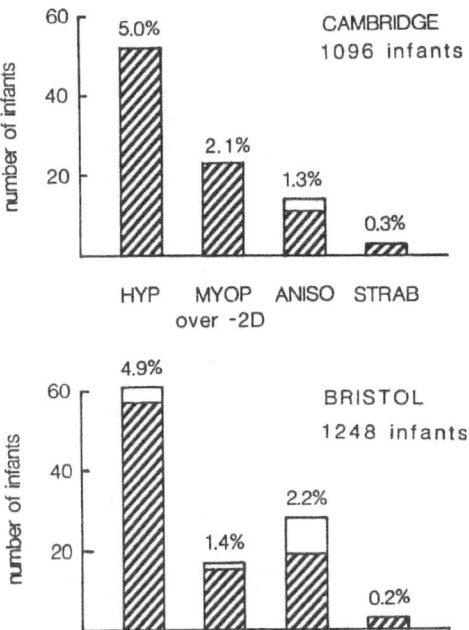

Figure 1. Refractive errors found in photorefractive screening at 6-9 months of age: initial data from Cambridge and Bristol programmes. HYP = hypermetropia +4 D or greater in at least one axis. MYOP = myopia -2 D or greater in at least one axis. ANISO = 1.5 D or greater difference between corresponding axes in the two eyes. STRAB = manifest strabismus. Shaded areas = refractive errors confirmed by subsequent retinoscopy.

The first hypermetropes detected in the Bristol and Cambridge screening programmes, and their control cases, have now reached the age of 3 1/2 years and completed these tests. Tables 1 and 2 show the percentage of these groups who are normal on our acuity and binocularity tests at 3 1/2 years. This is true for nearly all the controls but for very few of the hypermetropes. Thus from these early results it does appear that refractive errors picked up in infant screening are indeed an effective predictor of later visual problems. The relation of these results to refractive correction is discussed below.

Table 1. CAMBRIDGE SCREENING: HYPERMETROPES (N=22) AND CONTROLS (N=26) WHO HAD REACHED 3 1/2 YEARS BY NOVEMBER 1984

	Abnormal on :		
	acuity		binocular vision
	single	multiple	
hypermetropes	68%	83%	18%
controls	4%	7%	0%

Table 2. BRISTOL SCREENING PROGRAMME: HYPERMETROPES (N=58) AND CONTROLS (N=88) WHO HAD REACHED 3 1/2 YEARS BY NOVEMBER 1984

	Abnormal on acuity (single letter) and/or binocular vision
Hypermetropes	71%
Controls	6%

Table 3. REFERRALS SO FAR TO REGULAR EYE CLINIC FOR TREATMENT FROM ALL STAGES OF CAMBRIDGE SCREENING

(Incomplete: most children have not yet reached 3 1/2 years)

Strabismus	55
Anisometropia (1.5D or more)	20
Reduced acuity/amblyopia	19
Myopia (-3D or more)	10
Hypermetropia (over +7 D)	5
Ocular abnormality	6
Total	115 = 3.8% of 3016 in screened population

Table 3 shows the numbers of children who have already been referred for treatment out of the first 3016 screened in Cambridge, amounting to 3.8%. These 115 children include those who have failed our tests at the age of 3 1/2 years, but also others who have been referred at earlier ages. Since a number of children who have already been screened, but who are not yet 3 1/2, must be expected to be referred in the future, we estimate that the final percentage requiring treatment, by the age of 3 1/2 years will be around 5%.

Undoubtedly some of the strabismic children would have been detected in the absence of a screening programme. These figures suggest that they make up about half of the estimated 5% with vision problems. However, even if all those with manifest strabismus were identified and referred, there would still be 2-3% of the population who would have an identifiable visual problem and yet would not be picked up before 3 1/2 years. If leaving these cases unidentified and untreated until 3 1/2 years leads to irreversible problems, such as amblyopia, there would be a strong argument for screening at a younger age than 3 1/2. On the other hand, if in fact treatment of eye problems was as effective at 3 1/2 years as at 6-9 months, then the case for identifying problems in the younger age group would be much weaker.

To answer this question we would need to know in much more detail the extent and nature of plasticity in the visual system at different ages. It has been generally found that some binocularity can be restored only if strabismus is treated before the second year of life (Taylor, 1972) This suggests that the plasticity of the system for binocular function is nearing an end by two years of age. However the critical period in which amblyopia develops and can be reversed by treatment is highly contro-versial. In general it appears that plasticity is highest early in life but whether this really means that treatment is necessary in the first three years of life, rather than later, cannot be decided on the basis of present knowledge.

3. Study of natural history of development of refraction

Data from the screening of 6-9 month-olds shows that the average cycloplegic refraction at this age is between 1.0 and 1.5 D hypermetropic, and that approximately 50% of this population shows 1.0 D or more of astigmatism (confirming earlier findings of Howland et al (1978); Mohindra et al (1978)). Analysis of the axis of astigmatism in a sample of these infants indicates that different populations may show markedly different ratios of the different axes (see Atkinson & Braddick, 1983).

We have conducted a pilot analysis of the first 33 of those with significant degrees of hypermetropia (+4.0 D or more) but who have not worn spectacles. In this group hypermetropia reduces by an average 0.75 D between 1 and 2 years of age. There is also a reduction in astigmatism over this period (as found earlier by Atkinson et al (1980)); however this reduction appears to be at a slower rate in those with against-the-rule or oblique astigmatisms, than in with-the-rule astigmatisms. The reason for this difference is unknown, and it remains to be seen whether it will be substantiated by analysis of a larger group. If the course of the reduc-tion of astigmatism is found to be dependent on the axis, then it seems likely that this process is determined, or at least strongly constrained, by structural factors in the eye rather than being entirely under the control of a visual feedback process.

4. Randomised control trial of the prevention of strabismus and amblyopia

In this trial half the infants who had been identified in the screening as having a significantly hypermetropic refraction were offered a partial spectacle correction for their hyperopia. The correction given was not a full correction of the hypermetropia; rather it brought their corrected refraction close to the norm for their age group. The other half were uncorrected. However, after the trial had been running for 6 months it was decided to increase the proportion offered spectacles to 2/3, to equalise the groups allowing for the drop out of those who did not wear the spectacles prescribed.

Parents are carefully questioned at each follow-up examination about the time for which their children wear the spectacles, and a full record kept. This has often not been done in studies of refractive correction of children, but in our view it is essential if we are to evaluate the effectiveness of this treatment. At the present time we estimate that approximately 50% of those given a prescription at 6-9 months wear the glasses most or all of the time, with the other 50% ranging from intermittent wearing to "never worn". We have found that very few infants under 1 year of age will persistently not tolerate spectacles, but that there is more frequent non-compliance if the spectacles are first prescribed at 1 to 2 years. In general, we find that the parent's reluctance is the main factor leading to infants who do not wear their spectacles at all. Although undesirable this is understandable considering that these children show no obvious visual defect such as strabismus.

The number of hypermetropic children from the trial who have reached the age of 3 1/2 years is still too small for us to assess the outcome of these partial refractive corrections. However, the initial results are encouraging. In the data from Cambridge summarised in Table 1, of the 18 hypermetropic infants who had abnormal vision at 3 1/2 years, nearly all (16/18) had not worn spectacles. In contrast, 2 out of the 4 children with normal vision had worn spectacles.

5. Evaluation of the application of photorefraction in the context of community screening

In general the screening programme has been well accepted in its community setting, with an overall attendance of 72% of the total population called for screening in Cambridge, and 90% of the population in Bristol (where the screening is based in a selected set of clinics).

One additional merit of community vision screening is that it allows the examination for strabismus and refractive errors of children who are outside the screening population (either in terms of geographic location or age) by allowing referrals into the system. In many cases the anxieties of parents or health visitors about possible strabismus can be discussed and alleviated in their visit to the community clinic without requiring referral to a hospital outpatient department. Out of the first 120 such referrals from outside the screening population, 20 were found to require further examination or treatment. While this represents a higher proportion than from the unselected screening population, it also demonstrates the large number of children for whom there is uncertainty and concern about their eyes in the first year of life, but in fact no problem is present. An important benefit of screening early compared to 3 1/2 years, therefore, is that it can prevent false referrals of pseudostrabismus to outpatient clinics. Such false referrals are costly both in terms of anxiety to the parent and to the Health Service in terms of administrative costs and of valuable specialist time.

In general the vision screening programme has worked smoothly with good cooperation being established between those involved in different parts of the programme and its follow up. The final analysis of its outcome remains to be carried out over the next few years.

INDIVIDUAL ASSESSMENT OF VISION

In contrast to screening, individual assessment is carried out with specific groups for whom detailed knowledge of their visual function is required. One such group is infants and children with physical and mental handicaps, among whom there is well known to be a high level of visual disorders. Most of the previous studies (many of which are reviewed by Goble, 1985) have concentrated on specific isolated aspects of vision such as strabismus or acuity. Here we have taken a somewhat different approach, with an interdisciplinary team working together to look at a number of interrelated aspects of vision. The eventual aim is to help those involved in the care, treatment and education of these children to understand the effect of the child's visual deficits on everyday life, so that every effort can be made to help the child to develop strategies to deal with their problems. The details of many of the tests we use have already been published elsewhere (Atkinson, 1984) and so will only be briefly described here.

Clinical population

108 children were referred for assessment to the Visual Development Unit by paediatricians from the Child Development Centre and Addenbrooke's Hospital, Cambridge, between January 1983 and December 1984. The ages of these children ranged from 4 months to 12 years, but nearly all of them (100) were 4 years of age or younger. Many had the mental age of normal infants. In 30% of the cases a visual problem had already been diagnosed or was strongly suspected by the clinicians making the referral, while the remaining 70% were referred for a visual assessment as part of a more general battery of sensory and developmental tests. Children were referred with a wide variety of paediatric diagnoses; one third were cases of cerebral palsy and one third had general developmental delay with the other third having a range of disorders.

Procedure

Table 4 shows the tests that were used in the procedure. Each examination starts with a discussion with the parents (or other relevant caregiver) about their observations of the child's behaviour and what they think the child sees and perceives. Any relevant family history of eye problems is noted. We then watch the child playing and interacting with others in our small reception nursery. This is supplemented by informal testing of visually guided reaching and grasping for bright toys, visual attention to distance (e.g. awareness of parents entering or leaving the room, or response to peek-a-boo at 2 meters around the edge of a door) and informal field testing. For the latter test a visually conspicuous but silent toy is brought in laterally from either side of the child and we observe when the child first notices its appearance. When perceptual and cognitive deficits are suspected we sometimes informally test for the understanding of object permanence by hiding toys in different ways, and test for visual recognition of toys, objects and people.

TABLE 4. INDIVIDUAL ASSESSMENT OF VISION

1. Discussion of child's history, including family history of eye problems

2. Observation of general visuo-motor behaviour

3. Orthoptic examination

4. Isotropic photorefraction without cycloplegia

5. Acuity assessment (forced-choice preferential looking, STYCAR, Sheridan-Gardiner, "crowding")

6. Field testing (when necessary)

7. Optokinetic nystagmus (OKN)

8. Pattern VER (when necessary)

9. Binocular vision (monocular OKN; binocular VER)

10. Discussion of results

The other more formal tests are carried out in separate rooms away from the nursery, so that the child is not distracted by toys and other people. Frequent breaks are given between tests for playing so that the child does not become bored and the parents have time to relax and talk about their child's problems. The 'field testing' referred to in Table 4 has so far been carried out only when indicated by a history of hemiplegia or by observations on informal testing. It is done by bringing Stycar balls into the field of view from behind in a non-distracting environment, with the child's attention initially attracted forwards by an observer who then notes when the first fixation towards the target is made. We have been primarily concerned to identify children for whom there is a consistent asymmetry between the points at which attention is attracted in the two lateral half-fields.

Non-cycloplegic photorefraction

We use isotropic photorefraction without cycloplegia (Atkinson et al, 1981a), both to indicate possible refractive errors and to assess the child's ability to shift focus with changes in visual attention. J. Wattam-Bell in our unit has developed a method of recording video photo-refractive images in a digital frame store, which enables the images to be immediately examined after each flash exposure. This immediacy is essential for looking at children wih multiple problems since it allows the

tester to make several rapid assessments of focussing with minimum effort
on the child's part. From a series of photorefractive tests with targets
(large, noisy brightly illuminated toys) set at different distances from
the eyes, we can ascertain how reliably the child is able or willing to
change focus and accommodate accurately on nearby targets. Of course it
is necessary to compare the results of this test with those of cycloplegic
photorefraction to ascertain whether any lack of appropriate focussing is
due to a significant myopia or whether it a consequence of motor difficulties or deficits in the control of visual attention.   In non-myopic
children we find one of three kinds of behaviour when tested with target
distances of 20 to 200 cm:
(i) normal focussing over the entire range
(ii) fixed focus close to the position of cycloplegic refraction
(iii) appropriate changes of focus for nearby targets (e.g. 20 to 75 cm) with
little of change of accommodation for targets beyond these distances.
Behaviour of type (ii) or (iii) is taken to indicate deficits of visual
attention.

Measures of acuity

With many of these children we have used forced-choice preferential
looking (FPL; see Teller 1979, Atkinson and Braddick, 1981a, Atkinson et
al 1982, 1983, Atkinson et al 1985a). The method depends on the fact that
most children prefer to look at something (the grating pattern) rather
than nothing (a blank patternless screen) but sometimes handicapped
children do not even show this basic preference. It is as though the
blank bright screen competes for attention with the screen containing the
pattern. It may be that such children are showing the same kind of
'externality' effect found in very young normal infants of one month or
less, who will equate two patterns in terms of visual attention if both
have a similar outline or boundary (Milewski 1976, Bushnell 1979). In
this case both the patterned and unpatterned screen have a circular bright
edge with darker surround which could induce an 'externality effect'.

If a child does show a marked preference for looking at a coarse
grating pattern compared to the blank screen then we proceed in the normal
way to get an estimate of acuity (see Atkinson et al, 1985a). Sometimes a
child who will not cooperate in FPL can be tested with the Stycar Balls at
1, 2, or 3 metres (Sheridan, 1976). Such testing measures are of 'detection' rather than 'resolution' but can be used to gain a very crude idea
of the visual behaviour of the child. The shortcomings of such procedures
as Stycar Balls, rolling balls and Catford Drum have been explained more
fully by Atkinson et al (1981b).

With some children of over 3 years mental age an operant alley-
running technique can be used (Atkinson et al, 1981c; 1985b). The child
has to choose between two cubes, with a reward hidden under the cube
showing the target letter (e.g. a letter O). The discriminations of which
a particular child is capable will depend on the child's perceptual-
cognitive development as well as sensory factors. Sometimes a child will
be happy to give simple responses (when pointing to the stripes) in the
FPL set-up, but cannot cope with picking out one letter from a group on a
cube. By using several acuity tests such differences in ability and
flexibility can be discovered.

For some children, who show no responses for any of the acuity tasks
described, above we use a test of optokinetic nystagmus (OKN) to find out

whether an entire field of pattern can stimulate a response in the visual
system. In this test the infant sits in front of a very large screen
(preferably not less than 100 degrees visual angle) to avoid the possibility of suppression of OKN by fixation on an edge. A field of high
contrast random dots moves in front of the child. If no response is given
at a speed of approximately 20 degrees per second then higher or lower
speeds should be tested. If OKN is elicited for binocular viewing then
this can be taken as an indicator of a functioning pathway from the eyes
to subcortical centres at least. If the OKN is only triggered in one
direction and the direction is the same for the two eyes in monocular
viewing conditions then lateralised hemisphere damage is suspected. If
each eye will show OKN only for temporal-to-nasal pattern movement then
there is a deficit either of binocular function (see below) or of cortical
function more generally.

An indicator that a visual signal is reaching the primary visual
cortex may be obtainable from the visual evoked potential (VEP), time
locked to a phase reversing stripe pattern (for example see Atkinson et al
1979, Harris et al 1976, Pirchio et al 1978). For some children, in whom
responses involving eye or head movements are unreliable (e.g. severe
cerebral palsy), the VEP may provide one of the few feasible ways of
estimating acuity. However there are reported cases, where normal VEPs
have been recorded from adults who are functionally 'blind' (Bodis-
Wollner, 1977) and so caution should be used when interpreting a positive
VEP response as evidence of functional everyday vision. In any case, if a
child with cerebral palsy cannot control eye or head movements to fixate,
any vision that is demonstrated by a positive VEP can only be used in a
very abnormal way. It should also be remembered, that for measures of
VEPs to be reliable the child must be cooperative enough for electrode
attachment and willing to sit in front of a screen for a few minutes at a
time for signal averaging to take place. For many disabled children VEP
measures are not possible because of these practical drawbacks.

Tests of binocularity

For some children (particularly the hemiplegics) it is often desir-
able to know more about binocular vision than can be obtained from an
orthoptic examination. We have used two other methods. In the first we
measure the symmetry of monocularly viewed patterns in inducing OKN
(MOKN). Asymmetries of OKN in the two directions when patterns are viewed
with each eye alone can indicate a lack of binocularity (Atkinson, 1979;
Atkinson and Braddick, 1981b; van Hof-van Duin and Mohn, 1985) In general
it is easier to elicit OKN for patterns moved temporal-to-nasalward in the
visual field than vice versa. This is because this direction of movement
is likely to be controlled by a subcortical pathway, whereas OKN elicited
by temporalward pattern movement involves visual pathways in the binocular
cortex. A second test for binocularity depends on the fact that a VEP
specifically related to binocular vision can be elicited in infants with
normal visual development after the age of 4 months (Braddick et al 1980,
1985; Braddick and Atkinson, 1983). The method requires the child to wear
electrodes and red/green goggles and so again requires a cooperative
child for succesful testing.

Cycloplegic isotropic photorefraction

To complete our assessment it is necessary to know whether there is
any significant refractive error under cycloplegia. When tests of acuity

and binocularity are complete 1% cyclopentolate drops are administered and
isotropic photorefraction carried out once again. If a large refractive
error is present retinoscopic refraction may be needed to confirm its
size.

Results

The results of these various tests have been summarised in Table 5.
Many of the children failed more than one test and only 19% showed no
visual problems on any of the tests given.

**TABLE 5.   OUTCOME OF VISUAL ASSESSMENTS ON 108 CHILDREN REFERRED FROM
PAEDIATRICS AND CHILD DEVELOPMENT CENTRE**

Type of abnormal result	Proportion abnormal
Visual acuity / amblyopia	45%
Strabismus/abnormal eye movements	46%
Poor visual attention / perceptual deficits	47%
Abnormal refraction under cycloplegia	44%
'Cortically blind' - no confirmed ocular pathology	11%
Confirmed ocular pathology	4%
(Visual fields: 9 deficits out of 12 children tested)	

Children found to have one or more visual defects	81%

Almost half the children showed abnormal eye movements or strabismus
and almost half had significant refractive errors. For some of these
children the strabismus may be associated with the refractive error. In
at least some of these cases the disorder might be expected to be improved
by ophthalmological treatment.

The percentage of children with 'cortical blindness' without confirmed ocular pathology is worryingly high. However, four of this group
had been fitting and were still receiving anticonvulsant medication. It
has often been observed in our own studies and in the literature, that for
many of these cases of infantile convulsions there is a steady recovery of
some visual function when the convulsions have been controlled; and it is
also likely that the medication may reduce responsiveness.

Only a small group of children have been 'field' tested. Of the 9
showing a field deficit, 7 were hemiplegics. In future more extensive
field testing of those with cerebral palsy may reveal a higher incidence
of such problems.

A high percentage of these children suffered from attentional and perceptual deficits (47%). These were often non-specific and could not be clearly defined from the tests we were using. New methods will need to be developed to split this large group into subgroups whose problems can be defined more specifically. The different classes of behaviour in changing focus, found using non-cycloplegic photorefraction, might provide a starting point for categorising different types of deficit.

DISCUSSION AND CONCLUSIONS

In this paper we have briefly described both our screening programme and our methods of individual visual assessments for children suffering neurological impairments. It is apparent that there is a significant group of children in need of assessment and treatment both in the normal population and in those who are handicapped. While children with severe disability only represent a small percentage of the population, we have found that most of these children have visual problems, some of which might be treated successfully if identified at an early stage. In our view this group have not in the past received the ophthalmological attention they deserve, partly because adequate assessment of their visual function has not been available.

In considering population screening programmes there are still a number of major questions that need to be answered before any definite policy can be decided. We need to know the effectiveness with which clinical treatment (surgery, patching) for strabismus and amblyopia can achieve normal vision at different ages and stages of intervention. Although this is an old question it still cannot be adequately answered from published data. From our present screening programme it is clear that we can identify the 7% of the infant population with abnormal refractions, and that a high proportion of these children will have other visual problems later in life, but unless we understand how early refractive errors lead to visual problems, and how this can be prevented, early identification will not necessarily lead to improvements of vision in the preschool population. The question of cost effectiveness both in social and financial terms also needs to be answered and here we need to compare screening of the whole population with the selection of specific 'at risk' subgroups. One such subgroup we are currently investigating is infants (estimated to be about 10% of the population) with a strabismic or amblyopic first-degree relative. Table 6 shows the refractive and orthoptic problems found in a pilot group of such infants. The table shows that compared to the general population (see Figure 1) there is a high percentage with abnormally hypermetropic refractions. In addition, the numbers

TABLE 6. VISUAL DISORDERS IN INFANTS WITH FAMILY HISTORY OF SQUINT

(first-degree relative with strabismus/amblyopia: approx 10% of population)

Hypermetropia (+4D or more)	21%
Strabismus (manifest in first year)	5%
Anisometropia (1D or more)	5%
Myopia (-2D or more)	3%

in this group with manifest strabismus at 6-9 months are sufficient (5% of 10% of the population) that they must constitute a very large part of the incidence of early onset strabismus in the whole population (0.3% in the data of Figure 1). Thus one way to reduce the overall cost of screening might be to screen this subgroup, although this would mean that those in the other 90% of the population with visual defects in the abscence of strabismus might not be identified until later preschool or school ages, when treatment may prove less effective in the long run.

These questions need to be answered with careful longitudinal research. We are beginning to do this, but before firm conclusions on policy can be reached a good deal of collaborative scientific and clinical effort will be necessary.

ACKNOWLEDGEMENTS

We would like to thank John Wattam-Bell, Carol Evans, Shirley Anker, Ann MacIntyre, William Bobier, and Claire Towler, all of the the Visual Development Unit, for their help in both the visual assessment and screening work. We thank members of the Department of Community Health (Cambridge Health Authority) and of the Ophthalmology Department, Addenbrooke's Hospital for their collaboration in the Cambridge screening programme, especially Dr Fiona Griffith. The Bristol screening programme was initiated by Dr Sue Atkinson, Department of Community Medicine, Bristol Health Authority.

This work is supported by programme and project grants from the Medical Research Council.

REFERENCES

Atkinson J. Development of optokinetic nystagmus in the human infant and monkey infant: an analogue to development in kittens. In: Freeman RD ed. Developmental Neurobiology of Vision. New York: Plenum Press 1979:277-89.

Atkinson J. Assessment of vision in infants and young children. In Harel S, Anastasiow NJ eds. The At-Risk Infant. Baltimore: Paul H Brookes Publishing Co. 1984:341-52.

Atkinson J, Braddick OJ. Acuity, contrast sensitivity, and accommodation in infancy. In: Aslin RN, Alberts JR, and Peterson MR, eds. Development of Perception, Vol. 2: The Visual System. New York: Academic Press. 1981(a):245-77.

Atkinson J, Braddick OJ. Development of optokinetic nystagmus in infants: An indicator of cortical binocularity? In: Fisher DF, Monty RA, and Senders JW, eds. Eye movements: Cognitive and visual perception. Hillsdale, NJ: Lawrence Erlbaum. 1981(b):53-64

Atkinson J, Braddick OJ. The use of isotropic photrefraction for vision screening in infants. Acta Ophthal 1983; Suppl 157: 36-45.

Atkinson J, Braddick OJ, French J. Contrast sensitivity of the human neonate measured by the visual evoked potential. Invest Ophthal vis Sci 1979;18:210-13.

390

Atkinson J, Braddick OJ, French J. Infant astigmatism: Its disappearance with age. Vision Res 1980;20:891-93.

Atkinson J, Braddick OJ, Ayling L, Pimm-Smith E, Howland HC, Ingram RM. Isotropic photorefraction: A new method for refractive testing of infants. Doc Ophthal Proc Series 1981(a);30:217-23.

Atkinson J, Braddick OJ, Pimm-Smith E, Ayling L, Sawyer R. Does the Catford Drum give an accurate assessment of acuity? Brit J Ophthal 1981(b);65:652-56.

Atkinson J, French J, Braddick OJ. Contrast sensitivity function of pre-school children. Brit J Ophthal 1981(c); 65: 525-29.

Atkinson J, Braddick OJ, Pimm-Smith E. 'Preferential looking' for monocular and binocular acuity testing of infants. Brit J Ophthal 1982; 66:264-68.

Atkinson J, Pimm-Smith E, Evans C, Braddick OJ. The effects of screen size and eccentricity on acuity estimates in infants using preferential looking. Vision Res 1983;23: 1479-83.

Atkinson J, Braddick OJ, Durden K, Watson PG, Atkinson S. Screening for refractive errors in 6-9 month old infants by photorefraction. Brit J Ophthal 1984;68:105-12.

Atkinson J, Pimm-Smith E, Evans C, Harding G, Braddick OJ. Visual crowding in young children. This volume. 1985(a).

Atkinson J, Wattam-Bell J, Pimm-Smith E, Evans C, Braddick OJ. Comparison of rapid procedures in forced choice prefential looking for estimating acuity in infants and young children. This volume. 1985(b).

Bodis-Wollner I, Atkin A, Raab E, Wolkstein M. Visual association cortex and vision in man: pattern-evoked occcipital potentials in a blind boy. Science 1977;198:629-31.

Braddick OJ, Atkinson J. Some recent findings on the development of human binocularity: a review. Behav Brain Res 1983;10:71-80.

Braddick OJ, Atkinson J, Julesz B, Kropfl W, Bodis-Wollner I, Raab E. Cortical binocularity in infants. Nature 1980; 288: 363-65.

Braddick OJ, Atkinson J, Wattam-Bell J. VER testing of cortical binocularity and pattern detection in infancy. This volume. 1985

Bushnell IWR. Modification of the externality effect in young children. J exp Child Psychol 1979;28:211-29.

Goble JL. Visual Disorders in the Handicapped Child. New York: Marcel Dekker. 1985.

Harris L, Atkinson J, Braddick OJ. Visual contrast sensitivity of a 6-month-old infant measured by the evoked potential. Nature 1976; 264: 570-71.

Howland HC, Atkinson J, Braddick O, French J. Infant astigmatism measured by photorefraction. Science 1978;202:331-3.

Ingram RM, Traynar MJ, Walker C, Wilson JM. Screening for refractive errors at age 1 year: A pilot study. Brit J Ophthalmol 1979;63: 243-50.

Milewski, AE. Infants' discrimination of internal and external pattern elements. J exp Child Psychol 1976;22:229-46.

Mohindra I, Held R, Gwiazda J, Brill S. Astigmatism in infants. Science 1978;202:329-31.

Pirchio M, Spinelli D, Florentin A, Maffei L. Infant contrast sensitivity evaluated by evoked potentials. Brain Res 1978; 141: 179-84.

Sheridan MD. Manual for the STYCAR vision tests. Slough: NFER Publishing Co. 1976.

Teller DY. The forced-choice preferential looking procedure: A psychophysical technique for use with human infants. Infant Behav and Devel 1979;2:135-53.

Taylor DM. Is congenital esotropia functionally curable? Trans Am Ophthal Soc 1972;70:529-76.

van Hof-van Duin J, Mohn G. Vision in the preterm infant. In: Prechtl HFR, ed. Continuity of Neural Functions from Prenatal to Postnatal Life. Oxford: Blackwell, 1985;93-114.

DISCUSSION

Fells: In Mohn's paper, when using the Seattle cards, the first picture that was shown when doing the testing had a small grey screen. What was the function of that?

Mohn: That was to prevent the person holding the infant from seeing the grating, so that whoever is holding the infant can't point them towards the grating.

Fells: That seems to be quite important.

Mohn: I think it is a very good thing to have.

Warburg: We have just started using acuity cards and we are quite happy about them for mentally retarded children, even in age groups between 3 years and 7 years, and both in those in whom we can compare acuity tests in the ordinary way and in those who are too autistic or too disturbed; the children find the acuity cards much more pleasant. We have, out of 35, had 2 who were almost impossible to test, while 5 or 6 were doomed by the staff to be completely uncooperative. There was too little discrimination in the original acuity cards, so that we have obtained cards with finer gratings.

Atkinson: The one element that has been dropped using the acuity cards is the forced choice part of the procedure, because presumably the person who holds up the cards knows which side the stimulus is on. So I was very gratified to see your agreement with FPL. How do you feel about this having used both techniques? Do you think that you lose a little, or do you think that it doesn't make very much difference as long as you have trained observers doing it in either condition.

Mohn: We often use the forced choice procedure, presenting the gratings 'blind', and then making a forced choice about the position of the grating. Then we reverse the grating and look whether the infant switches fixation to the other side. If you present them blind like that, and you get them right 4 or 5 times in a row, then that is probably still the best way.

Atkinson: What I am worred about is that as half these infants are astigmatic to a degree, has anybody done any comparisons? We have studied different orientation with the stripes. It is going to make quite a difference with a significantly astigmatic infant at the age of 3 months. We have a difference of an octave between some of our astigmatic children.

Warburg: Doesn't that give you an error?

Atkinson: No. These are reliable results.

Warburg: How large is the range?

Atkinson: The range is quite large. These are individual children. We use two staircases using horizontal gratings and then two staircases for verticals, so we know what the reliability of their response is for each orientation, and they have got statistically reliable differences in acuity depending on whether they are horizontal or vertical astigmats, and it fits very nicely with their cycloplegic or their non-cycloplegic refractions showing big myopic astigmatism.

Warburg: Do you think that squinting is a hereditary disorder?

Atkinson: I don't know but this seemed to be the best way to look at that. All I know is about 10% of our Cambridge population have this family history of a first degree relative with strabismus, and out of that group they do have a much higher risk of refractive error. I wouldn't like to say whether it is a genetic or an environmental effect, or what it is exactly in this particular group but they obviously have a higher incidence and they would make up half of our population of infant hypermetropes.

Warburg: In this way you select for familial hypermetropia, I believe.

Warburg: You take out the risk for being hyperopic, through that selection.

Atkinson: We are taking out half of them that are in the population, by subdividing the population into that group.

Fielder: You are talking, Mohr, about brightness differences between the test grating and the grey stimulus. Do you put anything behind the grating card?

Mohn: Sometimes there is a difference in colour or luminance between the grating and the 'blank', and you can put in coloured paper behind one of the stimuli to improve the match.

Harcourt: I didn't get the point about the parental strabismus group. Were you saying that in congenital strabismus in first degree relatives it is an almost 100 per cent predictor?

Atkinson: I am saying that if you pick out the children, the 10% of the population who have a first degree relative with strabismus at birth, their refractions will tend to be at the abnormally hyperopic end of the normal distribution.

Braddick: I think Harcourt is asking about the group that is actually congenitally strabismic. Five per cent of those children did have strabismus and that was equal in number to the strabismics we found in our screening programme.

Atkinson: If we want to look for congenital strabismics it is highly likely that we will find a lot of them by asking about the family history.

Harcourt: You mean that there was a strong family history of strabismus in children who had congenital strabismus.

Atkinson: Five per cent of them, whereas within the total population there was only .3%. So if you take that as a percentage of the population, virtually all our congenital strabismic patients, manifest in the first year, picked up at 6 to 9 months, would have had a first degree relative with strabismus.

Harcourt: This is what I find so interesting because it was Lang who compared two populations with stabismus and found that a family history of strabismus was much rarer in patients with congenital strabismus.

Atkinson: I am not sure what their definition of positive family history was.

Harcourt: It is rare in early-onset strabismus to have a relative with strabismus than it is in later onset strabismus.

Atkinson: All I can say is that this is population data collected in 1984 and I have no explanation for it. All I am saying is that is the result.

Braddick: But they probably weren't conspicuously squinting at the neonatal examination.

Campos: I think there is a point in between. The existence of congenital strabmismus is very difficult to detect, because I don't think any ophthalmologist was able to see a child at the day of birth. Strabismus generally is a condition attributable to different causes. Probably one is putting together congenital strabismus with relatively early onset strabismus. The second condition can be of the accommodative type, ie related to hyperopia. Hyperopia can be hereditary.

Atkinson: Our group of 55 were referred before the age of 3.5 years, and many of those are identified at 6 or 9 months with hypermetropia and have then gone on to become either anisometropic, strabismic or both and have then been referred to the hospital for treatment. I would call those later onset strabismus, but I don't know how late is late. They are after the initial screening at 6 to 9 months. My main message is if we are going to look for squint, manifest strabismus in screening in the first year, we are not going to find very many.

FINAL DISCUSSION

Taylor: First of all I would like to say that I enjoyed this meeting immensely. Actually understanding sometimes what the scientists are saying in this sort of meeting is tremendous. I remember a meeting in Berkeley where there were 30 people: 15 eye-movement scientists and 15 doctors of various sorts. Fifteen talked within that group and 15 within the other. The wonderful thing about this meeting is the tremendous feeling between the two basic disciplines.

We have had a lot of suggestions for collaboration. These have included: some form of genetic register, ways of giving genetic advice, genetic or diagnostic advice for geneticists, and collaboration on diagnostic facilities. We have had a brief mention of epidemiological trends in a collaborative way. Campos has mentioned collaborative research, for instance, collecting human brains from amblyopes. I am not sure whether collaborative research is the right way of doing it, but research into the effects of early intervention and whether it is a useful means, it absolutely stunned me that anybody could even feel there is any real question about whether such a relatively harmless form of treatment needs scientific evaluation. Perhaps it does. That may be Harcourt's role.

Then, of course we had the whole thing about visual measurement. But for me the main thing has been about screening policy and seemed clear that there are 7 points about this. I would like to hear answered in the near future what we are we screening for, because we don't really have any ideas. There is a rather woolly feeling about what we screen for. Are we screening for serious visual disorder, are we screening for amblyopia, what are we looking for? What tests do we use? At what age do we screen? Will the results help us? If we think more about screening, will it help us to influence the child's vision in the long run. If we do screening, are we really going to help individuals reduce the impact and incidence of visual handicap? If we do, at what cost? The next question is the much more difficult one to answer, but nonetheless important. What social benefit is there really associated beyond the actual cost in mark, lire or whatever currency you are going to use? What I really don't think is terribly important, because it varies so much between each country, is that unless there is a European-wide policy, who is going to do it? I think that is the last question that needs to be answered.

All I can tell you is what is possible now, without great cost in the UK. The neonatal screening test performed by a paediatrician, usually a senior house officer or registrar, could be upgraded enormously by a very simple test in addition to the external inspection of the eyes, provided the child is kind enough to open his eyes. That is to teach them how to use an ophthalmoscope. Medical students should be taught how to do quick tests which will add only the cost of an ophthalmoscope, which I hope that their department already has. Then we have the well baby clinics. I think again in this country they do everything fine, they look at them at 6 weeks and 9 months, but those are the wrong times. I think these should be at 6 weeks, 6 months, and one year. You could make an even better case for repeating the neonatal test at 6 weeks, and doing a vision test at 3 months and 6 months. That would be more useful. We need a guideline as to when you are going to pick up the most serious defects, the ones that we think we are screening for.

We also have to educate the health visitors, that is the nurses who visit the children at home. We then have to make the school vision test better. In that way you are not committing yourself to what otherwise could be an absolutely enormous cost. The cost implications of screening are vast, and there are ways of doing it that are relatively inexpensive. We need to help the paediatricians understand the vision side of an 'at risk' concept. We need an 'at risk' concept for premature babies, for those with birth asphyxia, and for those with a family history of eye or systemic disease. We need to define what we are actually looking for, and· think about ways of doing it, but first decide whether it is really worthwhile.

Jay: Would you like to discuss further the general concept of screening? If we are talking in terms of a collaborative programme, the only way we could do this would be to try to define those centres that have a very definite screening programme. We could then get information on all these centres, arrange a meeting of interested people to see whether a pattern emerges which could be used throughout Europe, particularly in those areas that have not got a well defined screening programme. Because the points that Taylor has made are very important, cost effectiveness of any screening programme is suspect, and I think that this goes right the way through medicine. Screening of whole populations is not something that governments like because it is very expensive and it is not cost effective. Screening of 'at risk' populations is quite another matter. Now if you can build into a programme, as exists in a rudimentary state in this country where babies are looked at at these various times, simple tests which have very little effect on cost, then it is not so bad.

Hache: I would like to agree with Taylor about what he said regarding screening at the age of about 6 weeks. As I see it in our country they will refuse any additional screening programme. We have one programme in which they look at the baby in 8 steps and the health visitor is refused additional costs, but when we suggest that they should have some ophthalmic examinations we come into conflict with our professional organisation of ophthalmolgists. But that is politics! Nevertheless I would suggest minature programmes as a suggestion by the panel here to examine a baby at the age of 6 weeks by simple methods, but I would prefer a retinoscope to an ophthalmoscope, because with this instrument you can estimate roughly the refractive error and the whiteness of the fundus and so on.

Atkinson: Could I ask whether people here feel it would be possible for more population screening to occur on a small scale in different populations? One of the problems is that most of the data that comes from screening is from populations we cannot define. They are preselected when they walk into a hospital or a clinic or are referred by somebody. In some of the Scandinavian countries I think we get much more population screening. I would like to see small scale comparisons in different countries when we know the population that is being screened. I don't think it is adequate to look at the importance or outcome of a screening programme if you don't know the population that you are looking at. There seems to me to be very little population data at 6 weeks or at any age. I would be very happy to talk to other people with the possibility of setting up small-scale pilot population studies in other countries. At the moment there is very little comparison data. This would depend on the health facilities in other countries.

Warburg: It is generally not acceptable to do screening for any sort of disorder unless you can treat the disorder that is being found.

Campos: Adding to that, I think an important aspect is to underline exactly what we are looking for. It has been possible to collect some information from those countries where screening was done in an imperfect way. I also think we should get together again and decide which are the conditions we are going to treat. It is also true that we can do something without a lot of expense, but we do need the co-operation of other colleagues, including paediatricians. In Italy paediatricians lack knowledge as far as the eyes are concerned, so we should encourage a continuing education programme. I have been trying to do this both for paediatricians and for ophthalmologists in my area. Booklets or some other simple information should be provided for paediatricians in order to inform them on basic eye conditions in early childhood.

De Laey: Some answers to the questions put by Taylor. Most European countries have a screening programme. Perhaps not at an appropriate age, perhaps not of the appropriate population, perhaps not of the 'at risk' population. We do have it and we should be meeting to compare data. I can only think of the patients who are referred to my department from screening programmes. I don't think, of the children referred to my department, more than 5% come from screening programmes. This raises the question: are the screening programmes badly conducted, under the wrong leader, or done on the wrong population? If we are talking about cost I think that we have to be conscious of the fact that we cannot extend the screening programme, but that we have to maximise the existing programmes. But as Campos said, a few techniques taught to the paediatrician, and also to the school doctors, would be sufficient to solve a lot of problems. I don't think that we need orthoptists specifically doing the screening. Because screening is usually done by nurses or by doctors, and we need to teach them how to do simple diagnostic procedures. The orthoptists can help to train them. In the whole of Belgium we have only 65 orthoptists, and I don't think we have sufficient orthoptists to screen the whole Belgian population. I think the same problem may exist in other European countries. I think the problem lies in existing programmes, not in creating new programmes.

Loewer-Sieger: This is what we think is the most practical thing for the Netherlands. Not a special screening programme, but improvement in already existing programmes, and by health doctors.

Taylor: Also needed is enthusiasm and skill.

Jay: The impression I am getting is that people want information about what programmes are taking place throughout Europe. We will then want the interested people to meet to discuss the present programmes and how they can be adapted, with the minimum of expense, to the needs of whatever is required in screening. We want to know what screening programmes are available, and it will then be up to those who are interested to give some indication how they can be adapted for finding out what we want to screen for.

Harcourt: I would have thought that one of the important things about this meeting is that it should not allow itself to be swept away on a wave of enthusiasm. What I think is very important is that the experienced people at this meeting put the brakes on and don't allow themselves to be rolled along at a great speed into a large area of new territory which might be entirely inappropriate, and this is why Taylor bringing us down to earth is good. It is very easy to say that what is available is bad, and we have got to have something else. I think that is quite a wrong idea. I think what is available at this time from what we hear is very appropriate with some minor shifts. The programmes that are available in England and used are excellent, and when Fells talks about all his dense amblyopes turning up at 8, it isn't because the programme is not there to pick those children out, it is just that at a very simple level bad testing has been done. So it is a question of improving what is there rather than starting a great range of new things.

Taylor: In screening you have got to have some failures and anybody who says 'here is somebody who has slipped through the net' is going to do much more harm than good. We are looking for screening programmes, but to make any argument on any form of screening, whether to set up new ones or not, we need the advice of epidemiologists.

Jay: One of the more valuable things that has come out of European cooperation at the ophthalmic level was a study undertaken some years ago mainly in Holland, Belgium, Scandinavia on causes of blindness in childhood. We need the same sort of thing on the incidence of strabismus in early childhood, and this is something else we might think about.

Haase: I agree. We can approach this argument only once we have an understanding of what we are doing. Strabismus is a rather general term and we should define what we mean by it. Perhaps we could also insist on 'at risk' populations. This is something which can be done and which has already been done . The definition of this population is needed and we must adapt the screening programmes accordingly. I think of mentally handicapped children, and we can perhaps include the strabismic population as well.

De Laey: I should stress the point that Warburg made. Is it not also important to think of the consequences of screening programmes, there is a cataract problem, there is an amblyopia problem. Noone knows exactly what to do if there is screening.

Jay: I think that would come at a second stage in any such enquiry. The first stage is to define your parameters; the second stage is to look at what you are going to do with the various populations. The one you are talking about is one of the smaller populations.

Hache: In France we are screening by either a paediatrician or a generalist, at 2 months, 6 months and at one year. We examine all boys at 5 years of age and we have a programme when they enter primary school.

Harcourt: It was asked, and quite rightly, whether to use orthoptists for screening at any age, whether that was the best use of skilled manpower. It has been suggested that orthoptists should do the whole population screening in France. Orthoptists in this country are getting to the stage where they consider it appropriate for them to have a university education. We have a 3 year training programme for orthoptists, and they are very highly skilled and highly trained, and I think it would be totally inappropriate for people of that sort and range of skills to be used in whole population screening.

Jay: Wouldn't you think that that sort of discussion ought to take place after we have defined what we want to do.

Campos: At this point I have to make my point on this subject because I am also director of a training programme for orthoptists, even if it has nothing to do with our problem as Jay pointed out. We agree that orthoptists are highly skilled personnel. The problem is that changing the approach to the strabismic patient changes completely the role of the orthoptist. One has to ask why orthoptics was established as a profession and realise that its role is changing. Treatment, which was one of the main activities of the orthoptist, has now been abandoned in some countries, including Italy, and therefore trying to place the orthoptist in a position which makes her useful to society is not something to be disapproved.

Harcourt: That turns the whole argument on its head. Those that pay for any professionals to be trained are the state, either directly or indirectly, and the state would not wish to train a certain number of people who are going to be grossly underutilised. I don't think you train orthoptists and then try to find something for them to do. That is an absurdity.

Bagley: What I said this morning was trying to be objective. I am not looking at the problems as an orthoptist. This is not the forum to decide who is doing the screening.

Jay: It does appear that there is a need for some sort of coordinated interchange of information, and this is something that I think we can put down on paper.

Braddick: If there is going to be a coordinated interchange of information, the most important aspect of that is that our results should be presented in a comparable form. That is if we are going to look at different screening programmes elsewhere, to try and decide which is the most appropriate. Figures must be based on similar criteria.

Jay: It sounds fine, but I am not sure that it will work in practise, because so many different type of people will be providing the information.

Warburg: One of the things that made the original COMAC project on the prevalance of deafness in children so good was that it also led to an improvement in the EEC countries of hearing aids. This project led to improvement in industrial design and this is also what we have to bear in mind. Would some of the ideas that have been put forward, induce new industries within the EEC?

Jay: What about some of the other collaborative ideas?

Schulz: I have plenty that have not been mentioned. Concerning what Warburg said for some industry-producing things we need for our patients. Beginning with our congenital cataracts, what we badly need and what is an obstacle is a good contact lens for these small eyes with high refractive errors. I think this is a need that has some industrial potential. Concerning congenital cataract, there are rather few patients in any one clinic, so it takes rather long to evaluate them. There should be standardised data collection within European countries, so that whoever might be interested in these patients, whether one should operate or not, could get better information. This would prevent us having these waves of enthusiasm, whether to operate early or whether this is useless, and so on. I think we would benefit from the exchange of data.

Jay: You raise two points. One I know nothing about is contact lenses. Taylor, is there difficulty in getting appropriate contact lenses?

Taylor: Not now. In 1975 there was, but now they are made in Cambridge and two or three laboratories in London. But the cost is absolutely enormous. For one reason or another, one of the big manufacturers, because they have a near monopoly of the market, they seem to think they are much better than anybody else and therefore charge vast amounts more. I was interested to see you use mainly hard lenses. I am not a contact lens expert, but I should have thought that if you talked to the person making them, all their blades now will cut the appropriate contact lens buttons. You should be able to get them made locally. It costs us £7.50 a lens, which is quite a lot of money.

Fielder: I have no trouble at all getting lenses from a variety of sources.

Schulz: It is a question of the different producing systems the firms have so you might have some difficulties with very small eyes. It is not a problem with all our patients, but in some the contact lens fitting is one of the obstacles that might be improved.

Campos: I agree with Schulz. I have the same problem. I have been able to get some laboratories that make contact lenses for me on a one-to-one basis, but this is not a solution.

Jay: Bearing in mind that the COMAC that is concerned with this is the one on Biomedical Engineering I am surprised that electrophysiologists aren't suggesting that there ought to be standardisation of their techniques.

Vital-Durand: I think it is nice that several teams have tried several things with different goals. At least one point has emerged which I think is shared by everybody; it has brought to the eyes of the people here the possible interest to search for abnormalities at that early age which tended to be overlooked 5 years ago, and still possibly in some places. At least that is a positive achievement that has come out here. I don't think people have yet quite developed the best possible test, the easiest, cheapest, and fastest. There is now apparently a way to test visual acuity at an early age and fast. As a physiologist I had no idea at what precise age those tests should be made. Is screening a necessity just for children at risk who might constitute 95% of the pathological population? I do not know. There is also one thing which is of interest to me, I have seen practically no data about ocular movement abnormalities or visual abnormalities which have a long follow-up. Is that quite enough and in any case has there been one big study?

Harcourt: There is no doubt that strabismus and its natural history, and the way treatment has been modified, that is the one area which is the least understood. Children with severe bilateral handicaps are now discovered early in populations in Europe, even including the retarded population. But very little is known about the incidence, the natural history, the association of strabismus and its effects. I think this is an underexplored area, and such studies are going to be very interesting. In each of the screening programmes that has been mentioned, the number of children with serious visual deficit was tiny. This is not surprising, because severe bilateral visual deficit is a rare condition. What was mainly found was evidence of refractive errors with inequality between the two eyes, and evidence of strabismus.

Warburg: I don't see how the study would become better spread over all the European countries, rather than being done on a national scale.

Harcourt: I wasn't necessarily meaning on an EEC basis, but this is a very underexplored area.

Warburg: What we are coming back to is that we need new tests. We need them being put into production, and we will have to let other groups go into the logistics of their use. We have not yet decided if there are areas of technical development that need to be developed within the EEC.

Sargentini: I would like to remind you that this group is under the umbrella of Biomedical Engineering and we said before that the Committee that runs this emphasises that it is important to look at these problems in the light of standardisation of methods and equipment.

Braddick: We are here in a position of having described equipment not yet in general use which we have not been able to make available commercially. Is this the kind of issue on which the Bioengineering Committee can offer us any kind of advice?

Sargentini: I would like to emphasise that this is one of the points that this group has to make.

Jay: I think it is just as well that there is overlap, because otherwise the other group will not have adequate input of experts that are needed in the assessment of equipment on a very large scale. What about some other things that we should be thinking about?

Spekreijse: If we look at the screening programmes described for different countries, I think one thing is clear. Screening is done in a rather rough way and that is the way you have to do it because what we are lacking to make it more effective is normal data. Many of us have been presenting data which show how acuity develops and the best we could see was the acuity cards that were demonstrated today. I think we should analyse what are the differences and is it possible to have collaboration to do this? At the moment we know what the normal values are for acuity, and acuity might be an important parameter because it determines at an early age the signals.

Atkinson: I would be very much in support of this, because there are very few collaborative studies between people doing behavioural tests and VERs. We have done a few on isolated children where we have got reasonably compatible results between two techniques, but we could do with more collaboration in other places where there is some interchange between data and standardisation techniques. I think that might be one of the recommendations that we make. If we can possibly form in our own countries some kind of collaboration with other groups doing other types of testing procedures, there may be some interchange and there might be some standardisation of tests as well.

Hache: We tried to get some standardisation on several tests and COMAC helped us.

Jay: How would COMAC react to several suggestions about having groups of people looking at different aspects of things?

Sargentini: It is possible.

Jay: One of the first things that Taylor mentioned was the genetic registers. Is there any comment?

Warburg: It is irritating that paediatricians describe their hereditary diseases, even those with eye disorders, without making it easy for us to find them. I suggest that a group of interested people read through their journals and make a revised catalogue in which we go from the ophthalmic picture. It is a simple thing to do with computerised system. It would be a great help not only because we would have direct access to information about ophthalmogenetic disorders, but also because it would help us interact with paediatric geneticists. They would know that we had the information; we would be able to answer those questions that they don't know to ask us.

Jay: Who is interested in collaborating in an ophthalmological catalogue like that of McKusick?

Warburg: It isn't all that difficult. It has been done in biochemistry, it has been running in paediatrics. It could be copied.

Jay: It is time-consuming. One also wonders whether there should be interchange of ideas about specific diseases in regions. My worry there is of data protection but, having said that, if you were interested in this sort of thing it would be possible to exchange hospital numbers.

Warburg: What you could give would be the sum total of this or that disorder if you were asked. That would be simple.

Fielder: The potential for collaboration has been there for a long time, and why should we do it tomorrow more than we have done today? I hope that what has come out of this meeting is that we have met people, and got to know them better, and we can then collaborate by our own efforts rather than making formal proposals.